Springer

Tokyo
Berlin
Heidelberg
New York
Barcelona
Budapest
Hong Kong
London
Milan
Paris
Santa Clara
Singapore

S. Ikehara · F. Takaku · R.A. Good (Eds.)

Bone Marrow Transplantation

Basic and Clinical Studies

With 121 Figures

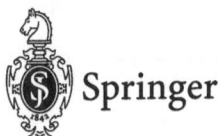 Springer

Susumu Ikehara, M.D., Ph.D.
Professor, First Department of Pathology, Kansai Medical University, 10-15 Fumizono-cho, Moriguchi, Osaka, 570 Japan

Fumimaro Takaku, M.D., Ph.D.
President, International Medical Center of Japan, 1-21-1 Toyama, Shinjuku-ku, Tokyo, 162 Japan

Robert A. Good, M.D., Ph.D., D.Sc., FACP
Distinguished Research Professor, University of South Florida
Head of Allergy and Clinical Immunology, Department of Pediatrics, University of South Florida, All Children's Hospital, 801 Sixth Street South Box 753, St. Petersburg, FL 33701, USA

Cover picture: Electron micrograph of a hemopoietic stem cell, taken by Dr. J. Toki. See p. 315.

ISBN 978-4-431-68322-3   ISBN 978-4-431-68320-9 (eBook)
DOI 10.1007/978-4-431-68320-9

Printed on acid-free paper

Preface

In the last decade, remarkable advances have been made in bone marrow transplantation (BMT), which is now becoming a powerful strategy in the treatment of diseases such as leukemia, aplastic anemia, and congenital immunodeficiency. However, because of the difficulty of obtaining HLA-matched donors, patients undergoing BMT have continued to suffer problems such as graft-versus-host disease and graft rejection.

This volume is a collection of the papers presented at the International Symposium on BMT - Basic and Clinical Studies, which was held in Tokyo on October 9 and 10, 1995. There are four sections: 1) Hematopoietic Stem Cells, 2) Growth Factors and Receptors, 3) Gene Regulation and Gene Therapy, and 4) BMT. Section 1 covers new methods for the purification of hematopoietic stem cells in mice, section 2 includes descriptions of new cytokines that regulate hematopoiesis, section 3 covers new gene therapies for metabolic disorders and cancer, and section 4 discusses the prospects for BMT.

The papers present the following new information: bone grafts to recruit donor stromal cells help prevent graft rejection: BMT plus bone grafts completely restores T cell functions, although their recovery after conventional BMT is incomplete in major histocompatible complex-incompatible combinations: performing BMT at the same time as organ allografts helps prevent the rejection of those allografts without recourse to immunosuppressive agents.

In animal experiments, it has been found that BMT can be used to treat not only systemic autoimmune diseases but also organ-specific diseases. In humans, it has recently been shown that rheumatoid arthritis, ulcerative colitis, and Crohn's disease can be successfully treated after BMT, which will therefore become an increasingly useful and powerful strategy in the treatment of various currently intractable diseases.

The Organizing Committee believes that this collection of papers will provide new insights into hematopoietic stem cells, growth factors and receptors, gene regulation and gene therapy, and BMT.

The Organizing Committee is grateful to the Japan Intractable Diseases Research Foundation and the Japanese Ministry of Health and Welfare for their support in holding the symposium. We would also like to thank Mr. Hilary Eastwick-Field, Ms. Keiko Ando, and the staff of Springer-Verlag Tokyo for their help in the preparation of this publication.

Susumu Ikehara
Chairman of the Organizing Committee

Acknowledgments

The editors gratefully acknowledge the support of the following organizations and individuals.

Host Organizations

The Japan Intractable Diseases Research Foundation
The Japanese Ministry of Health and Welfare

Organizing Committee

Susumu Ikehara, Shigetaka Asano, Ken-ichi Arai, Yukihiko Kitamura,
Masahisa Kyogoku, Yasusada Miura, Hideaki Mizoguchi,
Shin-ichi Nishikawa, Fumimaro Takaku
Takato O. Yoshida

Secretary-General

Muneo Inaba

Sponsors

Organizations

All Nippon Airways Co., Ltd.
Asahi Chemical Industry Co., Ltd.
Bristol - Myers Squibb Co., Ltd.
Chugai Pharmaceutical Co., Ltd.
Ciba-Geigy Japan Ltd.
Clea Japan, Inc.
Daiichi Pharmaceutical Co., Ltd.
Fast and Accurate Laboratories with Confidence
Fujisawa Pharmaceutical Co., Ltd.
Green Cross Corp.
Hayashibara Biochemical Laboratories Inc.
HESCO International Ltd.
Hosaka Children's Clinic
Hotel New Otani Co., Ltd.
Japan Rheumatism Association
Kanebo Ltd.
Kashimura Co., Ltd.
Kirin Brewery Co., Ltd.
Kit Chemical Co., Ltd.
Kiwa Laboratory Animals Co., Ltd.
Kogaku Ltd.
Kowa Co., Ltd.
Kureha Chemical Industry Co., Ltd.
Kyoto Medical Co., Ltd.
Kyoto Microbiological Institute
Laboratory of Chuo Medical Technology
Marubeni Corp.
Nacalai Tesque Co., Ltd.

Nikon Instech Co., Ltd.
Nihon Kohden Corp.
Nippon Boehringer Ingelheim Co., Ltd.
Nippon Kayaku Co., Ltd.
Nippon Pharmaceutical Co., Ltd.
Nippon Shinyaku Co., Ltd.
Nobeoka Hygienic Laboratory
Olympus Japan Co., Ltd.
Osaka Cytopathology Laboratories Inc.
Otsuka Pharmaceutical Co., Ltd.
Pfizer Pharmaceuticals Inc.
Sandoz Pharmaceuticals, Ltd.
Sanei Camera
Sankyo Co., Ltd.
Satouchi Co., Ltd.
Schering-Plough K. K.
Shimizu Laboratory Supplies Co., Ltd.
Shionogi & Co., Ltd.
Silk Kogei Inc.
Sumitomo Pharmaceuticals Co., Ltd.
Takeda Chemical Industries, Ltd.
Tokuyama Science
Tumura & Co.
Wakenyaku Co., Ltd.
Yashima Pure Chemicals Co., Ltd.
Yasuda Igaku Kinen Zaidan
Yoyodo Printing Kaisha Ltd.

Individuals

Kaname	ABE	Shinichiro	MORI
Yasuo	AMOH	Haruo	MORITA
Keiko	ANDO	Norikazu	NAGATA
Hiroshi	DOI	Takeshi	NINAGAWA
Yoh	FUKUBA	Nobuhiro	NISHIO
Hiroki	HARUNA	Ken	NOGUCHI
Futoshi	HASHIMOTO	Hajime	OGATA
Haruki	HAYASHI	Ryokei	OGAWA
Hiroko	HISHA	Koichi	OHTSUKA
Naoki	HOSAKA	Jiro	OKAMOTO
Tatsujiro	IKEHARA	Kazuya	SAKAMOTO
Susumu	IKEHARA	Toshimichi	SAWA
Muneo	INABA	Tadashi	SAWAME
Yasuko	INAFUKU	Yoshiko	SHINNO
Sadamitsu	INAFUKU	Akira	SUGIHARA
Yoko	INOUE	Kikuya	SUGIURA
Takahiro	ISHIDA	Sohei	SUZUKI
Kiyoshi	ITOH	Kozo	TAGUCHI
Hajime	IWAI	Yoshihisa	TAKAYAMA
Tienan	JIN	Mitsuyoshi	TAKEUCHI
Masayo	KAWAMURA	Kenji	TAKEUCHI
Jun	KAWASAKI	Fujiko	TANIGUCHI
Latt	KHIN MAUNG	Junko	TOKI
Mikio	KOHAMA	Takeo	UEDA
Takayuki	KUMAMOTO	Hisayo	WATANABE
Yongan	LI	Yoshihisa	YAMAMOTO
Zhexiong	LIAN	Takumi	YASUI
Yuki	MATSUI	Ryoji	YASUMIZU
Tuneo	MIYAKE	Cheng-Ze	YU
Shigeo	MIYASHIMA		

Contents

Growth Factors and Their Receptors

Gene Regulation and Gene Therapy

Bone Marrow Transplantation

Hematopoietic Stem Cells

The use of embryonic stem cells to study hematopoietic development in mammals

Michael V. Wiles* and Britt M. Johansson

Basel Institute for Immunology, Grenzacherstrasse 487, CH-4005 Basel, Switzerland.
*current address and corresponding author:
Max-Planck Institute für Molekulare Genetik, Ihnestrasse 73, D-14195 Berlin, Germany

Abstract

To study the process of mesoderm and subsequent hematopoietic cell development in mammals, we used embryonic stem (ES) cells in vitro differentiation. In fetal bovine serum containing medium, ES cell differentiation appears to be refractive to most exogenously added growth factors. Therefore to avoid the masking effects of serum we developed a serum-free, chemically defined medium (CDM). In CDM, ES cells grown as aggregates (known as embryoid bodies (EBs)), differentiate to neuroectoderm. If however activin A is added to CDM, both neuroectoderm and mesoderm develop. If bone morphogenetic protein 4 (BMP-4) is present in CDM, a process resembling primitive streak formation (at the molecular level) is induced, including the development of hematopoietic cells. These data combined with other reports strongly suggest that BMP-4 is intimately involved in mesoderm formation and possibly early hematopoietic development.

Introduction and discussion

In mouse, the primitive ectoderm begins to form the primary germ layers at around 6.5 days post coitum (p.c.). This process involves the formation of the primitive streak which is an 'outpouring' cells which form mesoderm between the primitive ectoderm and an outer layer of endoderm (i.e. mesoderm is fated to contribute to the embryo proper and 'ancillary' structures involved in its maintenance). Definitive endoderm and neuroectoderm also develop at this time. Slightly later, as the first somites form, hematopoietic precursor cells arise in the extraembryonic mesoderm and probably in the embryo proper in a region around the developing aorta, gonad, mesonephros (the AGM region, (1)). Although these processes

3

have been examined closely, there is little information regarding the actual factor/s which mediates these events. This paucity of information is due to the difficulty of manipulating the mouse embryo, which at this time is deeply imbedded in maternal tissues (the decidua) and is only 0.1 to 0.2 mm in length. Additionally, there has been no experiential amenable 'pathfinder' system with which to examine this process in vitro.

In contrast, using the amphibian Xenopus laevis (a kind of frog), pioneering work has clearly shown that a number of defined polypeptide factors can influence primary germ layer formation, and the formation of hematopoietic cells (see review and references therein (2)). This is due to the ease of access to the Xenopus's large multi-cellular egg (the blastula), which can be easily microsurgically divided into a number of tissue types. Using a portion of the blastula, known as the 'animal cap' region, in vitro assays were developed where the effects of specific factors of growth factors could be experimentally tested. These experiments showed, for example, that the TGF-β family member activin A can induce the animal cap region to become dorsal-anterior mesoderm (3, 4). Another member of the same family, bone morphogenetic protein 4 (BMP-4), can induce posterior mesoderm formation, including the development of hematopoietic cells (5, 6). These studies clearly showed that defined growth factors can influence the developmental pathway of competent cells. It should be noted that the TGF-β growth factor family is highly functionaily conserved, having members in all major animal phyla, from humans to insects (7). The use of the Xenopus blastual has been invaluable in the elucidation of the processes involved in early vertebrate development. However, 'man is not a frog' and although Xenopus is a vertebrate, its development is quite different from mammals (e.g. the Xenopus egg is essentially prepatterned by differential placement of RNAs and proteins before cell cleavage occurs).

In mammals, such an experimentally assessable and manipulatable system does not exist. However, there is a type of mouse cell line which has some functional resemblances to the animal cap cells of the Xenopus. These are embryonic stem cell (ES cells). These cells are isolated from the 3.5 day mouse blastocyst and in vitro maintain some similarities to the inner cell mass of the blastocyst (8, 9). ES cells are totipotent and can, if introduced into the 'correct' environment, develop into many different cell types. Furthermore, they appear to be 'immortal' but are not transformed, possessing a normal karyotype. They are maintained in culture in an undifferentiated state either on "feeder" cells (fibroblast cells which have been rendered mitotically inactive), or in the presence of an inhibitor of ES cell differentiation, known as leukemia inhibitory factor (LIF) (10).

ES cells have two current main uses:

i) They can be introduced back into a 3.5 day mouse blastocyst, which when placed into the uterus of a pseudopregnant mouse will give rise to mice which are derived partly from the ES cells and partly the host blastocyst. These animals are known as chimeras. If colonization of the chimeric animal includes those cells which will give rise to sperm or oocytes (i.e. the germ cells), transmission of the ES cell's genetic information will occur upon breeding (11).

Combined with homologous recombination, this unique ability makes ES cells the fundamental tool in the generation of genetically modified mice (e.g. as disease models).

ii) ES cells also have an innate ability to differentiate to many different cell types, including hematopoietic cells (12, 13). This occurs if they are grown in the absence of LIF and feeder cells, as cell aggregates (embroid bodies, (EBs)). This differentiation is rapid and apparently in normal tissue culture conditions, spontaneous.

It is this second aspect of ES cells which has potential in the study of growth factor involvement in the formation of mesoderm and hematopoietic cells. Unfortunately, the early ES cell differentiation experiments relied upon such esoteric reagents as human cord serum. Such reagents were of variable quality and gave rather inefficient and unreliable ES cell differentiation.

In 1991, we developed an approach which allowed the efficient and reproducible formation of yolk sac-like hematopoietic progenitors from ES cells grown as EBs. This was achieved using conventional tissue culture medium with batch selected fetal bovine serum (FBS), plus the presence of a reducing agent, monothioglycerol. This showed that ES cells had the potential to be used as a model system to study the factors involved in mesoderm and hematopoietic development (14, 15). However, we subsequently found that the factor which had the greatest effect upon mesoderm and hematopoietic cell development was FBS. Further, in the presence of FBS, ES cell differentiation was refractory to exogenously added growth factors (15).

Recently we developed a tissue culture medium which is serum free and chemically defined, CDM. This medium is composed of commercially available components and can support ES cell growth and differentiation (16).

As mentioned above ES cells can be maintained in an undifferentiated state in the presence of LIF and FBS. Upon removal of LIF, but still in the presence of FBS, they rapidly differentiate, forming predominantly endoderm and mesoderm. This differentiation is caused by the absence of LIF and by undefined factors present in FBS. In contrast, if ES cells are grown in serum free medium (i.e. CDM) they rapidly loose their ES cell phenotype without forming mesoderm (16), and that under these conditions neuroectodermal develops (as indicated by Pax-6 expression).

If, however, the TGF-β family members activin A or BMP-4 are present in CDM, mesoderm-development occurs in a factor concentration dependent manner. For example, activin A will mediate the formation of dorsoanterior-like mesoderm, whilst bone morphogenetic protein's 2 or 4 (BMP -2 or -4) facilitate the formation of posterior-ventral mesoderm (16). This posterior-ventral mesoderm contains hematopoietic precursor cells and expresses hematopoietic markers, including GATA-1 and -2, embryonic and adult globins, Ikaros and the endothelial markers Flk-1 and its ligand VEGF. Hematopoietic differentiation can be further augmented by the addition of VEGF, possibly indicative of a link between endothelial cells and hematopoiesis (i.e. possibly the haemangioblast).

Although we reported that ES/EBs respond to both activin A and BMP-4 in vitro, this does not formally prove thier active involvement in mesoderm induction and hematopoiesis in vivo. To answer this we examined the expression of both activin A and BMP-4 in vivo. Activin βA is present in the decidua at days 6 to 7 of development (15, 17). Additionally, BMP-4 RNA is detectable in both the day mouse egg cylinder and in undifferentiated ES cells, although the expression level is highly variable (16). Thus these factors are present at the correct time and place to be involved in mesoderm and for BMP-4, hematopoietic development.

Life, however, is not simple. It is becoming obvious, as more data is acquired, that mesoderm formation involves a coalition of many factors, with no single element being the prime instigator of mesoderm or hematopoietic development. For example, the BMP-4 locus has been disrupted in mice by homologous recombination, yet anterior mesoderm still forms in null mutant embryos (18). Thus, although BMP-4 is crucial for the proper formation of posterior structures, it is probably only one of a number of factors which act in concert to either induce and/or pattern the entire mesoderm. There is however, in the case of hematopoietic development a strong possibility that the formation of hematopoietic cells from (competent) mesoderm is achieved with only a few growth factors - and although the data is not yet conclusive, it would appear that BMP-4 (or another close member of the BMP family) is a candidate hematopoietic factor.

In conclusion, the studies outlined in this brief review suggest that ES cell differentiation can be influenced by specific growth factors. Further, that BMP-4 (or a very similar molecule) is probably a key factor in the formation of hematopoietic cells from ventral-posture mesoderm.
It is also clear from many studies that embryonic development involves transient combinations of factors which operate as a network. These control networks function as an integrated whole, and provides a high degree of developmental assurance and compensation and also reflects the evolutionary nature of life. Integrated networks are also difficult to analyze, and although ES cell in vitro differentiation is not a simplification of the mechanisms involved, the approach offers the potential to break the processes down into experimentally amenable units. If this approach is used with care, it can both validate and extend the information we learn from nonmammals to mammals.

References

1. A. L. Medvinsky, N. L. Samoylina, A. M. Muller, E. A. Dzierzak, *Nature* **364**, 64-7 (1993).

2. D. S. Kessler, D. A. Melton, *Science* **266**, 596-604 (1994).

3. A. J. van den Eijnden-Van Raaij, et al., *Nature* **345**, 732-4 (1990).

4. J. C. Smith, B. M. Price, N. K. Van, D. Huylebroeck, *Nature* **345**, 729-31 (1990).

5. C. M. Jones, K. M. Lyons, B. L. Hogan, *Development* **111**, 531-42 (1991).

6. M. Köster, et al., *Mech Dev* **33**, 191-9 (1991).

7. R. W. Padgett, J. M. Wozney, W. M. Gelbart, *Proc Natl Acad Sci U S A* **90**, 2905-9 (1993).

8. M. J. Evans, M. H. Kaufman, *Nature* **292**, 154-6 (1981).

9. G. R. Martin, *Proc Natl Acad Sci U S A* **78**, 7634-8 (1981).

10. R. L. Williams, et al., *Nature* **336**, 684-7 (1988).

11. A. Bradley, M. Evans, M. H. Kaufman, E. Robertson, *Nature* **309**, 255-6 (1984).

12. A. M. Wobus, H. Holzhausen, P. Jakel, J. Schoneich, *Exp Cell Res* **152**, 212-9 Issn: 0014-4827 (1984).

13. T. C. Doetschman, H. Eistetter, M. Katz, W. Schmidt, R. Kemler, *J Embryol Exp Morphol* **87**, 27-45 (1985).

14. M. V. Wiles, G. Keller, *Development* **111**, 259-67 (1991).

15. G. Keller, M. Kennedy, T. Papayannopoulou, M. V. Wiles, *Molecular And Cellular Biology* **13**, 473-486 (1993).

16. B. M. Johansson, M. V. Wiles, *Mol Cell Biol* **15**, 141-51 (1995).

17. K. Manova, B. V. Paynton, R. F. Bachvarova, *Mech Dev* **36**, 141-52 (1992).

18. G. Winnier, M. Blessing, P. A. Labosky, B. L. M. Hogan, *Genes & Development* **9**, 2105-2116 (1995).

Development of Blood Cells from Mouse Embryonic Stem Cells in Culture

Toru Nakano[1], Takumi Era[1], Hiroaki Kodama[2], and Tasuku Honjo[3]

[1]Department of Molecular Cell Biology, Research Institute for Microbial Diseases, Osaka University, Yamada-Oka 3-1, Suita, Osaka 565 Japan, [2]Department of Anatomy, Ohu University School of Dentistry, Tomitamachi, Koriyama, Fukushima 963 Japan, and [3]Department of Medical Chemistry, Faculty of Medicine, Kyoto University, Yoshida-Konoe, Sakyo-ku, Kyoto 606 Japan

SUMMARY

We developed an efficient differentiation induction system from mouse embryonic stem (ES) cells into blood cells by coculture on a novel stromal cell line named OP9. ES cells could give rise to adult type definitive erythrocytes, myeloid and B lineage cells, when the cells were simply cocultured with the OP9 stromal cells. This stromal cell line does not produce functional macrophage colony-stimulating factor (M-CSF) and presumably the deficiency of M-CSF production of OP9 cells might induce preferential differentiation into hematopoietic cells other than monocyte-macrophage lineage. Unfortunately, there did not appear to be any self-renewing hematopoietic stem cells to produce spleen colonies or bring about long term reconstitution of hematopoiesis in lethally irradiated mice during the differentiation induction. Several systems of *in vitro* differentiation induction from ES cells to lympho-hematopoietic cells are summarized. The usefulness and the limitation of the *in vitro* differentiation induction systems are discussed.

KEY WORDS: cell differentiation, hematopoietic stem cells, stromal cell, embryogenesis, embryonic stem cells

INTRODUCTION

Development of blood cells is a sequential cell fate determination process from fertilized eggs to mature blood cells of various lineages through mesoderm and lymphohematopoietic progenitor cells. Though the cells and regulators governing lymphohematopoiesis in mouse bone marrow or fetal liver have been defined, the molecular mechanisms of lymphohematopoietic cell development largely remain to be elucidated. One main reason why there are only a few satisfied studies of the developmental process is the difficulty of obtaining *in vivo* materials from the developing mouse embryos. Mouse embryonic stem (ES) cells can be regarded as a substitute for the *in vivo* source, since they are pluripotent cells derived from the inner cell mass of blastocysts and can contribute to all lineages including germlines in chimeric animals once reintroduced into eight-cell or blastocyst embryos [1]. Several groups have reported methods of inducing differentiation from ES cells to hematopoietic cells *in vitro* [2-11]. However, these systems required formation of complex embryoid structures, the addition of exogenous growth factors, or both. Other limitations of these systems were the inability to analyze the

9

developmental processes from ES cells to blood cells and the lack of simultaneous induction of both myeloid and lymphoid lineage cells.   To overcome these limitations, we developed an efficient differentiation induction system by simple coculture of ES cells on a novel stromal cell line OP9 [12, 13] which does not produce functional M-CSF [14, 15].

Unfortunately, the coculture of ES cells on the stromal cell lines expressing M-CSF induced only macrophage like cells [8].   The study of pre-B lymphoid cells expressing *fms* (M-CSF receptor) gene, however, showed that interleukin-7 (IL-7) ostensibly inhibited the differentiation into macrophage lineages and signal transduction through *fms* induced the differentiation or lineage switch into macrophage lineage reciprocally [16].   We naively hypothesized that preferential differentiation into the macrophage lineage and no obvious differentiation into other lineage cells might be mainly due to signal transduction of the M-CSF/fms system.   We then decided to use the novel stromal cell line OP9 which had been established from new born calvaria of B6C3F2-*op/op* mice, which lack functional M-CSF because these mutant mice have a mutation in the coding sequence of the M-CSF gene [15].   The strategy for the induction is as follows; 1) Elimination of LIF and feeder cells, which keep the ES cells immature;   2) Utilization of M-CSF deficient stromal cells to avoid the M-CSF/c-fms signaling pathway discussed above; 3) Reduction of ES cell growth by removal of reducing agents such as 2-mercaptoethanol (2ME) or methyl-thyogalactoside (MTG), on which ES cell growth is partially dependent.

MATERIALS AND METHODS

ES cells were maintained on embryonic fibroblasts in the presence of leukemia inhibitory factor (LIF) under the standard procedures [1].   OP9 cells were cultured and the induction was carried out in α-MEM supplemented with 20% FCS and standard antibiotics [14].   OP9 cells were passed every four days (just around reaching confluence) and the culture medium were changed once between passages.   For differentiation induction, ES cells were trypsinized, dispersed into single cell suspensions and seeded at a cell density of 10^4/ 35 mm culture dish covered with confluent OP9 cells.   In the usual experiments, whole culture was trypsinized 5 days after the initiation of the induction, and suspended as a single cell suspension and 10^5 of the day 5 cells reseeded onto a fresh OP9 cell layer in a 35 mm culture dish.   The first passage at day 5 is obligatory, unlike the second passage at day 10.   However, in most experiments, the induced cells were harvested and reseeded at day 10 of the induction to remove residual differentiated and undifferentiated colonies.   No trypsin was used for the harvest and only vigorous pipetting gave rise to a good number of hematopoietic progenitor cells at the second passage.   For pro-B cell production, 100 U/ml interleukin-7 and 10^{-4} M 2-ME were added.   Most of the differentiation induction experiments were carried out with D3 ES cells derived from 129/Sv mouse strain [1].

For the examination of hematopoietic stem cell activity, ES cells derived from C57BL/6 mice were used for the differentiation induction and injected into lethally (9.5 Gray) irradiated C57BL/6 mice or sublethally irradiated (2.0 Gray) WBXC57BL/6-*W/W*^{v} mice [17].   The induced cells were trypsinized, harvested, and the harvested cells then left on the culture dish for 30 minutes to remove the stromal cells.   The removal of OP9 cells was obligatory because even relatively small numbers of OP9 cells caused apoplexy when injected. 10^7 cells in 0.5 ml α-medium supplemented with heparin were injected into individual irradiated mice via the tail vein.

RESULTS

Differentiation of Embryonic Stem Cells into "Differentiated" Colonies

ES cells grew slow and flat after their transfer onto OP9 cells.   Undifferentiated ES cell colonies or "non-ES" cell colonies became detectable 3 days after the induction at a cloning efficiency of 200-400 colonies per 10^4 ES cells (Fig. 1).   The clusters grew flat until day 4 and then piled up without producing any complex structure.   Undifferentiated ES cell colonies on OP9 cells resemble those on embryonic fibroblasts in the presence of LIF.   The "non-ES" cell colonies were much larger than the ES cell colonies and consisted of very immature blastic cells larger than ES cells, however the cells did not have any morphologically differentiated characteristics.   In some special experiments, individual undifferentiated ES cell colonies and non-ES cell colonies were picked, trypsinized, suspended and transferred onto OP9 cells at day 5.   In those experiments, only non-ES cell colonies gave rise to hematopoietic cell clusters in the following 5 days, as described below.   We tentatively regard non-ES cell colonies as differentiated mesodermal colonies because of their capacity to differentiate into hematopoietic cells during the following 5 days.

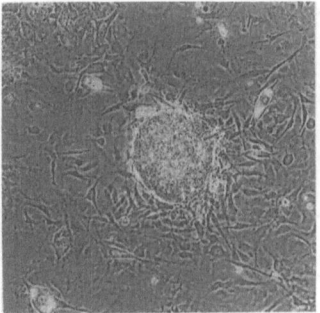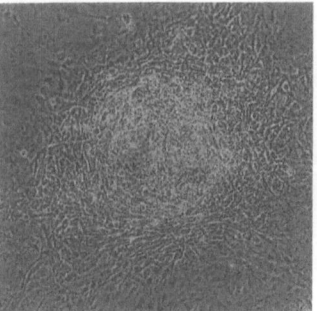

Fig. 1 Undifferentiated and differentiated colonies at day 5 of the differentiation induction
Five days after the coculture of D3 ES cells on OP9 stromal cells, undifferentiated ES cell colonies (left) and differentiated colonies (right) appeared.

Appearance of Hematopoietic Cell Clusters

The first passage should be carried out at day 5, otherwise hematopoietic cells would be buried in the differentiated colonies and subsequent analysis of hematopoietic cells would become impossible.   Usually, mixtures of undifferentiated ES cell colonies and differentiated non-ES cell colonies were trypsinized together and used for the first passage.   After the first passage, there appeared and proliferated round cell clusters (Fig. 2, left).   Various numbers of the cells of day 5 induced cells were replated onto OP9 cells and the numbers of small round cell clusters at day 5 were counted.   As shown in Fig. 2 (right), a linear relationship was observed between the numbers of the seeded day 5 cells and those of day 10 small round cell clusters.   This linear relationship shows that the day 10 small round cell clusters were of clonal origin.   There was about one clonogenic cell per 10^3 day 5 induced cells.

12

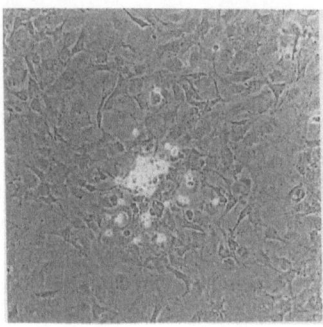 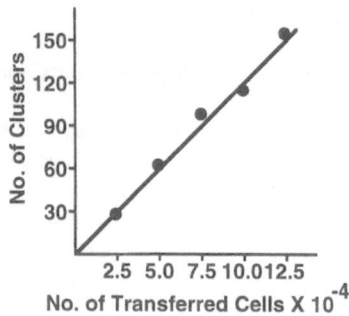

No. of Clusters

No. of Transferred Cells X 10^{-4}

Fig. 2 <u>Hematopoietic cluster at day 10 and the clonal nature of the clusters.</u>
After the first passage at day 5, hematopoietic cell clusters appeared (left). When various numbers of day 5 cells were seeded onto OP9 cells, a linear relationship between the number of the seeded cells and the number of day 10 hematopoietic cell clusters was observed (right).

Next, we examined the differentiation capacity of day 10 small round cell clusters to erythroid and myeloid lineage cells. Individual day 10 small round cell clusters were picked and put into methyl-cellulose semisolid medium containing erythropoietin and interleukin-3 (IL-3) as growth factors to stimulate the erythroid and myeloid lineage cells.

Table 1. <u>Differentiation capacity of day 10 hematopoietic clusters.</u>

Colony Type	Numbers
n m E mast M blast	2
n m E blast	2
m E M blast	1
m E blast	1
m blast	1
n m E mast	1
m E M	2
m E	5
n m	2
m	1
E	1
none	1
Total	20

Individual day 10 clusters were picked and transferred into methylcellulose semisolid medium containing IL-3 and Epo. Colonies appearing 8 days after the transfer were picked and stained with May-Grunwald Giemsa. Types of cells are n, neutrophil; m, macrophage; E, erythroid; mast, mast cell; M, megakaryocyte; and blast, blastic cell.

Nineteen out of 20 picked clusters produced colonies of hematopoietic cells in the semisolid culture.   More than 75 percent of the colonies contained multiple lineages of hematopoietic cells (Table 1).   In conclusion, the cells which produce day 8 small round cell clusters were multipotential hematopoietic progenitor cells and the small round cell clusters appearing after the first passage could be designated as hematopoietic cell clusters.

The second passage is usually carried out at day 10 in order to eliminate the undifferentiated ES cell and the differentiated non-ES colonies.   Proliferation and differentiation into mature blood cells occurred after day 10, regardless of whether the second passage was carried out.   Cells in hematopoietic clusters continued to proliferate and differentiate.   Cells obtained at day 14 were characterized with lineage and stage specific monoclonal antibodies combined with flow cytometric analysis.   More than 25% of the cells expressed a surface marker characteristic of erythroid lineage cells (TER-119), and about 5% of the cells expressed the granulocyte/macrophage lineage marker (Mac-1).   The B cell lineage marker B220 was also expressed on about 7% of the cells; however significant expression of surface IgM could not be detected.   Morphological analysis showed the emergence of megakaryocytes and mast cells. Taken together, all myeloid lineage cells and B lymphoid lineage cells appeared at day 14 of the induction.

Differentiation into B lineage Cells

The majority of the cells started detaching from the stromal cells after day 14, presumably due to

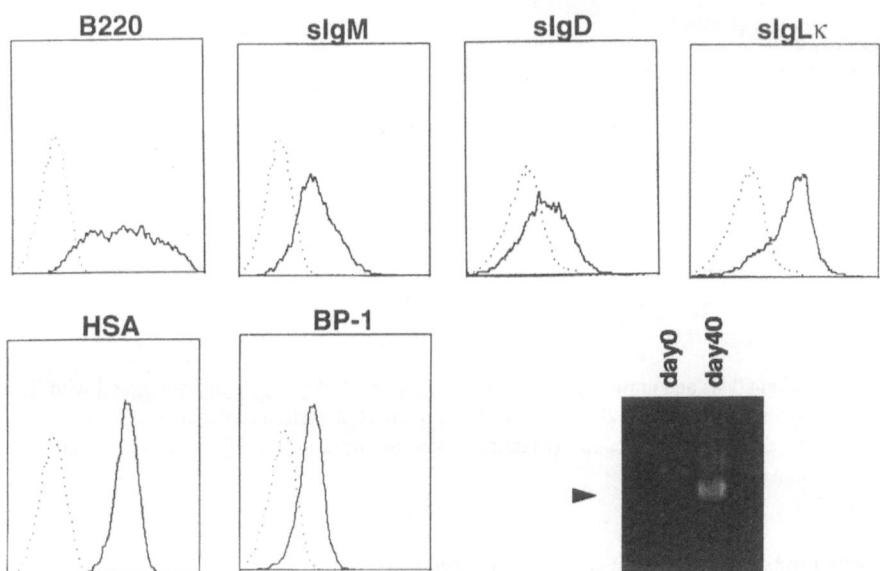

Fig. 3 <u>FACS analysis of day 40 induced B lineage cells.</u>
Expression of B220, IgM, IgD, Igκ, Heat stable antigen (HSA) and BP-1 are shown.   RT PCR analysis shows that immunoglobuin VDJ transcript is undetectable in undifferentiated D3 cells but detectable in day 40 cells.

completing terminal differentiation.   There remained scattered macrophages and mast cells. Meanwhile, very small proportion (1/500-1000) of day 14 clusters continued to proliferate until day 40 through several passages although cell growth was slow.   Such day 40 cells were morphologically very homogeneous and expressed B220, IgM, IgD, Igκ, Heat stable antigen (HSA) and BP-1 on their surface.   Furthermore, immunoglobulin VDJ rearrangement was detectable by RT-PCR (Figure 4).

An alternative and more efficient way to obtain B lineage cells is the addition of IL-7 and 2ME. When IL-7 and 2ME were added to the coculture after day 10, there was a burst in the proliferation of B lymphoid lineage cells.   The earlier administration of IL-7 and 2ME since day 5 stimulated the growth of only the undifferentiated colonies and the differentiated colonies but did not stimulate that of B lineage cells.   Presumably, there were no progenitor cells committed to the B lineage which could respond to IL-7 at day 5.   At day 20, which was 10 days after the addition of IL-7 and 2ME, more than 95% of the cells were B220 and HSA positive.   Day 20 B lineage cells did not show surface expression of IgM or BP-1; however, DJ rearrangement was detected by Southern blot analysis using a JH probe (Figure 5).   These data show that the day 20 cells obtained in the presence of IL7 and 2ME are B lineage cells in the early Pro-B cell stage.

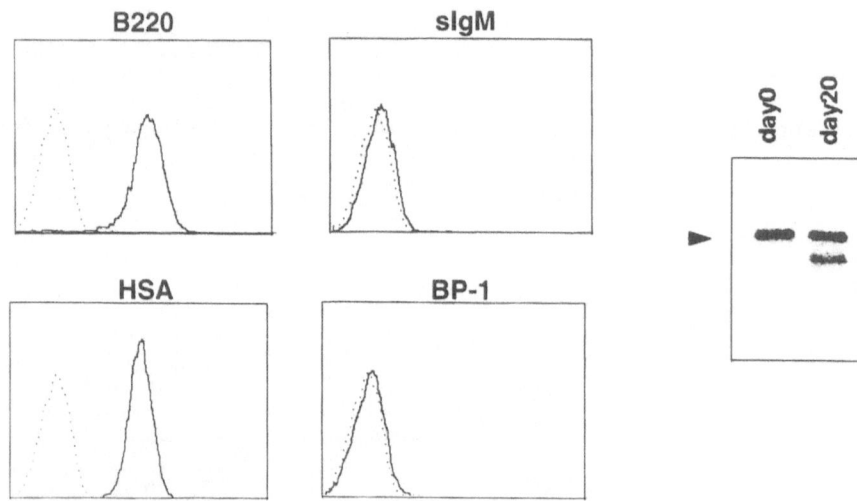

Fig. 4 FACS analysis and immunoglobulin DJ rearrangement of day 20 cells stimulated with IL 7. FACS analysis shows that B220 and HSA were positive but surface expression of IgM and BP-1 were negative.   Immunoglobulin DJ rearrangement occurred in day 20 induced cells but not in undifferentiated D3 ES cells.

In vivo Transfer of the Differentiation Induced Cells

More than 10^8 cells of the day 5 to day 10 induced cells were injected into lethally irradiated mice or sublethally irradiated *W/W^v* mice.   However, neither spleen colonies nor long term hematopoietic reconstitution occurred.   This suggests that no self-renewing hematopoietic stem cells during the early phase of the ES cell differentiation induction on OP9 cells.   Considering that OP9 stromal cells possess the ability to maintain self-renewing hematopoietic stem cell activity in the long term, the disappearance of the differentiation induced cells after day 14 of induction seems to support the notion that no hematopoietic stem cells with any self-renewing capacity appear during the differentiation induction.

DISCUSSION

In vitro Differentiation Capacity of Embryonic Stem Cells to Myeloid and Erythloid Cells

ES cells resemble inner cell mass cells or the primitive ectoderm of the very early postimplantation embryo and have the ability to contribute to all lineages including germline in chimeric animals once reintroduced into eight-cell or blastocyst embryos.   Although *in vitro* differentiation capacity of ES cells is not so broad as the *in vivo* capacity, hematopoietic cells can be easily obtained from ES cells in culture.   Doetschman et al. found that ES cells formed aggregates in suspension, grew into complex embryoid bodies (EBs) with endoderm, basal lamina, mesoderm and ectoderm, which were morphologically similar to embryos of the 6- to 8- day egg-cylinder stage [2].   Thereafter EBs expanded into large cystic structures and differentiated into various cell lineages spontaneously.   Very low percentages of EBs gave rise to blood island containing primitive erythrocytes inside.   Human cord serum, however, dramatically improved the blood island development and 30% of the cysts finally contained blood island.

Schmitt et al. also used human cord serum as a differentiation inducing agent and revealed that EBs contained not only primitive erythrocytes but also hematopoietic precursors which could differentiate into all myeloid lineage cells [3].   As a matter of course, human cord serum is very difficult to collect and batches vary in induction capacity.   Two groups improved the differentiation induction method by using a methylcellulose semisolid medium to support the EB development [4, 5].   Using their systems, ES cells differentiated into hematopoietic cells along various myeloid lineages, and the kinetics of differentiation were similar to those found in mouse embryogenesis.

In vitro Differentiation Capacity of Embryonic Stem Cells to Lymphoid Cells

Differentiation induction from ES cells to lymphoid precursors has been reported by four independent groups based on different strategies.   Two systems are essentially identical to the induction method of EB formation discussed above.   Chen et al. reported that a significant proportion of EBs became "ES cell fetuses", which contained pulsating cardiac muscle, yolk sac blood islands and cup-shaped structures containing lymphoid cells [6, 7].   Meanwhile the development of "ES cell fetuses" occurred rather asynchronously between days 11 and 30. Although phenotypes of lymphoid cells in "ES cell fetuses" were not characterized, those lymphoid cells presumably possessed the capacity to differentiate into mature B and T cells. When ES fetuses were cultured in the presence of Interleukin-2 (IL-2), IL-3 and ConA or infected with retroviruses such as Abelson murine leukemia (v-abl), J2 (v-raf/mil + myc), or RIM (Ig-myc + v-Ha-ras) viruses, mixed populations containing erythrocytes, macrophages, megakaryocytes and lymphocytes emerged in various ratios.   ES cell fetus-derived mature B cells, T cells and macrophage/granulocyte lineage cells appeared when these mixed populations were transferred into lethally irradiated mice.   Potocnik et al. reported a much simpler method for lymphohematopoietic differentiation from ES cells [11].   By their system, ES cells underwent lymphohematopoietic differentiation in EB under a low-oxygen (5% CO_2) atmosphere without additional exogenous factors.   After 15-20 days of the differentiation induction, lymphoid lineage cells (Thy-1[+], Pgp-1[+], c-kit[+] and B-220[+]) appeared.   Productive immunoglobulin VDJ rearrangement paralleled by light chain VκJκ recombination then occurred, which indicates a developmental stage of pre-B cells.   Furthermore, rearrangements of the T cell receptor γ as well as δ chain segments were observed.

The coculturing of lymphohematopoietic stem or progenitor cells with bone marrow stromal cell lines has been very useful in analyzing lympho-hematopoieis *in vitro*, and this system is also applicable for the *in vitro* lymphopoietic differentiation induction from ES cells.   Gutierrez-Ramos et al. cocultured ES cells on bone marrow stromal cell line RP010 in the presence of a mixture of saturated doses of exogenous IL-3, 6, and 7 [8].   Mononuclear cells with the immature hematopoietic blast cells appeared by day 10 and differentiated.   By days 20 and 25, B-220 positive B lineage cells and Joro75 positive T lineage cells appeared, although no surface IgM positive cells or CD3, 4 or 8 positive cells were detected.   In addition to immature lymphoid lineage cells, less-differentiated hematopoietic cells were also detected.   ES cells induced for 25 days differentiated into mature B and T cells in sublethally irradiated scid mice or normal mice.   One notable point in their system is the role(s) of exogenous cytokines. Coculture with IL-6 alone generated only macrophage-like and fibroblast-like cells which could not differentiate into B or T cells *in vivo*.   There are two explanations for the synergistic effects of IL-3 and 7.   One possibility is that IL-3 and 7 induced differentiation into and/or proliferation of immature lymphoid lineage cells.   The other is that the IL's prevented the differentiation into macrophage lineage cells.   The result obtained by coculturing ES cells on an M-CSF deficient stromal cell line seems to agree with the latter possibility although cannot rule out the former.

The third system is a combination of EB formation and coculture on stromal cells.   EBs were formed by culturing ES cells in methylcellulose and then transferred onto bone marrow stromal cell line ST2 in the presence of IL-7 [10, 18].   Mononuclear cells appeared 10 days after the transfer (7 days for EB formation and 3 days on ST2 cells) and proliferated up to 8 weeks. The result that a significant percentage of the day 21 cells (i.e.; 7 days in methylcellulose and 14 days on ST2 cells) expressed Ly-5, Sca-1 or c-kit on their surface suggests that at least a part of the day 21 cells belong to hematopoietic lineage cells.   However, lineage specific surface markers such as B220, T200 and Mac-1, which are expressed on the surface of B, T, or macrophage lineage cells, respectively, were not detectable.   Expressions of RAG-1, RAG-2 and TCRδ were but those of λ5, mb-1 were not detectable by RT-PCR.   And RT-PCR showed that a small percentage of the cells completed rearrangement of immunoglobulin DJ. Furthermore, *in vivo* transfer of the induced cells into sublethally irradiated RAG-2 deficient mice gave rise to both B and T cells.   Taken together, the authors argued that the induced cells should be very immature lineage marker negative lymphoid precursors.   Macrophage lineage cells which must have existed in EBs were not maintained on ST2 stromal cells in the presence of IL-7, which suggests again the inhibitory effect of IL-7 on proliferation and/or differentiation of macrophage lineage cells.

Development of Self-Renewing Hematopoietic Stem Cells from Embryonic Stem Cells

The hierarchy of hematopoietic cells in adult mice is generally considered to be as follows. There are long-term reconstituting cells at the top of the hierarchy, followed by colony forming unit of the spleen (CFU-S), both of which possess the capacity for self-renew. Below these hematopoietic stem cells, are non-self renewing multipotential hematopoietic progenitor cells and mature blood cells. If hematopoietic cell hierarchy of adult mice were applicable to the developmental order of blood cells during the mouse ontogeny, hematopoietic stem cells should exist somewhere between the embryonic stem cells and differentiated blood cells. However, no hematopoietic stem cells could be detected during the early phase of the differentiation induction with OP9 cells or EB systems [19]. There are two possible explanations for this discrepancy; one is that the *in vitro* differentiation induction systems produced blood cells via an artificial differentiation pathway. The other is that the order of hematopoietic cell development during the mouse ontogeny is different from the hierarchy in the adult hematopoietic system. The excellent series of Dzierzak's papers regarding the development of hematopoietic stem cell activity in the mouse embryo seems to support the latter notion. Dzierzak et al. reported that the order of the appearance of hematopoietic cells during the mouse ontogeny is the reverse of the steady state hierarchy of hematopoietic cells found in adult mice [20-22]. That is, hematopoietic progenitors appear first followed by CFU-S, and finally long term repopulating cells. Considering these results, the OP9 differentiation induction system seems to mimic until the production of non-self-renewing hematopoietic progenitors but cannot reproduce the further stage of self-renewing hematopoietic stem cell development.

Recently, Palacios et al. reported that self-renewing hematopoietic stem cells developed from ES cells when ES cells were cocultured on the stromal cell line RP010 in addition of the combination of IL-3, IL-6 and "F" factor (cell free supernatants from cultures of the FLS4.1 fetal liver stromal cell line) [20]. The cell-sorter-purified PgP-1[+], lineage marker (Lin)[-] cells produced by induced ES cells could repopulate the lymphoid, myeloid, and erythroid lineages of irradiated mice. Moreover, marrow cells from irradiated mice reconstituted with PgP-1[+], Lin[-] cell-sorter-purified cells by induced ES cells repopulated the lymphoid, myeloid and erythroid lineages in secondary mouse recipients after their transfer into irradiated secondary mice. The EB and OP9 might lack an unknown factor "F", which seems to be necessary for the development of self-renewing hematopoietic stem cells from ES cells [20].

CONCLUSION

Both recessive and dominant genetic alterations to hematopoietic cells, which are necessary for a complete analysis of the gene function in development and differentiation of hematopoieitc cells, can be generated through genetic manipulations of ES cells. The mechanisms of differentiation from genetically manipulated ES cells to blood cells can be easily examined *in vitro* without passage of germ line or chimera formation. The *in vitro* differentiation induction system should be especially useful for studying the gene functions essential for the development and differentiation of lymphohematopoietic cells because the targeted disruption of such genes often causes a lethal phenotype during ontogeny. Differentiation induction of ES cells in which a special gene function is knocked out and complemented with conditionally controllable and/or structurally modified genes must be the best system for elucidating the development and differentiation programme of lymphohematopoiesis.

REFERENCES

1. Wurst W, Joyner AL. (1992) Production of targeted embryonic stem cell clones. In : Gene Targeting, a practical approach. Joyner, AL (ed) IRL Press, Oxford; pp33-62
2. Doetschman TC, Eistetter H, Katz M, Schmidt W, Kemler R. (1985) The in vitro development of blastocyst-derived embryonic stem cell lines: formation of visceral yolk sac, blood islands and myocardium. J Embryol exp Morph 87:27-45
3. Scmitt RM, Bruyns E, Snodgrass HR. (1991) Hematopoietic development of embryonic stem cells in vitro: cytokine and receptor gene expression. Genes & Dev 5:728-740
4. Wiles MV, Keller G. (1991) Multiple hematopoietic lineages develop from embryonic stem (ES) cells in culture. Development 111:259-267
5. Burkert U, von Ruden T, Wagner EF. (1991) Early fetal hematopoietic development from in vitro differentiated embryonic stem cells. New Biologist 3:698-708
6. Chen U. (1992) Differentiation of mouse embryonic stem cells to lympho-hematopoietic lineages *in vitro*. Dev Immunol 2:29-50
7. Chen U, Kosco M, Staerz U. (1992) Establishment and characterization of lymphoid and myeloid mixed-cell populations from mouse late embryoid bodies, "embryonic-stem-cell fetuses". Proc Natl Acad Sci USA 89:2541-2545
8. Guiterrez-Ramos JC, Palacios R. (1992) *In vitro* differentiation of embryonic stem cells into lymphocyte precursors able to generate T and B lymphocytes *in vivo*. Proc Natl Acad Sci USA 89:9171-9175
9. Keller G, Kennedy M, Papayannopoulou T, Wiles MV. (1993) Hematopoietic commitment during embryonic stem cell differentiation in culture. Mol Cell Biol 13:473-486
10. Nisitani S, Tsubata T, Honjo T. (1994) Lineage marker-negative lymphocyte precursors derived from embryonic stem cells *in vitro* differentiate into mature lymphocytes *in vivo*. Int Immunol 6:909-916
11. Potocnik AJ, Nielsen PJ, Eichman K. (1994) *In vitro* generation of lymphoid precursors from embryonic stem cells. EMBO J 13:5274-5283
12. Nakano T, Kodama H, Honjo T. (1994) Generation of lymphohematopoietic cells from embryonic stem cells in culture. Science 265:1098-1101
13. Nakano T. (1995) Lymphohematopoietic development of embryonic stem cells *in vitro*. Sem Immunol 7:197-203
14. Kodama H, Nose M, Niida S, Nishikawa S, Nishikawa S-I. (1994) Involvement of the c-*kit* receptor in the adhesion of hematopoietic stem cells to stromal cells. Exp Hematol 22:979-984
15. Yoshida H, Hayashi S, Kunisada T, Ogawa M, Nishikawa S, Okamura H,Sudo T, Shultz LD, Nishikawa S. (1990) The murine mutation osteopetrosis is in the coding region of the macrophage colony stimulating factor gene. Nature 345:442-444
16. Borzillo GV, Ashmun RA, Sherr CJ. (1990) Macrophage lineage switching of murine early pre-B lymphoid cells expressing transduced fms genes. Mol Cell Biol 10:2703-2714.
17. Nakano T, Waki N, Asai H, Kitamura Y. (1987) Long-term monoclonal reconstitution of erythropoiesis in genetically anemic W/W^v mice by injection of 5-fluorouracil-treated bone marrow cells of $Pgk-1^b/Pgk-1^a$ mice. Blood 70: 1758-1763
18. Ogawa M, Nishikawa S, Ikuta K, Yamamura K, Naito F, Takahashi M, Nishikawa SI. (1989) B cell ontogeny in murine embryo studied by a culture system with the monolayer of a stromal cell clone, ST2: B cell progenitor develops first in the embryonal body rather than in the yolk sac. EMBO J 7:1337-1343
19. Muller AM, Dzierzak EA. (1993) ES cells have only a limited lymphopoietic potential after adoptive transfer into mouse recipients. Development 118: 1343-1351

20. Medvinsky AL, Samoyina NL, Muller AM, Dzierzak EA. (1993) An early pre-liver intraembryonic source of CFU-S in the developing mouse. Nature 364:64-67
21. Dzierzak E, Medvinsky A. (1995) Mouse embryonic hematopoiesis. TIG 11:359-366
22. Muller AM, Medvinsky A, Strouboulis J, Grosveld F, Dzierzak E. (1994) Development of hematopoietic stem cell activity in the mouse embryo. Immunity 1: 291-301
23. Palacios R, Golunski E, Samaridis J. (1995) *In vitro* generation of hematopoietic stem cells from an embryonic stem cell line. Proc Natl Aca Sci USA 92:7530-7534

Stem cells for lymphocytes: comments on the time and place of commitment of precursors for the T lineage

Roland Scollay[1] and Mariastefania Antica[2]

[1] Centenary Institute of Cancer Medicine and Cell Biology, Sydney. Locked Bag No. 6, Newtown, NSW 2042, Australia

[2] R. Boskovic Institute, Bijenicka 54, 41000 Zagreb, Croatia

SUMMARY

T cell development occurs predominantly in the thymus, although some thymus independent T cells certainly occur in tissues such as the gut. Thymic development is dependent on continual replacement of intrathymic precursors with new precursors from the bone marrow, but it is still unclear whether the cells that migrate into the thymus are multi potential or committed to the T or lymphoid pathways. Although a T cell precursor with limited potential has not been found in adult murine bone marrow, the presence of such a cell in human bone marrow and the absence of a multi potent stem cell inside the thymus of the mouse, suggests that lineage commitment (or at least partial commitment) occurs prior to migration of precursors to the thymus. The identification of the pre-thymic but committed precursor in the murine bone marrow awaits better markers and more refined experimental strategies.

KEY WORDS: Thymic stem cells, lymphoid precursors, lineage commitment, thymus, T lymphocytes, multi potent stem cells

INTRODUCTION

All the cells of the blood and lymphoid systems are derived from multi potential haemopoietic stem cells. These precursors eventually give rise to progeny which are committed to particular lineages. Many of these commitment steps occur in the complex micro environments of the bone marrow (in the adult), and it is also in the bone marrow that production of the functional end cells of many lineages occurs. Production of T cells, in contrast, occurs at a remote and specialised site, the thymus. The isolated and specialised nature of the thymus has facilitated study of the processes of T cell development, and many aspects of T cell development can now be clearly described. For example, it is clear that bone marrow derived precursors are carried by the blood to the thymus, at least in the adult thymus. A number of strands of evidence indicate that continual provision of these blood born, bone marrow derived precursors is essential for the thymus, since precursors within the thymus have only limited proliferative potential [1, reviewed in 2]. For example in thymic organ culture, expansion ceases after about two weeks and the organ then degenerates. Similarly, in a variety of systems (bone marrow chimeras [3,4], thymic organ grafts [5,6], parabiotic mice [1]) the endogenous thymocytes are almost completely replaced by progeny of externally derived precursors within 3-5 weeks. Although all these systems are artefactual, and hence the data circumstantial rather than definitive, the body of data has led to the view that the thymus needs continual input of new precursors, and this view is probably correct. For more detailed discussion and reviews on stem cell entry to the thymus see refs

2, 7.
This leads to the question of the nature of this precursor. Is it already committed to the T cell lineage when it reaches the thymus, or does it only become committed once inside the thymus? In other words, does commitment occur before or after thymic entry. In this paper we will briefly review some of our data and see to what extent we can discriminate these possibilities. As is often the case, it seems most likely that an intermediate position is correct, with partial commitment occurring prior to thymic entry, and full commitment occurring inside the thymus.

RESULTS AND DISCUSSION

The possibilities for the way precursor cell commitment might occur relative to thymic entry are shown in Figure 1. Each of the models shown makes a very clear prediction about the kind of cells that should be found in different tissues. Thus in model A, precursors committed to the T lineage ought to be detectable in bone marrow and blood. In model B, multi potent cells should be detected in the thymus. In model C, a partially committed or intermediate precursor is postulated, which should be present in both the thymus and the bone marrow.

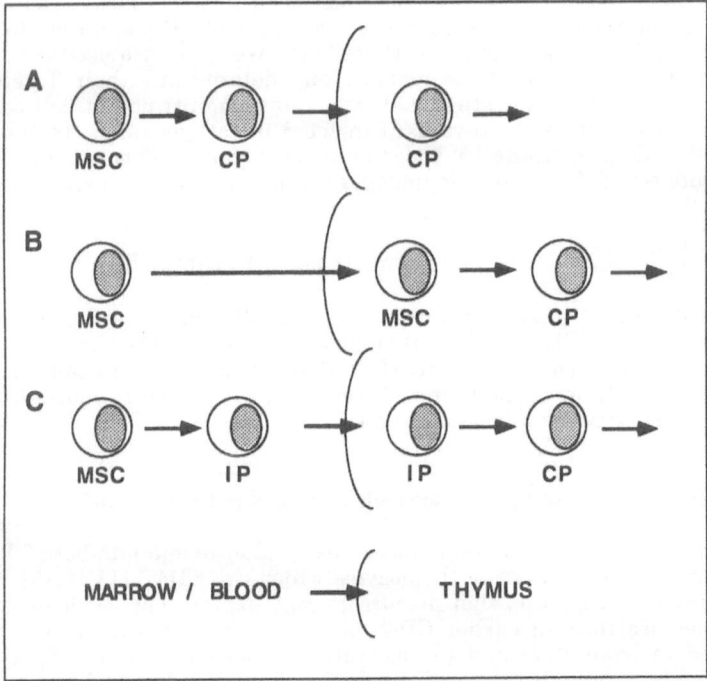

FIGURE 1. This diagram shows the possible ways that stem cells might colonise the thymus. The cells left of the arc represent cells in the bone marrow and migrating through the blood. Cells to the right represent cells inside the thymus. MSC = multi potent stem cell. CP = committed T cell precursor. IP = intermediate precursor, partially committed or committed to the lymphoid lineages, but not specifically to the T lineage.

However, note that in all possible models, there must be a cell type which is both inside and outside the thymus, ie. the migrating cell as it leaves the bone marrow or travels through the blood, and at the moment it enters the thymus. In practice this may not be the case if the migrating cell changes its state the very moment it enters the thymus or very soon after, in which case it would be almost impossible to detect.

It is well documented that there are multi potent stem cells in the bone marrow and that under appropriate circumstances these can colonise the thymus, either directly or by the production of progeny which can [8,9]. Similarly there are clearly precursors in the thymus which are fully committed to the T lineage [10,11]. So what are the data which could give weight to any of the models A, B or C? The questions are simple to ask, but difficult to answer experimentally.

1. Can intermediate or partially committed precursor cells be found in either the thymus or the bone marrow?

2. Can completely T committed precursors be found in bone marrow or blood?

3. Can multi potent cells be found in the thymus?

Our own approach as T cell biologists has been to work backwards through the thymus, to find the earliest precursor we can there [11-13], and then to look in the bone marrow for an equivalent cell there [14]. We have also used the approach of purifying stem cells from bone marrow and determining their T cell precursor function [9]. These latter studies showed that a multi potent cell could, at the single cell level, colonise a thymus if injected intrathymically. In this system, a single cell could give rise to 10^7 progeny in the thymus. This same cell type could reconstitute all the heamopoietic lineages if injected intravenously. The phenotype of this cell was:

Lin⁻ Thy1^lo Sca1⁺ Sca2⁻ CD4⁻ (multi potent stem cell in bone marrow)

However it seems unlikely that this cell normally colonises the thymus since it generates myeloid cells inside the thymus at early times after injection; a situation not normally seen. These data only show that this multi potent cell can give rise to T cells. Probably in normal circumstances, it gives rise to more differentiated progeny which actually migrate to the thymus.

Can partially committed precursor cells be found in the thymus?

Inside the thymus, we and others have clearly identified a number of T committed precursors among the 2-3% of thymocytes which are CD4⁻8⁻ [11,12,15]. However, it was only upon recognition that precursors may express low levels of the CD4 and CD8 molecules that an earlier CD4^lo precursor was identified and its function confirmed in irradiation and reconstitution experiments [16]. This cell proved able to make T cells, B cells and dendritic cells (DC), but had lost the ability to make myeloid cells [13,16,17]. This was an intermediate precursor. Its ability to generate T cells was reduced relative to the bone marrow stem cell. The phenotype of the intrathymic cell was:

Lin⁻ Thy1^lo Sca1⁺ Sca2⁺ CD4^lo (intermediate precursor in thymus)

Thus it differed phenotypically from the multi potent cell in bone marrow in being

Sca2$^+$ and CD4^b, but was otherwise very similar. One must qualify the conclusion that this cell is oligopotential, because although the population of CD4^b precursors is homogenous for a wide range of markers, reconstitution assays have not been performed at the single cell level. This is for the very good reason that clonal expansion from these cells is rather small, so single cell assays are extremely difficult. Nonetheless it remains a possibility that the T, B and DC precursor activities reside in different cells that have co-purified within this population, although this becomes increasingly less likely as more antibodies are tested and shown unable to separate the T and B precursor activities.

Still, taken at face value, these data imply that model A (Fig. 1) is not correct, if one assumes a committed precursor is limited to the T lineage. The data favour model C, with the intermediate precursor having retained B and DC activity, but lost myeloid and erythroid precursor activity. This being the case, there should be an equivalent or very similar cell in the bone marrow.

Can partially committed precursor cells be found in the bone marrow?

We then went back to the bone marrow to see if the Sca2$^+$ CD4^b phenotype would help us find a partially committed precursor there and separate it from the mutipotential cell. Indeed we did find a cell with the same phenotype as the intrathymic CD4^b precursor, but it turned out to be multi potent, although with less expansion potential than the Sca2$^-$ stem cell [14]. However, these experiments are technically demanding and it has to be admitted that one could not absolutely exclude the possibility of a multi potent cell contaminant, or a multi potent cell co-purifying with a genuine committed cell. Since, as we have mentioned, a single multi potent cell can colonise a thymus, or give rise to all the myeloid lineages, a single contaminant can affect the apparent function of any population. It is very difficult to exclude the possibility of a single contaminant when 10^4 or 10^5 cells are being assayed.

In contrast, it has been reported by Galy and colleagues [18 and Immunity, in press)] that in the adult human bone marrow a cell can be isolated which has very similar potential to the murine intrathymic CD4^b precursor. This cell has precursor potential limited to T, B, DC (and NK) lineages. The phenotype of this cell is:

$$\textbf{CD34}^+\textbf{Lin}^-\ \textbf{CD10}^+\textbf{CD45R}^+ \quad \text{(intermediate precursor in adult human}$$
$$\text{bone marrow)}$$

This provides the missing link we were unable to detect in adult mouse bone marrow, and further supports model C (Fig. 1). Although it is possible that there are differences between human and mouse precursors, we believe that this is not likely. With different or better markers, an intermediate precursor of this kind will probably be found in due course in the mouse bone marrow.

Does a multi potent cell exist in the thymus?

Our own studies of adult murine thymus suggest such a cell must be extremely rare [13,14]. Other studies have generally found the same; for example, in foetal thymus [19] stem cells were detected, but at less than one cell per thymus. If multi potent cells are present, they are extremely rare in the normal thymus of both adult and foetus, although they may persist in the thymus in certain experimental situations, for example after injection of bone marrow cells into irradiated thymuses

[20]. If there are indeed no multi potent stem cells in the normal thymus, it seems to rule out model B (Figure 1).

These data should probably be given more weight than those derived from experiments which could not detect a committed cell in the bone marrow, since the presence of multi potent stem cell would be "dominant" while absence of a committed cell is "recessive" in the sense that it could be easily obscured by contaminating multi potent cells.

Can precursors committed to the T lineage only be found outside the thymus?

This has not been possible in either human or mouse, with one exception. In the mouse, Rodewald [21] detected a precursor cell in foetal blood which was fully committed to the T lineage; that is, only able to make T cells and hence even more committed than the intra-thymic precursor which retains B and DC precursor activity. It is not clear quite how this cell fits into the picture, and it is not yet certain whether it is indeed a natural precursor. It has only been detected in the embryo. Given the presence of intermediate precursors inside the thymus, it is tempting to dismiss this cell. However, it is possible to imagine a model which incorporates such a cell as a real precursor and part of the process of T cell development.

A composite model of T cell development.

Figure 2 shows a possible alternative to those shown in Figure 1.

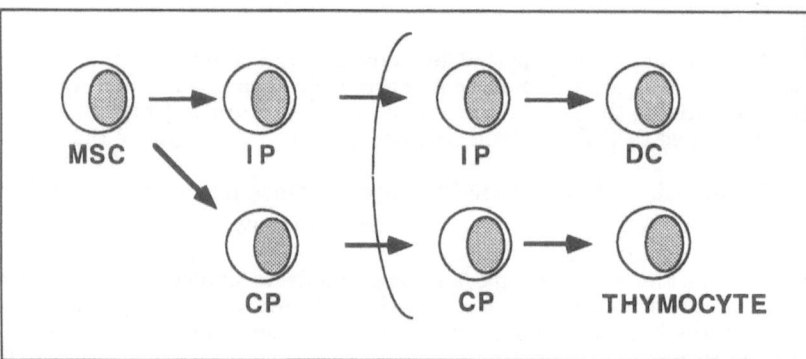

FIGURE 2. This shows an alternative model in which the intermediate precursor in the thymus gives rise to DC but not T cells. The T cells are derived from a truly committed precursor also present in the thymus. This allows for both intermediate and fully committed precursors in the thymus, but requires both to be present outside the thymus as well. By this model, the T precursor activity of the IP is an artefact of the assay systems, and would not occur in the normal thymus.
MSC = multi potent stem cell. IP = intermediate precursor. CP = committed T cell precursor. Thymocyte = all the T lineage cells.

This model suggests that perhaps the intrathymic CD4^b precursor is not the usual (or perhaps not the only) source of lymphocytes in the thymus, but that it would use its DC precursor potential (or even B cell) under normal circumstances. Its pre T potential would only be apparent in the rather artificial purification and transfer systems we have used. By this argument, some other, more T committed precursor (eg Rodewald's) would normally provide the pre T activity. Although this model incorporates all the data, it has less appeal to us than model C, as it requires the considerable pre T activity of the CD4^b precursor to be deemed an artefact. It might be preferable to assume that the Rodewald cell is specific to the embryo, and retain model C. There are other reasons for thinking the situation in the embryo is different, as we will now discuss.

Precursor Cells in the embryo.

While trying to understand the ontogeny of T cell development, we looked in the early thymus for precursor cells like the adult intrathymic, intermediate CD4^b precursor. Indeed we found a cell of this type in foetal thymus, or at least of this phenotype [22]. In fact functional analysis by the same intrathymic transfer approach showed that these foetal "precursors" had very poor pre T activity. This low activity continued after birth, and full reconstitution potential was not reached until four weeks of age. These data lead to the conclusion that foetal development may be quite different from adult development, and that different precursors may be involved. Again this brings into question the relevance of the cell identified by Rodewald to adult T cell development.

These data also highlight the caution that cells of apparently identical phenotype may be functionally different at different stages of development. As we all know, but often forget, phenotypic identity is not a guarantee of functional identity.

A final cautionary note.

A final point to keep in mind in the context of precursor cell analysis is that purified precursor cells may behave differently than those in mixed populations. The specific example we shall discuss here concerns the bone marrow multi potent stem cell discussed above [9]. In purified form this cell saturates for T cell development at 100 cells or less [9] upon intrathymic injection. Since it has a frequency of about 1 in 10^3 cells in whole bone marrow, 10^5 whole bone marrow cells should also saturate. In fact even 10^6 whole marrow cells injected intrathymically do not saturate (unpublished data), while in intravenous injections, 5×10^7 cells have faster kinetics than 5×10^6 cells [2,23], (indeed 5×10^8 is faster still - unpublished data), suggesting that saturation has not been reached here, 5×10^3 times the level predicted from data with purified cells. These results again require a cautionary note, that purified and non-purified stem cells may not behave in exactly the same way.

CONCLUSIONS

In this paper we have briefly reviewed data pertaining to precursor cell colonisation of the thymus. We have discussed the reasons why we favour the model in which partial lineage commitment occurs in the bone marrow, prior to migration to the thymus. Partial in this context means loss of myeloid and erythroid precursor activity but maintenance of lymphoid and dendritic cell precursor activity. Final complete commitment to the T lineage occurs inside the thymus.

The remaining unanswered question is whether the lymphoid/DC precursor is the natural precursor of both B cells and DC (ie do both these lineages also go through this stage) as well as T cells, or is this a genuine committed pre T cell which has not yet lost all of its other potential (ie this cell would not normally become a B cell or DC in the normal animal)? If the latter is true, do B cells go through a stage in which they are truly committed to the B lineage but retain the ability to make T cells and DC when pushed in an experimental situation? These questions await further experiment and perhaps new reagents and approaches.

ACKNOWLEDGEMENTS

The authors acknowledge the many discussions and joint experiments performed with our friends and colleagues Ken Shortman and Wu Li. RS would like to thank the Japan Intractable Disease Foundation and Professor Susumu Ikehara for the opportunity to attend this conference.

REFERENCES

1. Donskoy E, Goldschneider I. (1992) Thymocytopoiesis is maintained by blood-born precursors throughout postnatal life. A study in parabiotic mice. J Immunol 148: 1604-1612
2. Scollay R, Smith J, Stauffer V. (1986) Dynamics of early T cells: Prothymocyte migration and proliferation in the adult mouse thymus. Immunol Rev 91:129-157
3. Micklem HS, Ford CE, Evans EP, Gray J. (1966) Interrelationships of myeloid and lymphoid cells: Studies with chromosomally marked cells transferred in lethally irradiated mice. Proc Roy Soc London Series 3 165:78
4. Boersma W, Betel I, Daculsi R, van der Wester G (1981) Post irradiation thymocyte regeneration after bone marrow transplantation. I. Regeneration and quantification of thymocyte progenitor cells n the bone marrow. Cell Tissue Kinet 14:179
5. Metcalf D (1966) Its role in immune responses, leukemia development and carcinogenesis. Springer-Verlag, New York thymectomised and normal mice. Nature 214:801
7. Scollay R, Shortman K. (1985) Cell traffic in the adult thymus: Cell entry and exit, cell birth and death. In:Recognition and regulation in cell-mediated immunity. Eds JD Watson and J Marbrook, Marcel Dekker Inc, New York and Basel
8. Spangrude GJ, Smith L, Uchida N, Ikuta K, Heimfeld S, Friedman J, Weissman IL (1991) Mouse hematopoietic stem cells. Blood 78:1395-1402
9. Spangrude GJ, Scollay R. (1990) Differentiation of hematopoietic stem cells in irradiated mouse thymic lobes: kinetics and phenotype of progeny. J Immunol 145:3661-3668
10. Godfrey DI, Kennedy J, Suda T, Zlotnik A. (1993) A developmental pathway involving four phenotypically and functionally distinct subsets of CD3-CD4-CD8-triple-negative adult mouse thymocytes defined by CD44 and CD25. J Immunol 150:4244-4252
11. Scollay R, Wilson A, D'Amico A, Kelly K, Egerton M, Pearse M, Wu L, Shortman W. (1988) Developmental status and reconstitution potential of subpopulation of murine thymocytes. Immunol Rev 104:81

12. Pearse M, Wu L, Egerton M, Wilson A, Shortman K, Scollay R. (1989) A murine early thymocyte developmental sequence is marked by transient expression of the interleukin 2 receptor. Proc Natl Acad Sci USA 86:1614-1618
13. Wu L, Antica M, Johnson GR, Scollay R, Shortman K. (1991) Developmental potential of the earliest precursor cells from the adult thymus. J Exp Med 174: 1617-1627
14. Antica M, Wu L, Shortman K, Scollay R. (1994) Thymic stem cells in the mouse bone marrow. Blood 84:111-117
15. Godfrey DI, Zlotnik A. (1993) Control points in early T-cell development. Immunol Today 14:547-553
16. Wu L, Scollay R, Egerton M, Pearse M, Spangrude GJ, Shortman K. (1991) The earliest T-lineage precursor cells in the adult murine thymus express low levels of CD4. Nature 349:71-74
17. Ardavin C, Wu L, Li C-L, Shortman K. (1993) Thymic dendritic cells and T cells develop simultaneously within the thymus from a common precursor population. Nature 362:761-763
18. Galy AHM, Cen D, Travis M, Chen S, Chen BP (1995) Delineation of T progenitor cell activity within the CD34+ compartment of adult bone marrow. Blood 85:2770-2778
19. Barg M, Mandel TE, Johnson GR. (1978) Haemopoietic cells in foetal mouse thymus. Aust J Exp Biol & Med Sci 56:195-200
20. Ezine S, Papiernik M, Lepault F. (1991) Persistence of stem cell activity within the murine thymus after transfer of a bone marrow fraction enriched in CFU-S. Int Immunol 3:237-243
21. Rodewald H-R, Kretzschmar K, Takeda S, Itohl C, Dessing M. (1994) Identification of pro-thymocytes in murine fetal blood: T lineage commitment can precede thymus colonization. EMBO J 13:4229-4240
22. Antica M, Wu L, Shortman K, Scollay R. (1993) Intrathymic lymphoid precursor cells during fetal thymus development. J Immunol 151:5887-5895
23. Wallis V, Leuchars E, Chwalinski S, Davies AJS. (1975) On the sparse seeding of bone marrow and thymus in radiation chimeras. Transplantation 19:2

Effects of Interleukin 12 on Hematopoietic Stem and Progenitor Cells

Steven Neben[1], John Leonard[2], Samuel Goldman[2], and Rob E. Ploemacher[3]

[1]Department of Immunology and Hematopoiesis and [2]Pre-clinical Pharmacology, Genetics Institute, Inc., 87 CambridgePark Dr., Cambridge, MA, USA, and [3]Department of Hematology, Erasmus University, 3000 DR Rotterdam, The Netherlands

SUMMARY

Interleukin-12 (IL-12) has been shown to possess potent immunomodulatory activity. It has a unique structure among cytokines, consisting of two covalently linked subunits, one with homology to other members of the cytokine superfamily, the other being highly homologous to gp130, the signalling subunit of a number of cytokine receptors. Here we summarize studies showing that IL-12 is a hematopoietic growth factor with potent activity on hematopoietic stem and progenitor cells. In clonal and liquid culture assays, IL-12 synergizes with IL-3 and Steel Factor to increase the number of colonies as well as to expand both stem and progenitor cell content in the cultures. In stroma-dependent long-term bone marrow cultures, IL-12 addition causes a decrease in cell production in the first week after inoculation of whole bone marrow cells, followed by an increase in both mature cells and progenitor cells over the next 3 weeks. The initial decrease appears to be mediated by IL-12-induced production of IFN-γ, possibly by natural killer cells and/or T cells which do not persist in these cultures. Studies in naive mice demonstrate a similar acute decrease in peripheral leukocyte count, mediated by IFN-γ, upon administration of IL-12. In contrast, despite a significant decrease in peripheral platelet count, reticulated platelets become elevated and mean megakaryocyte ploidy in the bone marrow shifts from 16N to 32N during IL-12 treatment. These IL-12-mediated effects on megakaryopoiesis are abrogated by simultaneous treatment of mice with antibodies against IFN-γ. These studies provide further information on the potential physiological role and applications of IL-12 outside the immune system.

KEY WORDS: Interleukin-12, hematopoiesis, stem cells, megakaryocytes

INTRODUCTION

In the adult mammal, hematopoietic stem cells (HSC) reside in the bone marrow, where they serve to maintain a continuous output of functional circulating blood cells for an entire lifetime. HSC are capable of differentiating into both myeloid and lymphoid elements, as well as maintaining their own numbers either through a process of self-renewal or by conserving a quiescent stem cell reserve compartment with relatively few stem cell clones actually contributing to daily blood cell production. Although the exact mechanisms by which HSC self-maintenance and differentiation occur in vivo are not known, it is clear that these processes are heavily influenced by a network of stromal cells, extracellular matrix molecules, and cytokines that surround and bathe the HSC in the marrow cavity.

Murine HSC can be enriched from adult bone marrow using various combinations of density gradient materials, dyes, lectins, and antibodies. Near homogeneity, as assessed by both in vivo reconstitution of lethally irradiated mice with limiting numbers of cells and limiting dilution analysis of clonagenicity in long-term stroma-dependent culture systems, has been achieved by combining prior administration of cycle-active drugs, such as 5-fluorouracil (5-FU), density gradient centrifugation, immunomagnetic bead depletion with lineage-specific antibodies, and positive selection for one or more "stem cell antigens" using the fluorescence activated cell sorter. There is general agreement that HSC in the adult mouse have the phenotype lineage-marker negative to low,

28

Sca-1 positive or wheat germ aglutinin (WGA) positive, c-kit receptor positive, and rhodamine and Hoechst 33342 dull.

Studies over the past decade using enriched HSC populations and purified recombinant cytokines have led to the conclusion that these primitive cells are capable of responding, either by proliferating or differentiating, to a large number of known cytokines. Cytokines can be divided into three catagories based on their effects on different HSC and progenitor cell populations: 1) differentiation factors, which include erythropoietin, thrombopoietin, M-CSF, and IL-5, acting on erythroid lineage, megakaryocytes/platelets, monocytes/macrophages, and eosinophils, respectively; 2) proliferation factors such as IL-3, GM-CSF, and IL-4, which can stimulate HSC mitosis, but only after entry into the cell cycle; and 3) competence factors, like IL-6, IL-11, G-CSF, Steel Factor (SF), and FLT3 ligand, which affect entry of HSC into the cell cycle and act synergistically with the proliferation factors to support colony formation [1]. Here we review work by ourselves and others on a recently discovered cytokine, interleukin-12, which falls into the same category as IL-6, IL-11, and G-CSF with regard to its effects on HSC and hematopoietic progenitors.

Interleukin 12 (IL-12), also known as natural killer cell stimulatory factor (NKSF) or cytotoxic lymphocyte maturation factor (CMLF), was originally identified in the conditioned medium of Epstein-Barr virus (EBV) transformed human B cell lines by its ability to enhance cytotoxic activity and induce IFN-γ, TNF-α, and GM-CSF production from T and natural killer (NK) cells and to synergize with IL-2 in stimulating the generation of lymphokine activated killer (LAK) cells in vitro [2]. Subsequently, IL-12 has been shown to play a central role in cell-mediated immune responses by promoting the development of CD4+ T helper 1 (TH1) cells and antagonizing the development of TH2 cells [2]. The active form of IL-12 is secreted as a covalently-linked heterodimer consisting of a 40 kD heavy chain (p40) and a 35 kD light chain (p35) [3]. It has a unique structure among cytokines, in that the p40 chain shows significant sequence homology to the extracellular domain of the IL-6 receptor [4], and the p35 chain shows homology with both IL-6 and G-CSF [5]. Since both G-CSF [6] and IL-6 [7] had previously been shown to regulate the proliferation and differentiation of primitive hematopoietic progenitor cells, we reasoned that IL-12 might also be active on these cells.

IN VITRO ACTIVITIES OF IL-12 ON MURINE HSC

Several investigators have examined the effects of IL-12 on human and murine HSC and committed progenitors in clonal assay systems. Although similar studies with human HSC have been reported [2], in this review we will discuss only murine studies. Ogawa and colleagues studied the effects of IL-12 on colony formation from bone marrow mononuclear cells of normal mice and on cell cycle-dormant lymphohemopoietic progenitors (Lin-Sca-1+ HSC) from 5-FU treated mice [8]. IL-12 alone did not support colony formation, but significantly enhanced colony formation stimulated by Steel Factor (SF). Total colony formation was increased 1.5-fold, with a 5-fold increase in multilineage (GEMM) colonies. Similar to IL-6 [1], IL-12 synergized with SF or IL-3, but not with IL-4 or IL-11, to promote colony formation from primitive HSC. These results suggested that IL-12 belongs to a group of cytokines which includes IL-6, IL-11, and G-CSF, that can act synergistically with SF or IL-3 in support of proliferation of primitive HSC. In retrospect, this was not surprising given the similarities in protein structure between the p40 chain of IL-12 and the extracellular binding domain of the IL-6 receptor [4] and among IL-12 p35, IL-6, and G-CSF [5]. In addition it has been shown that IL-6 and IL-11 can combine extracellularly with soluble forms of their respective receptor binding chains and signal through a second, signal transducing receptor component, gp130, at the cell surface ([9] and V. Ling, S. Neben, unpublished). Recent cloning of a human IL-12 receptor, in fact, reveals close homology to gp130 [10]. In Ogawa's investigation, the combination of IL-12 + SF supported about 1/2 the number of colonies supported by IL-11 + SF, and the primary colonies induced by IL-12 + SF were only about 10-15% the size of those formed in the presence of IL-11 + SF [8], suggesting that the mechanism of action of IL-12 and IL-11 on HSC are not the same. IL-12 did, however, support the production of a significant number of pre-B cell progenitors in SF-stimulated primary colonies, a property previously noted for IL-11, IL-6, and G-CSF, but not for IL-3 or IL-4 [11], proving that all of these cytokines act on the same primitive lymphohemopoietic progenitor.

Similar studies have been performed by Jacobsen et al. using Lin-Sca-1+ cells from normal mice. In their studies, IL-12 was shown to synergistically enhance both colony number and colony size in the presence of M-CSF, G-CSF, IL-3, or SF [12]. The growth stimulating effects of IL-12 on HSC were also observed in single-cell cloning assays in microtiter wells, suggesting a direct effect not mediated by contaminating accessory cells. In addition, Jacobsen and colleagues have demonstrated an effect of IL12 on erythroid colony formation, with slight enhancement of Epo + IL4 and Epo + SF induced BFU-E [13]. Surprisingly, IL-12 showed no ability to increase BFU-E numbers stimulated by Epo + IL-3. Recently, Jacobsen et al. have demonstrated synergy between IL-12 and the recently cloned FLT3 ligand [14]. Morphological analysis of colonies derived from Lin-Sca-1+ cells grown in IL-12 + FLT3 ligand revealed more primitive blast cell types compared to the mainly granulocytic colonies which appeared in IL-12 + SF. It will be interesting to see whether these primitive blast cell colonies contain primitive marrow repopulating HSC.

We have performed a variety of experiments to determine the effect of IL-12 on colony formation as well as on the maintenance or expansion of progenitors in liquid culture [15, 16]. In addition, we have examined the role of secondary factors, such as IFN-γ, on IL-12 induced stimulation of HSC in vitro. The target cells for our experiments were either low-density cells from 6-day post 5-fluorouracil bone marrow (LD/FU6dBM) which we have shown previously to be 85-fold enriched in primitive long-term repopulating HSC [17], or LD/FU6dBM cells further separated by wheat germ agglutinin affinity into a WGA-dim, which are 400-800 fold enriched in long-term repopulating ability (LTRA) and only 1-3 fold enriched in day 12 CFU-S, and WGA-bright, which are only 10-20 fold enriched in LTRA but 200-250 fold enriched in day 12 CFU-S [18]. In a dose-response study, IL-12 was tested on LD/FU6dBM cells in concentrations ranging from 0.03 to 30 ng/ml in the presence of IL-3 alone or IL-3 + SF. The highest dose (30 ng/ml) was required to enhance colony formation with IL-3 alone. However, 100-fold less IL-12 (0.3 ng/ml) was sufficient to enhance colony formation 1.5 fold in the presence of IL-3 + SF, demonstrating an ability of SF to increase the sensitivity of progenitors to IL-12 stimulation. Similar to effects described by Jacobsen et al. with IL-12 + FL, we observed a significant increase in colonies containing small blast cells in the presence of IL-12 + IL-3. In cultures containing IL-3 + IL-11 or IL-3 + SF, addition of IL-12 increased both the percentage and absolute number of colonies with multiple lineages (CFU-Mix). IL-12 was able to stimulate colony formation from both WGA-dim and WGA-bright cells in the presence of combinations of IL-3, IL-11, and SF, suggesting that it can act on both primitive and more committed progenitors. Colony formation from LD/FU6dBM cells grown in either IL-3 + IL-12 or IL-3 + SF + IL-12 was not affected by anti-IFN-γ antibody added to the cultures, indicating that the observed stimulatory effects of IL-12 on HSC were not not mediated induction of IFN-γ. Whether other cytokines, such as GM-CSF, known to be elaborated by IL-12-activated NK cells, are involved in the IL-12 induced stimulation of HSC, remains to be determined.

Along with colony formation, we also tested IL-12 in combination with IL-3, IL-11, and SF for its ability to stimulate the production of hematopoietic progenitors and enhance the recovery of LTRA cells in liquid cultures [16]. Using LD/FU6dBM cells as targets, we first tested various concentrations of IL-12 in an 8-day liquid culture in the presence of SF + IL-3, the endpoint being the generation of CFU-C, determined by replating into methylcellulose with pokeweed mitogen stimulated spleen conditioned medium as a stimulus. At least 10 ng/ml IL-12 was required to enhance CFU-C generation in liquid culture; about 30 times more than that needed for enhancing primary colony formation in methylcellulose with the same synergistic cytokines (see above). IL-12 at 10 ng/ml increased approximately 2 fold the generation of CFU-C in liquid cultures in the presence of IL-3 + SF. Cobblestone area forming cell (CAFC) assays andsex-mismatched long-term chimerism in lethally irradiated mice were used to determine the generation and/or maintenance of more primitive progenitors. IL-12 synergized with IL-3 + SF in liquid suspension cultures to increase the number of CAFC day 28/35 (representing LTRA cells) 3.7-fold over input, and produced a similar increase in cells giving stable 50% chimerism in mice. Exogenous TGF-β, present in some media components, especially BSA, tended to mask the synergistic effects of IL-12 and SF in the absence of IL-3 in our ealry experiments [15, 16]. In the presence of neutralizing anti-TGF-β1 antibodies, however, SF gives about a 10-fold expansion of CFU-C and CAFC day 10 in 5-7 days of liquid cultures, while IL-12 synergizes with SF to produce a total 100-fold expansion.

EFFECT OF IL-12 IN LONG-TERM BONE MARROW CULTURES

In vivo, hematopoietic progenitors reside in complex microenvironments where they interact with a variety of stromal cells, extracellular matrix molecules, and cytokines. Although not completely analogous to in vivo hematopoiesis, the long-term liquid bone marrow culture (LTBMC) system, first described by Dexter [19], can be used to study HSC-microenvironmental interactions and allow detailed analysis of myelopoiesis under the influence of various types of manipulation. We have used this system to study the effects of exogenously added IL-12 on hematopoietic progenitor cell proliferation and differentiation in the context of a hematopoietic microenvironment. LTBMCs were established by inoculating normal bone marrow cells onto 20 Gy irradiated normal marrow stroma. Twice weekly addition of IL-12 to these cultures caused a decrease in total non-adherent cell production in the first 1-2 weeks, followed by an increase of up to 5-fold over the next several weeks compared to control cultures. Non-adherent (NA) CFU-C numbers were increased 12-fold except in the first week, when they were depressed as much as 80%. Both the inhibitory and stimulatory effects were seen at IL-12 doses between 10 and 100 pg/ml; low compared to effective concentrations in colony assays and stroma-independent liquid cultures. The greater stimulatory effect on CFU-C compared to NA cell counts suggests a differential effect on more primitive, compared to more differentiated myeloid cells. CFU-C in the adherent stromal layer were increased at week 4 in IL-12 supplemented cultures, but only at the higher dose of 10 ng/ml. Consistent with this finding, CAFC frequencies of all day types (6-42) were only slightly increased in IL-12 supplemented CAFC cultures. One possibility for the dramatically different effects of IL-12 on hematopoiesis at different time points in LTBMC is the induction of secondary stimulators and/or inhibitors from either the stromal cells or accessory cells present in the bone marrow inoculum. To this end, neutralizing antibodies against IFN-γ abrogated the early decrease in total NA cell and CFU-C production in IL-12 supplemented LTBMC and lead to increased numbers of stroma-associated CFU-C, suggesting that IFN-γ production mediated the early inhibitory effects. Other factors may also play a role. Semi-quantitative rt-PCR of cytokines in IL-12 stimulated stromal layers showed significant increases in GM-CSF and G-CSF mRNA levels. IFN-γ mRNA was not detected in either non-induced or IL-12 induced stromal layers, suggesting that the IFN-γ present in active LTBMC is probably produced by NK or T cells present in the inoculum. Recently, we have produced data indicating that IFN-γ is not exclusively inhibitory for hematopoietic cells, but may as well act as a synergistic activity on enriched HSC when combined with either SF or IL-3. IFN-γ enhanced SF- or IL-3-mediated colony formation two-fold from LD/FU6dBM and enhanced SF-induced proliferation of single sorted LD/FU6dBM WGA-bright cells 4-fold. This stresses the complex nature of the observed effects of IL-12 in LTBMC, in which there may be direct and indirect effects of IL-12 on stroma and/or hematopoietic cells, with IFN-γ clearly suppressing progenitor and mature cell production, but on the HSC level having the ability to stimulate proliferation in synergy with other cytokines.

IN VIVO EFFECTS OF IL-12 ON HEMATOPOIESIS

IL-12 demonstrates potent immunomodulatory activity when administered to normal mice, inducing a wide range of responses including induction of allo-specific CTL [20], augmentation of CD4+ TH1-type helper T cell development [21], and inhibition of IgE secretion [22]. Many of these in vivo activities are mediated, at least in part, by induction of IFN-γ from T and NK cells [23].

C57BL/6 mice injected with 1 μg murine IL-12 per day produced high levels of serum IFN-γ starting 48 hours after the first injection and lasting through the end of IL-12 administration. The effects of IL-12 administration on hematopoiesis in normal mice are consistant with high circulating levels of IFN-γ which has been shown to be an inhibitor of hematopoiesis both in vitro [24-26] and in vivo [27]. Mice given as little as 0.1 ug mIL-12/day demonstrated anemia, leukopenia, and thrombocytopoenia, with decreased numbers of mature neutrophils and red blood cell precursors in the marrow [28]. In contrast, IL-12 treated mice develop splenomegaly, attributable to extramedullary hematopoiesis of erythroid, myeloid, and megakaryocytic lineages [28, 29]. Decreased hematopoeisis in the bone marrow and increased hematopoiesis in the spleen were reflected in similar changes in progenitor cell (CFU-GM, CFU-E, and BFU-E) numbers in these two sites [28].

Jackson et al. have extended these studies to show differential effects of in vivo IL-12 treatment on primitive (HPP-CFC) versus committed (CFU-GM) progenitors in the bone marrow [30]. A single bolus injection of 1 μg per mouse resulted in a significant decrease in marrow CFU-GM content 4 days after treatment and a significant increase in marrow HPP-CFC 3 days after treatment. These results are compatible with our in vitro findings in both clonal cultures and LTBMC showing IFN-γ-independent stimulatory effects on primitive HSC and inhibitory effects, mediated by IFN-γ, on committed progenitor cells. Jackson et al. also showed that, like a number of other cytokines with activity on hematopoietic progenitors, chronic exposure to IL-12 can induce mobilization of hematopoietic progenitors into the peripheral blood [30]. It is not known whether IL-12 mobilizes progenitors possessing long-term marrow repopulating ability and further studies in a murine transplantation model [31, 32] are clearly warranted.

The role of IFN-γ in IL-12 induced changes in hematopoiesis in vivo has been addressed by Quesniaux and colleagues through the use of IFN-γ receptor knock out mice [33]. As with previous studies [28, 29], IL-12 injection into wild-type mice led to significant reductions in bone marrow cellularity, attributable to reductions in identifiable myeloid, erythroid, and lymphoid elements, reductions in bone marrow hematopoietic colony-forming cells, and a siginficant increase in splenic cellularity due mainly to macrophage infiltration. In IFN-γ receptor deficient mice, IL-12 did not cause a reduction in bone marrow cellularity, but instead produced an increase in immature blast cells and colony-forming cells. Splenic hematopoiesis was also increased in IFN-γ receptor knock-out mice with almost a 4-fold increase in splenic hematopoietic progenitor cells. These findings are again compatible with our in vitro results showing IL-12 induced IFN-γ-mediated reductions in hematopoiesis in LTBMC and IFN-γ-independent stimulation of primitive HSC in both clonal cultures and LTBMC.

In vivo studies performed in our own laboratory have confirmed the results of Tare et al. [28], Jackson et al. [30], and Quesniaux and colleagues [33], showing similar dose- and time-dependent decreases in peripheral counts and marrow progenitor cell numbers in IL-12 treated mice. In addition, we have observed dramatic changes in megakaryopoiesis following IL-12 administration in normal mice. In these studies, recombinant murine IL-12 was administered for 5 days at doses of 0.03, 0.3, or 1.0 μg/mouse/day by i.p. injection. At doses of 0.3 and 1.0 μg, an approximately 25% decrease in platelet counts occurred, whereas a dose of 0.03 μg had no effect on platelet count. In contrast, Thiazole Orange staining and flow cytometric analysis demonstrated a significant dose-dependent increase in both the percentage and absolute number of reticulated platelets (16.6%, 36.2%, and 37.1% for 0.03, 0.3, and 1.0 μg compared to 9.2% in controls) in the blood, suggesting an increase in thrombopoietic activity. Analysis of bone marrow megakaryocytes from rmIL-12 treated mice revealed a shift to higher ploidy at all three doses, with the majority of megakaryocytes having 32N DNA content at 0.3 μg/day. This ploidy shift is comparable, if not slightly better, than that seen with 7 days of IL-11 administration to normal mice [34]. Megakaryocyte progenitors were increased approximately 2-fold in the marrow and reached numbers greater than 1000 in the spleen of rmIL-12 treated mice, compared to undetectable levels in the spleens of control mice. Administration of antibodies to IFN-γ during rmIL-12 treatment completely abrogated the decrease in WBC, RBC, and HCT, dramatically reduced the increase in absolute reticulated platelets, and completely reversed the shift towards higher megakayocyte ploidy in the marrow. Paradoxically, the anti-IFN-γ treatment had no effect on the IL-12 induced decrease in platelet count, suggesting a mechanism, probably consumptive, that is not mediated by IFN-γ.

CONCLUSION

It is clear from both in vitro and in vivo studies that IL-12 is a potent stimulator of hematopoietic stem cell proliferation. Because it is also a potent inducer of other growth factors, most prominently IFN-γ from NK cells and T cells, its effects on hematopoiesis in cultures containing heterogenous cell populations and in vivo are complex, showing both stimulatory and inhibitory activity. In cultures containing highly enriched HSC, free of accessory cells, IL-12 acts much like IL-6, IL-11,

33

and G-CSF, synergizing with the same factors to promote myeloid colony formation. In liquid cultures, IL-12, when combined with other synergistic factors, appears to be capable of enhancing the production of more primitive progenitors, possibly even HSC with long-term repopulating ability. More work is needed to establish the true potential, both proliferative and differentiative, of HSC produced in IL-12 supplemented culture, especially in the context of ex vivo stem cell expansion for transplantation and gene therapy. It is difficult to determine at present whether IL-12 plays a physiological role in hematopoiesis in vivo either in the steady-state or during periods of stress. More studies with in vivo models, including models of chemotherapy and bone marrow transplantation in normal mice, and, in the future, in IL-12 knock-out or overexpressing mutant mice, will clarify its role in the physiology of hematopoiesis and as a pharmacologic agent for hematologic diseases.

REFERENCES

1. Ogawa M (1993). Differentiation and proliferation of hematopoietic stem cells. Blood 81:2844-2853.

2. Trinchieri G (1994). Interleukin-12: A Cytokine Produced by Antigen-Presenting Cells With Immunoregulatory Functions in the Generation of T-Helper Cells Type 1 and Cytotoxic Lymphocytes. Blood 84:4008-4027.

3. Kobayashi M, Fitz L, Ryan M, Hewick RM, Clark SC, Chan S, Loudon R, Sherman F, Perussia B, Trinchieri G (1989). Identification and purification of natural killer stimulatory factor (NKSF), a cytokine with multiple biologic effects on human lymphocytes. J. Exp. Med. 170:827-845.

4. Gearing DP,Cosman D (1991). Homology of the p40 subunit of NKSF with the extracellular domain of the IL6 receptor. Cell 66:9-10.

5. Merberg DM, Wolf SW, Clark SC (1992). Sequence similarity between NKSF and the IL6/G-CSF family. Immunology Today 13:77-78.

6. Ikebuchi K, Clark S, Ihle J, Souza L, Ogawa M (1988). Granulocyte colony-stimulating factor enhances interleukin-3-dependent proliferation of multipotential hemopoietic progenitors. Proc Natl Acad Sci USA 85:3445.

7. Ikebuchi K, Wong G, Clark S, Ihle J, Hirai Y, Ogawa M (1987). Interleukin-6 enhancement of interleukin-3 dependent proliferation of multipotent hemopoietic progenitors. Proc Natl Acad Sci USA 84:9035.

8. Hirayama F, Katayama N, Neben S, Donaldson D, Nickbarg EB, Clark SC, Ogawa M (1994). Synergistic interaction between IL-12 and steel factor in support of proliferation of murine lymphohematopoietic progenitors in culture. Blood 83:92-98.

9. Taga T,Kishimoto T (1993). Cytokine receptors and signal transduction. FASEB J 7:3387.

10. Chua AO, Chizzonite R, Desai BB, Truitt TP, Nunes P, Minetti LJ, Warrier RR, Presky DH, Levine JF, Gately MK, Gubler U (1994). Expression cloning of a human IL-12 receptor component. A new member of the cytokine receptor superfamily with strong homology to gp130. J Immunology 153:128-136.

11. Hirayama F, Shih J, Awgulewitsch A, Warr G, Clark S, Ogawa M (1992). Clonal proliferation of lymphohemopoietic progenitors in culture. Proc Natl Acad Sci USA 89:5907.

12. Jacobsen SEW, Veiby OP, Smeland EB (1993). Cytotoxic lymphocyte maturation factor (IL12) is a synergistic growth factor for hematopoietic stem cells. J. Exp. Med. 178:413-418.

13. Dybedal I, Larsen S, Jacobsen SEW (1995). IL12 directly enhances in vitro murine erythropoiesis in combination with IL-4 and stem cell factor. J. Immunol. 154:4950-4955.

14. Jacobsen SEW, Okkenhaug C, Myklebust J, Veiby OP, Lyman SD (1995). The FLK-2/FLT3 ligand potently and directly stimulates the growth and expansion of primitive murine bone marrow progenitor cells in vitro: synergistic interactions with interleukin (IL)-11, IL-12, and other hematopoietic growth factors. J. Exp. Med. 181:1357-1363.

15. Ploemacher RE, van Soest PL, Boudewijn A, Neben S (1993). IL12 enhances IL3 dependent multiplineage hematopoetic colony formation stimulated by IL11 or steel factor. Leukemia 7:1374-1380.

16. Ploemacher RE, van Soest PL, Vorrwinden H, Boudewijn A (1993). IL12 synergizes with IL3 and steel factor to enhance recovery of murine hemopoietic stem cells in liquid culture. Leukemia 7:1381-1388.

17. Ploemacher R, Van der Loo J, Van Beurden C, Baert M (1993). Wheat germ agglutinin affinity of murine hemopoietic stem cell subpopulations is an inverse function of their long-term repopulating ability in vitro and in vivo. Leukemia 7:120-130.

18. Ploemacher R, Van der Sluijs J, Van Beurden C, Baert M, Chan P (1991). Use of limiting dilution type long term marrow cultures in frequency analysis of marrow repopulating and spleen colony-forming hematopoietic stem cells in the mouse. Blood 78:2527-2533.

19. Dexter T, Allen T, Lajtha L (1977). Conditions controlling the proliferation of haemopoietic stem cells in vitro. J Cell Physiol 91:335-344.

20. Brunda MJ, Luistro L, Warrier RR, Wright RB, Hubbard BR, Murphy M, Wolf SF, Gately MK (1993). Antitumor and antimetastatic activity of IL12 against murine tumors. J Exp. Med. 178:1223-30.

21. Sypek JP, Chung CL, Mayor SEH, Subramanyam JM, Goldnam SJ, Sieburth DS, Wolf SF, Schaub RG (1993). Resolution of cutaneous leishmaniasis: IL12 initiates a protective T helper Type 1 immune response. J. Exp. Med. 177:1797-1802.

22. Morris SC, Madden KB, Adamovicz JJ, Gause WC, Hubbard BR, Gately MK, Finkelman FD (1994). Effects of IL-12 on in vivo cytokine gene expression and Ig isotype selection. Journal of Immunology 152:1047-1056.

23. Brunda MJ (1994). Interleukin-12. J of Leukocyte Biology 55:280-288.

24. Broxmeyer H, Lu L, Platzer E, Feit C, Juliano L, Rubin B (1983). Comparative analysis of the influences of human gamma, alpha, and beta interferons on human multipotential (CFU-GEMM), erythroid (BFU-E), and granulocyte-macrophage (CFU-GM) progenitor cells. J Immunol 131:1300-1305.

25. Means R, Krantz S (1991). Inhibition of murine erythroid colony forming units by g interferon can be corrected by recombinant human erythropoietin. Blood 78:2546-2567.

26. Gimble J, Medina K, Hudson J, Robinson M, Kincade P (1993). Modulation of lymphohematopoiesis in long-term cultures by gamma interferon: direct and indirect action on lymphoid and stromal cells. Exp Hematol 21:224-230.

27. Terrell T, Green J (1993). Comparative pathology of recombinant murine interferon-g in mice and recombinant human interferon-g in cynomolgus monkeys. Int Rev Exp Pathol 34:73-101.

28. Tare N, Bowen S, Warrier R, Carvajal D, Benjamin W, Riley J, Anderson T, Gately M (1995). Administration of recombinant interleukin-12 to mice suppresses hematopoiesis in the bone marrow but enhances hematopoiesis in the spleen. J Inter. Cyto. Res. 15:377-383.

29. Gately MK, Warrier RR, Honasoge S, Carvajal DM, Gaherty DA, Connaughton SE, Anderson TD, Sarmiento U, Hubbard BR, Murphy M (1994). Administration of recombinant IL-12 to

normal mice enhances cytolytic lynphocyte activity and induces production of IFN-γ in vivo. International Immunology 6:157-167.

30. Jackson J, Yan Y, Brunda M, Kelsey L, Talmage J (1995). Interleukin-12 enhances peripheral hematopoiesis in vivo. Blood 85:2371-2376.

31. Molineux G, Pojda Z, Hampson I, Lord B, Dexter T (1990). Transplantation potential of peripheral blood stem cells induced by colony-stimulating factor. Blood 76:2153-2158.

32. Neben S, Marcus K, Mauch P (1993). Mobilization of hematopoietic stem and progenitor cell subpopulations from the marrow to the blood of mice following cyclophosphamide and/or granulocyte colony-stimulating factor. Blood 81:1960-1967.

33. Eng V, Car B, Schnyder B, Lorenz M, Lugli S, Aguet M, Anderson T, Ryffel B, Quesniaux F (1995). The stimulatory effects of IL-12 on hematopoiesis are antagonized by IL-12-induced interferon g in vivo. J. Exp. Med 181:1893-1898.

34. Neben T, Loebelenz J, Hayes L, McCarthy K, Stoudemire J, Schaub R, Goldman S (1993). Recombinant human interleukin-11 stimulates megakarocytopoiesis and increases peripheral platelets in normal and splenectomized mice. Blood 81:901-908.

Identification and Characterization of a Ligand for Receptor Protein-Tyrosine Kinase HTK Expressed in Hematopoietic Cells

Seiji Sakano[1,3], Atsushi Iwama[3], Akira Ito[1], Chihiro Kato[2], Yukiko Shimizu[2], Renshi Shimizu[2], Ryo Serizawa[1], Tomohisa Inada[3], Shuuhei Kondo[2], Mituharu Ohno[1], and Toshio Suda[3]

[1]Fundamental Research Laboratory of Life Science, and [2]Laboratory for Biological Research, Institute for Life Science Research, Asahi Chemical Industry Co. Ltd., 2-1, Samejima, Fuji, Shizuoka-ken 416 Japan; [3]Department of Cell Differentiation, Institute of Molecular Embryology and Genetics, Kumamoto University School of Medicine, 2-2-1, Honjo, Kumamoto, 860 Japan

KEY WORDS: receptor tyrosine kinase, HTK, ligand, BIAcore, hematopoietic cells

SUMMARY

HTK is a receptor tyrosine kinase (RTK) which belongs to the Eph subfamily of RTK. Using a BIAcore, a surface plasmon resonance detection system, it was determined that a colon cancer cell line C-1 expressed HTK ligand (HTKL). From the conditioned medium of C-1 cells, a soluble form of HTKL was purified by receptor affinity chromatography. The N-terminal amino acid sequence of purified HTKL was determined and the full-length cDNA of HTKL was isolated from a C-1 cell cDNA library. HTKL is a type I transmembrane protein which consists of 333 amino acids. HTK receptor tyrosine phosphorylation was induced by membrane-bound or clustered soluble ligands but not by unclustered soluble ligands, indicating that HTKL requires cell-to-cell interaction for receptor phosphorylation. FACS analysis of human bone marrow mononuclear cells showed that HTK receptor was expressed in CD34^{low}c-KIT$^+$ hematopoietic progenitor cell fraction. These findings suggest the interaction of hematopoietic progenitor cells with HTKL-expressing cells in bone marrow and the involvement of HTKL in the differentiation and/or proliferation of these progenitor cells.

INTRODUCTION

The function of receptor tyrosine kinases (RTKs) includes cell growth and differentiation [1]. Recently, many researchers have tried to isolate novel tyrosine kinase genes from various cells and organs using the polymerase chain reaction (PCR) [2,3]. These trials have led to the identification of many novel RTK genes, including HTK, which belongs to the Eph subfamily of RTK[4]. We have also isolated a partial HTK cDNA from the human immature hematopoietic cell line, UT-7 [5], and determined its full-length cDNA sequence and characterized the expression in hematopoietic cells. Eph family kinases compose the largest subfamily of RTK, which includes Eph, Eck, Elk, Sek, Ehk-1, Ehk-2, Eek, TK2, Hek, Hek2, Cek5, Cek9, and HTK [6]. Among Eph family kinases, Eck and Hek are also reported to be expressed in hematopoietic cells [7, 8]. However, the functional involvement of these kinases in the hematopoietic system has not been determined.

To further understand the function of HTK in hematopoiesis, we have identified the HTK ligand (HTKL). Although the cloning of HTKL has already been reported by other groups [9, 10], here we show a different cloning approach using a BIAcore instrument, a bio-sensor system based on the surface plasmon resonance.

MATERIALS AND METHODS

Expression of HTK protein

A partial cDNA encoding the entire extracellular domain of HTK was fused in-frame to a sequence

36

of human IgG1Fc (HTKex-Fc) [11]. This HTKex-Fc cDNA was inserted into pMKITNeo expression vector (kindly provided by Dr Kazuo Maruyama, Tokyo Medical and Dental University) and transfected into COS7 cells by electroporation for transient production. HTKex-Fc protein was purified from the conditioned medium of transfected COS7 cells using a protein-G-Sepharose column (Pharmacia, Uppsala, Sweden). The partial cDNA encoding the entire extracellular domain of HTK was tagged with a FLAG octapeptide (DYKDDDDK)(HTKex-FLAG) and inserted into the pMKITNeo expression vector. HTKex-FLAG protein was purified from the conditioned medium of transfected COS7 cells using the anti-FLAG MoAb M2 affinity gel (Eastman-Kodak, New Haven, CT). A full-length HTK cDNA was tagged with a FLAG octapeptide (HTK-FLAG) and was inserted into the pMKITNeo expression vector. This expression vector was introduced into Ba/F3 cells by electroporation. Cells were selected in the presence of G418. Among several resistant clones, the clone with the highest HTK expression, designated as Ba/F3/HTK-FLAG cells, was selected by Western blotting with the anti-FLAG MoAb M2.

Generation of monoclonal antibodies against HTK

Hybridomas were produced by fusion of mouse myeloma cells with spleen cells from a Balb/c mouse immunized with purified HTKex-FLAG protein. All procedures were performed according to the method of Harlow and Lane [12]. Three positive hybridomas were selected by flow cytometric analysis, using Ba/F3/HTK-FLAG cells as indicators. The antibody produced by one of the hybridomas, named 38-1E (IgG1a, κ), was used in this study.

Flow cytometric analysis

Bone marrow mononuclear cells were stained with 5 μg/ml of biotinylated anti-HTK monoclonal antibody, followed by allophycocyanin (APC)-conjugated streptavidin (Becton Dickinson Immunocytometry Systems, San Jose, CA) with fluorescein isothiocyanate (FITC)-conjugated 4A1 (anti-CD34 MoAb; Nichirei Corporation, Tokyo) or with FITC-conjugated NU-c-kit (anti-KIT MoAb; Nichirei Corporation). To detect the expression of HTKL in cell lines, cell lines were stained with HTKex-Fc protein, followed by FITC-conjugated mouse anti-human Fc MoAb (Becton Dickinson Immunocytometry Systems). Stained cells were analyzed by FACSvantage (Becton Dickinson Immunocytometry Systems).

BIAcore binding analysis

Various human cell lines were cultured under serum free conditions in the presence or absence of 100U/ml of tumor necrosis factor α (TNFα, kindly provided by Mr Takao Kiyota, Asahi Chemical Industry Co. Ltd.) or 10 ng/ml of phorbol 12-myristate 13-acetate (PMA, Sigma Chemical Co:, St. Louis, MO). Conditioned mediums were concentrated 40-80 times with the Centricon 10 (Amicon, Danvers, MA) and applied to BIAcore (Pharmacia) analysis. HTKex-Fc protein was immobilized onto the dextran surface of a BIAcore sensorchip by the amino coupling method. Receptor binding activity (response units; RU) was measured and analyzed according to manufacturer's instructions and the method of Bartley et al. [13]. Binding profiles of recombinant HTKLex-FLAG and LERK-2ex-FLAG [14] proteins (see below) to immobilized HTKex-Fc protein were measured by BIAcore and their Kd values were calculated by the BIAevaluation2.1 program.

Purification and cDNA cloning of HTKL

Two liters of conditioned medium from C-1 cells was loaded directly onto a receptor affinity column of immobilized HTKex-Fc. After washing the column with phosphate-buffered saline (PBS), the bound proteins were eluted from the column with 0.1M glycine-HCl (pH 3.0). The eluate was concentrated and separated with a Superdex 75 gel filtration column (Pharmacia). The fractions containing the HTKL were re-loaded onto a smaller-sized receptor affinity column. N-terminal amino acid sequences of purified proteins were determined using ABI protein sequencer Model 1492. A partial cDNA probe (107 bp) encoding the N-terminal amino acid sequence of HTKL was amplified from C-1 cDNA by PCR using degenerate oligonucleotide primers. Using this cDNA probe, a C-1 cDNA library was screened. Three clones were isolated and their sequences were determined using ABI DNA sequencer Model 375S.

Expression of HTKL and LERK2 proteins

Coding region of human LERK-2 cDNA [14] was isolated from human placenta cDNA (Clontech, Palo Alto, CA) by PCR. HTKL and LERK-2 extracellular domain-human IgG1Fc fusion proteins (HTKLex-Fc and LERK-2ex-Fc, respectively) were expressed and purified by the same procedure as HTKex-Fc fusion protein. HTKL and LERK-2 extracellular domain-FLAG octapeptide fusion protein (HTKLex-FLAG and LERK-2ex-FLAG, respectively) were also expressed and purified by the same procedure as HTKex-FLAG fusion protein.

Induction of tyrosine phosphorylation of HTK

Ba/F3/HTK-FLAG cells were co-cultured with HTKL-expressing cells or incubated with clustered HTKLex-Fc with goat anti-human IgG Fc antibody (Organon Teknika Corp, West Chester, PA) for 20 mins at 37°C. The cells were then solubilized with lysis buffer [50 mM HEPES (pH 7.0), 1 % Triton X-100, 10 % glycerol, 10 mM sodium pyrophosphate, 100 mM sodium fluoride, 4 mM EDTA, 2 mM sodium orthovanadate, 50 µg/ml aprotinin, 1 mM PMSF] and HTK was immunoprecipitated with anti-FLAG M2 affinity gel (Eastman-Kodak). Immunoprecipitates were resolved by SDS/PAGE. After electrophoresis, proteins were transferred to PVDF membranes (Bio-Rad Japan), which were probed with the anti-phosphotyrosine antibody, 4G10 (Upstate Biotechnology Inc., Lake Placid, NY) or anti-FLAG M2 MoAb (Eastman-Kodak), and then peroxidase-conjugated goat anti-mouse IgG polyclonal antibody. Specific binding was detected using the enhanced chemiluminescencesystem (Amersham).

RESULTS

Expression of HTK in hematopoietic cell lines

In our previous study of a PCR-based cloning, we cloned a novel RTK gene, mek-1, from a human immature hematopoietic cell line, UT-7 [5]. Afterward, mek-1 was revealed to be identical to HTK. Table 1 shows the profile of protein tyrosine kinases cloned by the PCR-based cloning from UT-7 cells.

Table1 Profile of PTKs isolated from UT-7

Treatment	None	PMA	BA
ECK	30	14	6
HEK			2
HTK	1		1
FGFR-3	2		1
FGFR-4	7	3	21
IGF-1R	2		1
FLT-4			2
TIE	2	9	
c-abl	6	1	
c-fes	32	10	9
CSK	14	1	2
HYL	1	8	7
TYK2			1
JAK3	1	6	
	98	52	53

UT-7 cells were cultured with and without treatment of 10 ng/ml PMA or 1.3 mM n-butyric acid (BA) for 3 days. The method of PCR-based cloning has been described previously [5].

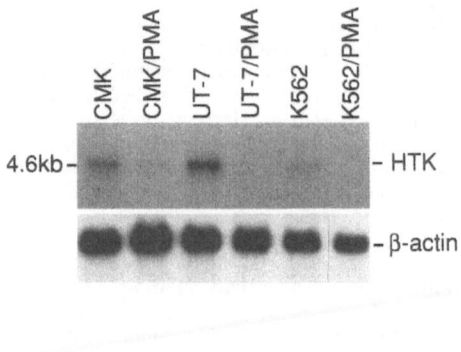

Fig.1 Northern blot analysis of HTK expression in hematopoietic cell lines. Two micrograms of poly(A)+RNA was loaded per lane. SmaI-SmaI fragment of HTK cDNA (7 46 bps) was used as a probe.

HTK was isolated from UT-7 cells both with and without n-butyric acid treatment (which induces erythroid differentiation), but not with PMA treatment (megakaryocytic differentiation). Northern blot analysis showed the down-regulated expression of HTK mRNA during megakaryocytic differentiation induced by PMA (Fig. 1). These data suggested the restricted expression of HTK in immature hematopoietic cells.

Expression of HTK in human bone marrow mononuclear cells

Figure 2 shows the FACS profiles of HTK expression in human bone marrow mononuclear cells (BMMNCs). HTK was expressed in three percent of BMMNCs, which also expressed c-kit and a low level of CD34.

Identification of human cell lines which express HTKL

For the screening of cell lines which express HTKL, we employed BIAcore analysis. Significant binding activities were observed in the conditioned media from four cell lines, C-1, KATO-III, COLO205, and H-1 (Fig. 3, indicated by arrows). Although the conditioned media from these four cell lines failed to induce tyrosine phosphorylation of HTK in Ba/F3/HTK-FLAG cells (data not shown), the phosphorylation of HTK was induced by co-culture of Ba/F3/HTK-FLAG cells with C-1 and KATO-III cells (Fig. 4). This autophosphorylation was inhibited by the addition of an excess molar of HTKex-Fc protein in the medium. Furthermore, specific binding of HTKex-Fc to C-1 cells, but not to BT-20 cells, was demonstrated by FACS analysis (Fig. 5). BT-20 cells were used as a negative control, because the conditioned medium failed to show significant binding activity in BIAcore analysis. These data suggested that the functional HTKL is expressed on the cell surface of C-1 cells and KATO-III cells, and that the HTKL is also secreted into the conditioned medium.

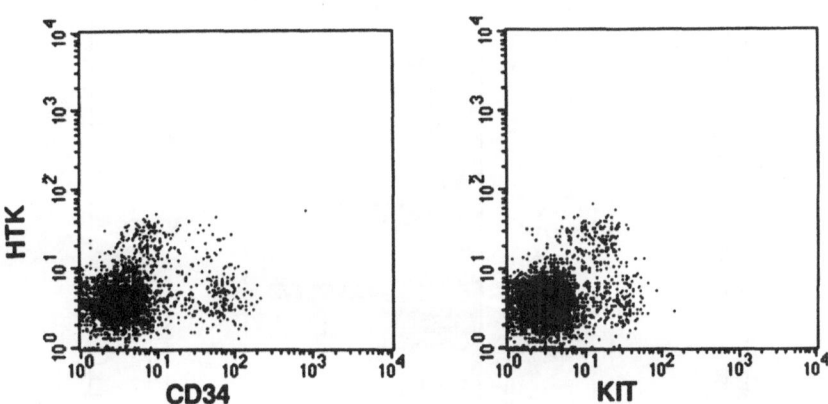

Fig. 2 <u>FACS analysis of HTK expression in human bone marrow mononuclear cells.</u> Cells were stained with monoclonal antibodies against HTK (38-1E) and (A) c-KIT or (B) CD34.

40

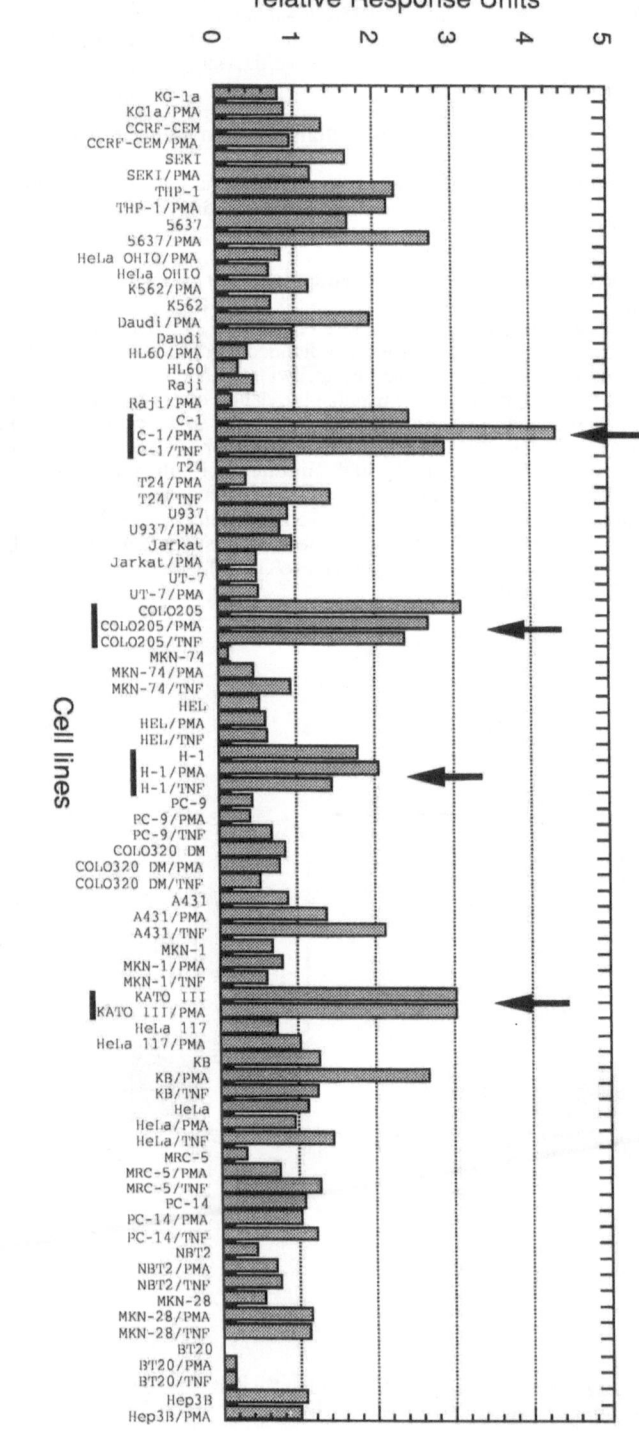

Fig. 3 Screening of conditioned mediums from various cell lines for binding activity to immobilized HTKex-Fc using BIAcore system. Relative response units (RU) were obtained by dividing an absolute BIAcore RU by the degree of concentration for each conditioned medium. The cell lines with high relative RU were indicated by arrows.

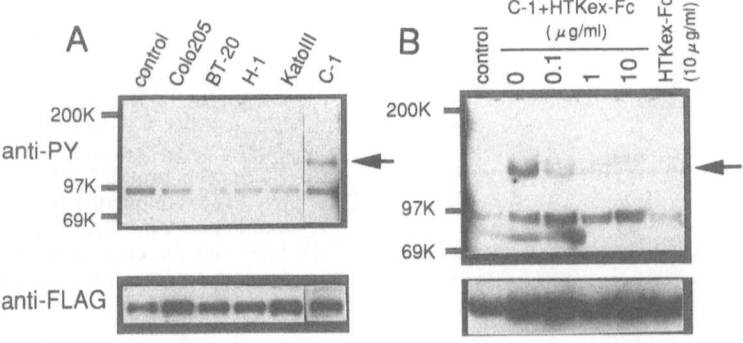

Fig.4 <u>Induction of receptor phosphorylation by co-culture with cell lines.</u> A: The phosphorylation of HTK in Ba/F3/HTK-FLAG cells was induced by co-culture with C-1 and KATO-III cells. B: The phosphorylation of HTK was inhibited by the addition of an excess molar of HTKex-Fc protein in the medium.

Purification and cDNA cloning of HTKL

Figure 6A summarizes the strategy for the purification and cDNA cloning of HTKL. Using a receptor affinity column of immobilized HTKex-Fc, HTKL was purified from the conditioned medium of C-1 cells, and was fractionated by gel filtration. Receptor binding activities were detected in two fractions with the molecular weights around 40 kDa and 20 kDa in BIAcore analysis. After the second purification, silver staining of the protein separated by SDS-PAGE showed highly purified proteins with the molecular weights of 41.5 kDa (Fig. 6B) and 23.5 kDa. These two proteins had the same N-terminal amino acid sequence of KSIVLEPIYWNSSNSKFLPGQGL VLYPQIGDKLDIIXPKVD. It is likely that the lower molecular weight protein is a degradation product of HTKL still having the receptor binding activity. Using degenerate oligonucleotide primers corresponding to the N-terminal amino acid sequence, 107 bps of partial cDNA of HTKL was amplified from C-1 cDNA by PCR, and full-length cDNA was cloned by screening a C-1 cDNA library. The deduced amino acid sequence of HTKL completely matches with that of Bennett et al. [9], which was cloned by expression cloning. Although the cleavage site of signal sequence in their report differs from ours, we confirmed this site by amino acid sequencing of the purified protein.

Characterization of recombinant HTKL

Because purified soluble HTKL does not induce autophosphorylation of the HTK receptor, we prepared HTKL extracellular domain-human IgG1Fc fusion protein (HTKLex-Fc). The autophosphorylation of HTK in Ba/F3/HTK-FLAG cells was induced by the stimulation of clustered HTKLex-Fc (Fig. 7) or by the co-culture with COS7 cells which were transiently transfected with HTKL (data not shown). However, clustered LERK-2ex-Fc proteins, the other transmembrane-type ligand for the Eph family, induced very low levels of HTK autophosphorylation. Figure 8 shows the binding profiles of HTKL and LERK-2 to HTK in BIAcore analysis. In this experiment, the monomer type of recombinant soluble ligands tagged with FLAG octapeptide were used. The Kd value between HTKL and HTK was calculated as 1.23 nM, as compared to 1.35 mM for LERK-2 and HTK. This data confirmed that HTKL is a specific ligand for the HTK receptor.

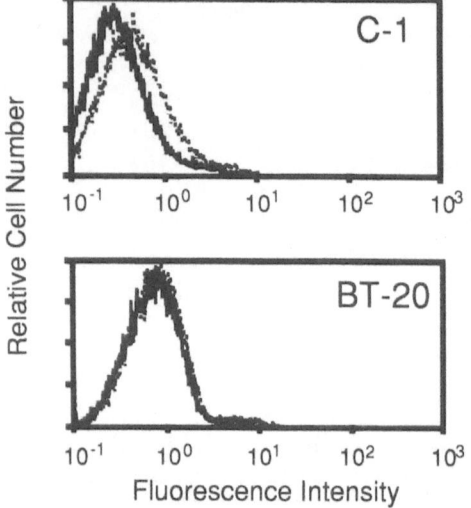

Fig. 5 <u>Detection of specific binding of HTKex-Fc protein to C-1 cells.</u> C-1 and BT-20 cells were stained with HTKex-Fc protein, followed by FITC-conjugated mouse anti-human Fc MoAb. Solid lines denote control; dotted lines denote samples stained with HTKex-Fc.

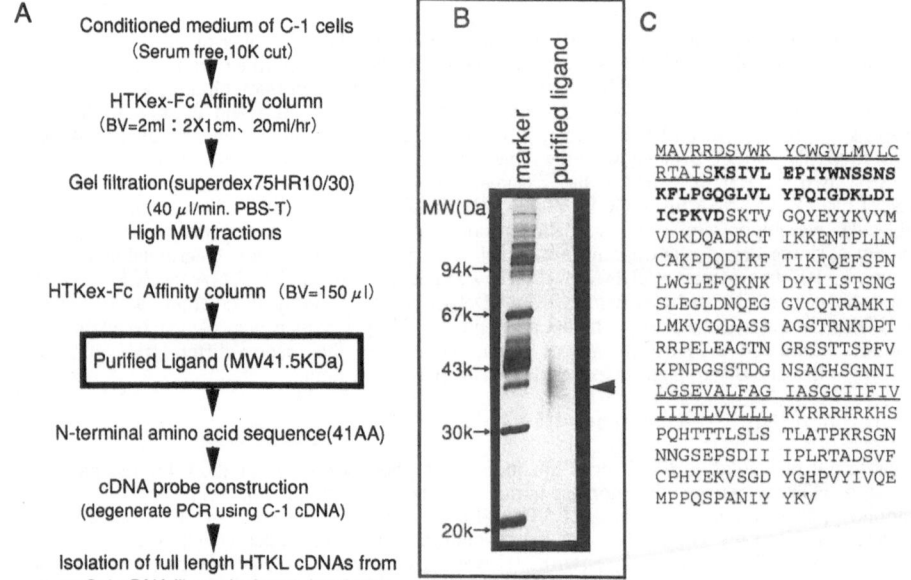

Fig. 6 <u>Purification and cDNA cloning of HTKL</u>.A: Summary of the strategy for the purification and cDNA cloning of HTKL. B: SDS-PAGE analysis of purified HTKL. Protein was visualized by silver staining. C: Deduced amino acid sequence of human HTKL. Signal sequence and transmembrane domain are underlined. The amino acid sequence determined by N-terminal sequence analysis of purified protein is presented in bold type.

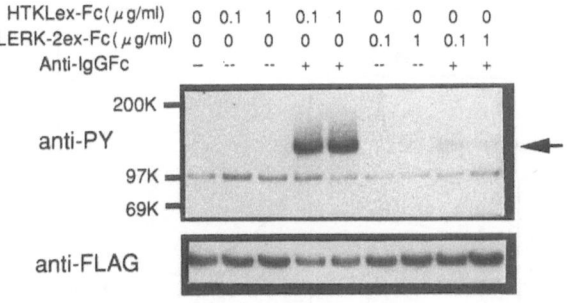

Fig.7 Induction of receptor phosphorylation by the stimulation of recombinant HTKL and LERK-2. HTKex-Fc and LERK-2ex-Fc proteins were clustered by incubation with 10 times excess molar of goat anti-human IgG Fc at 37°C for 10 min. The phosphorylation of HTK in Ba/F3/HTK-FLAG cells was induced by the clustered HTKL.

DISCUSSION

Recently, many different ligands for Eph family RTKs have been identified [15]. These ligands can be divided into two groups: the glycophosphatidylinositol (GPI)-anchored protein such as ELF-1, AL-1/RAGS, EHK-L/LERK-3, B61/ECK-L and LERK4 and the type I transmembrane protein such as LERK-2.

In this study, we have cloned an additional type I transmembrane ligand, HTKL from C-1 cells. HTKL cDNA encodes a transmembrane protein of 333 amino acids with a short cytoplasmic domain. The predicted molecular weight of the extracellular domain is 22 kDa. Since the molecular weight of a native, soluble HTKL is 41.5 kDa, it contains about 20 kDa sugar portion, which may consist of N- and O-linked glycosylated residues and probably contain some glycosaminoglycans. HTKL shows 55% identity with the other transmembrane-type ligand for EPH family, LERK-2 [14]. We have shown that HTKL binds to HTK with a much higher affinity and induces a higher level of HTK autophosphorylation than LERK-2 does. This suggests that HTKL is a specific ligand for the HTK receptor.

HTK was phosphorylated by the HTKL-expressing cells, C-1, or the addition of clustered soluble HTKL. Interestingly, unclustered soluble HTKL did not induce the phosphorylation. These results, similar to those of Davis et al.[16] on other ligands for the Eph sub-family, indicated that membrane-attachment of HTKL may be critical to activate its receptors. HTK receptor is expressed in hematopoietic progenitor cells. Therefore, it is likely that HTKL functions in the cell-to-cell interaction of progenitor cells to stromal cells (Fig. 9). We are now searching for the biological functions of HTK and its ligand on hematopoiesis.

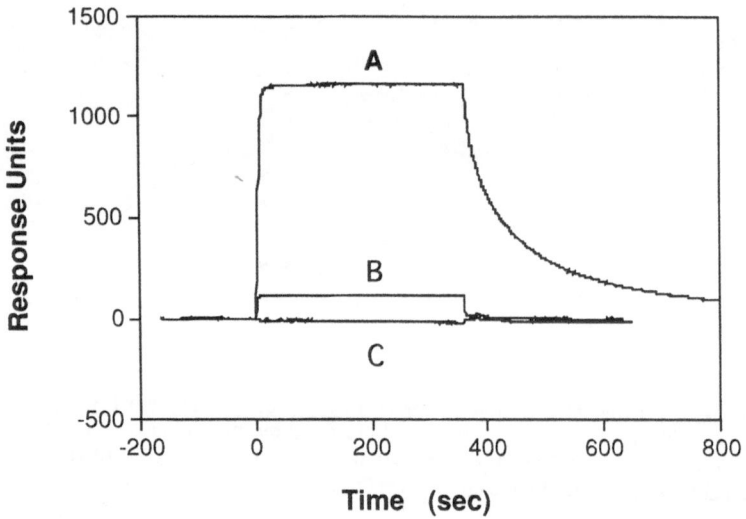

Fig.8 <u>Specific binding of extracellular domain of HTKL to HTK and comparison with LERK-2.</u> A sensor chip was immobilized with HTKex-Fc. Thirty microliter of samples were injected at zero time at flow rate of 5μl/min. A: HTKLex-FLAG (5μg/ml). B: LERK-2ex-FLAG(50μg/ml). C: BSA(100μg/ml)

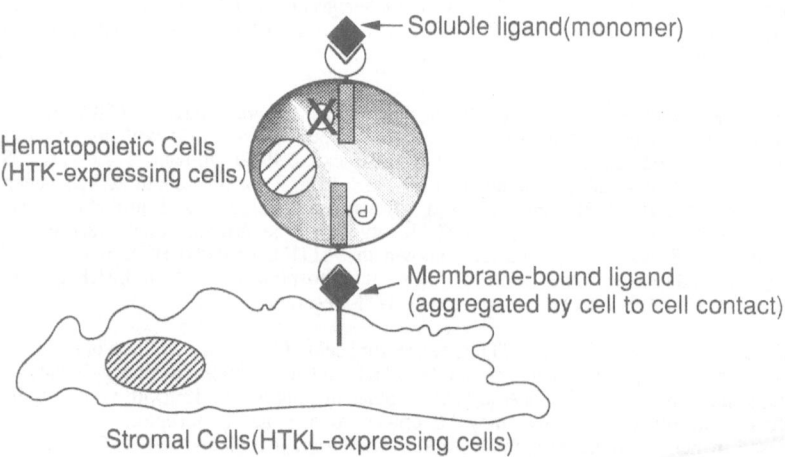

Fig.9 <u>Schematic representation of HTK-HTKL interaction.</u> Receptor auto-phosphorylation is induced only by the aggregation of membrane-bound ligand but not by the monomeric soluble ligand.

The Eph-related RTKs are abundantly expressed in the developing and adult nervous system. Recently, thebiological functions of ligands for Eph-related receptors, such as AL-1/RAGS, were elucidated in neuronal development. AL-1/RAGS contributes to the guidance of neuronal cells from retina to tectum in chick brain development [17,18] and axon bundle formation *in vitro* [19]. Surprisingly, the migration of growth corn of neuronal cells expressing Eph-related receptors was suppressed and collapsed on contact with the cells expressing the RAGS ligand. Pandey et al. [20] have shown that ECK and its ligand B61 are involved in the TNF-induced angiogenesis and migration of endothelial cells. It has been indicated that TNF-induced B61 stimulates the ECK kinase activity by an autocrine or paracrine manner in endothelial cells.

Very recently, Bergemann et al. [10] have reported that ELF-2/HTKL is segmentally expressed in mouse embryos in the region of the hindbrain and newly forming somites. From these findings, it is suggested that HTKL plays an important role in organogenesis, in which signals transduced by cell-to-cell contact are very important. Although the biological functions of Eph family RTKs on hematopoiesis have not been determined, the HTKL/HTK system could be a good model to clarify the significance of cell-to-cell interaction between hematopoietic cells and stromal cells.

Regarding the methodology of ligand cloning, although many methods have been employed including a general protein purification and an expression cloning for identification of ligands for orphan receptors, it is expected that the BIAcore system will be shown to be very useful for the identification of ligands for orphan receptors.

CONCLUSION

We isolated the ligand for HTK which showed unique and interesting characteristics in expression patterns and required cell-to-cell interactions for receptor activation. It is expected that biological functions of HTK/HTKL would be involved in hematopoietic cell differentiation as well as early organogenesis and neuronal development.

REFERENCES

[1]Ullrich A, Schlessinger J (1990) Signal transduction by receptors with tyrosine kinase activity. Cell 61:203-212

[2]Wilks AF (1989) Two putative protein-tyrosine kinases identified by application of the polymerase chain reaction. Proc Natl Acad Sci USA 86:1603-1607

[3]Partanen J, Makela TP, Alitalo R, Lehvaslaiho H, Alitalo K (1990) Putative tyrosine kinases expressed in K-562 human leukemia cells. Proc Natl Acad Sci USA 87:8913-8917

[4]Bennett BD, Wang Z, Kuang W-J, Wang A, Groopman JE, Goeddel DV, Scadden DT (1994) Cloning and characterization of HTK, a novel transmembrane tyrosine kinase of the Eph subfamily. J Biol Chem 269:14211-14218

[5]Sakano S, Iwama A, Inazawa J, Ariyama T, Ohno M, Suda T (1994) Molecular cloning of a novel non-receptor tyrosine kinase, *HYL* (hematopoietic consensus tyrosine-lacking kinase). Oncogene 9:1155-1161

[6]Tuzi NL, GullickWJ (1994) eph, the largest known family of putative growth factor receptors Br J Cancer 69:417-421

[7]Iwama A, Okano K, Sudo T, Matsuda Y, Suda T (1994) Molecular cloning of a novel receptor tyrosine kinase gene, STK, derived from enriched hematopoietic stem cells. Blood 83:3160-3169

[8]Wicks IP, Wilkinson D, Salvaris E, Boyd AW (1992) Molecular cloning of HEK, the gene encoding a receptor tyrosine kinase expressed by human lymphoid tumor cell lines. Proc Natl Acad Sci USA 89:1611-1615

[9]Bennett BD, Zeigler FC, Gu Q, Fendly B, Goddard AD, Gillett N, Matthews W (1995) Molecular cloning of a ligand for the Eph-related receptor protein tyrosine kinase Htk. Proc Natl Acad Sci USA 92:1866-1870

[10]Bergemann AD, Cheng H-J, Brambilla R, Klein R, Flanagan JG (1995) ELF-2, a new member of the Eph ligand family, is segmentally expressed in mouse embryos in the region of the hindbrain and newly forming somites. Mol Cell Biol 15:4921-4929

[11]Zettlmeissl G, Gręgersen J-P, Duport JM, Mehdi S, Reiner G, Seed B (1990) Expression and characterization of human CD4: Immunoglobulin fusion proteins. DNA Cell Biol 9:347-353

[12]Harlow E, Lane D (1988) Antibodies:a laboratory manual. Cold Spring Harbor Laboratry Press, Cold Spring Harbor, NY

[13]Bartly TD, Hunt RW, Welcher AA, Boyle WJ, Parker VP, Lindberg RA, Lu HS, Colombero AM, Elliott RL, Guthrie BA, Holst PL, Skrine JD, Toso RJ, Zhang M, Fernandez E, Trail G, Varnum B, Yarden Y, Hunter T, Fox GM (1994) B61 is a ligand for the ECK receptor protein-tyrosine kinase. Nature 368: 558-560

[14]Beckmann MP, Cerretti DP, Baum P, Bos TV, James L, Farrah T, Kozosky C, Hollingsworth T, Shilling H, Maraskovsky E, Fletcher FA, Lhotak V, Pawson T, Lyman SD (1994) Molecular characterization of a family of ligands for eph-related tyrosine kinase receptors. EMBO J 13:3757-3762

[15]Tessier-Lavigne M (1995) Eph receptor tyrosine kinases, axon repulsion, and the development of topographic maps. Cell 82:345-348

[16]Davis S, Gale NW, Aldrich TH, Maisonpierre PC, Lhotak V, Pawson T, Goldfarb M, Yancopoulos GD (1994) Ligands for EPH-related receptor tyrosine kinases that require membrane attachment or clustering for activity. Science 266: 816-819

[17]Drescher U, Kremoser C, Handwerker C, Loschinger J, Noda M, Bonhoeffer F (1995) In vitro guidance of retinal ganglion cells axons by RAGS, a 25 kDa tectal protein related to ligands for Eph receptor tyrosine kinases. Cell 82:359-370

[18]Chang H-J, Nakamoto M, Bergemann AD, Flanagan JG (1995) Complementary gradients in expression and binding of ELF-1 and MEK4 in development of the topographic retiotectal projection map. Cell 82:371-381

[19]Winslow JW, Moran P, Vaverde J, Shih A, Yuan JQ, Wong SC, Tsai SP, Goddard A, Henzel WJ, Hefti F, Beck KD, Caras IW (1995) Cloning of AL-1, a ligand for an Eph-related tyrosine kinase receptor involved in axon bundle formation. Neuron 14:973-981

[20]Pandey A, Shao H, Marks RM, Polverini PJ, Dixit VM (1995) Role of B61, the ligand of the Eck receptor tyrosine kinase, in TNF-a-induced angiogenesis. Science 268:567-569

EX VIVO EXPANSION OF HUMAN PRIMITIVE HEMOPOIETIC PROGENITORS

Tatsutoshi Nakahata*[1], Xingwei Sui*, Sakura Tajima*, Kohichiro Tsuji*, Kiyoshi Yasukawa†, Tetsuya Taga‡ and Tadamitsu Kishimoto§

*Department of Clinical Oncology, The Institute of Medical Science, The University of Tokyo, 4-6-1 Shirokanedai, Minato-ku Tokyo 108, Japan, †Biotechnology Research Laboratory, TOSOH Corporation, 2743-1 Hayakawa, Ayase, Kanagawa 252, Japan, ‡Institute for Molecular and Cellular Biology, Osaka University, 1-3 Yamada-oka, Suita, Osaka 565, Japan, §Department of Medicine III, Osaka University Medical School, 2-2 Yamada-oka, Suita, Osaka 565, Japan

*[1] To whom correspondence and reprints should be addressed.
Tatsutoshi Nakahata MD, DMSci, Department of Clinical Oncology, The Institute of Medical Science, The University of Tokyo, 4-6-1 Shirokanedai, Minato-ku Tokyo 108, Japan
FAX 81-3-5449-5428 , Phone 81-3-5449-5694

Introduction

The hemopoietic system is characterized by continuous cell turnover supported by a small populations of cells termed hemopoietic stem cells. It is generally held that multipotential hemopoietic stem cells possess extensive capabilities to self-renew and generate various committed progenitor cells(1). Intercellular communication in the hemopoietic system is mediated by soluble factors called cytokines, whose functional characteristics are now partly explained by their receptor system (2-5). Most cytokine receptor systems consist of a multi-chain complex, a ligand-specific receptor chain (α-chain) and a signal transducing chain (β-chain), the latter of which is often utilized in common by several receptor complexes(2,6).

IL-6, IL-11, LIF, OSM, CNTF and cardiotrophin (CT) are a subset of cytokines with structural and functional similarities. The functional redundancy of these cytokines is now well explained by the nature of their receptors (6,7,8). This subset shares gp130, a 130 kd transmembrane glycoprotein with a large intracytoplasmic domain, as a signal transducing receptor component. Receptor systems sharing gp130 are schematically depicted in Figure 1. In the IL-6-receptor interaction, IL-6 first binds to IL-6R, and this complex then associates with gp130 leading to its homodimerization. IL-6R has a very short cytoplasmic domain, which has been demonstrated to be dispensable for signaling. In contrast, the cytoplasmic region of gp130 is required for signal transduction and gp130 homodimerization results in the juxtaposition of the cytoplasmic regions of the two gp130 molecules that appear to initiate a downstream signaling cascade such as RAS/MAPK and JAK/STAT leading to cellular response(2, 6). This shared receptor model is a well accepted explanation of the redundancy of these cytokines in the IL-6 family. Although gp130 is found in almost all tissues, ligand-specific receptor components display a more limited expression, suggesting that cellular responsiveness is largely determined by the regulated expression of the ligand-specific receptors. Interestingly, a soluble form of IL-6R (sIL-6R), which lacks transmembrane and cytoplasmic region, can also induce homodimerization of gp130 upon IL-6 binding. More importantly, the IL-6-sIL6R complex confers IL-6 responsiveness of the cells on which gp130, but not lignad-specific membrane receptor (IL-6R), is expressed (2, 6). gp130 is ubiquitously expressed in various tissues and cells examined (7), but the role of gp130 in relation to normal human cells remains largely unknown, since gp130 has been studied primarily in cultured cell lines. In the human hemopoietic system, information on what cytokine receptors are normally expressed on stem cells remains incomplete and the effect of gp130 signaling initiated by the sIL-6R/IL-6 complex on stem/progenitor cells has so far not been reported. IL-6 has been shown to act on murine primitive hematopoietic progenitors and, together with IL-3, induces the proliferation of murine multipotential hemopoietic progenitor cells (9). However, this is not the case with human hemopoietic progenitor cells, in which the effect of IL-6 in combination with other cytokines, including IL-3 and SCF, is barely detectable.

There has recently been great interest in the *ex vivo* expansion of human hemopoietic stem/progenitor cells in a variety of clinical applications such as BMT and gene therapy. Although the expansion of relatively mature hemopoietic progenitors such as CFU-GM are often obtained using various combinations of cytokines or stromal cells, the magnitude of multipotential progenitors is usually low. To investigate the potential role of gp130 in human hemopoiesis *in vitro*, we have examined the effect of gp130 activation stimulated by a complex consisting of sIL-6R and IL-6 on proliferation, differentiation and expansion of normal human hemopoietic stem/progenitor cells using suspension and clonal cultures of purified human CD34$^+$ cells. Our recent studies have revealed that gp130 signaling initiated by sIL-6R/IL-6 in association with c-Kit activation by SCF may play a important role in human hemopoiesis and may be useful for ex vivo expansion of human hemopoietic stem/progenitors (10, 11, unpublished data).

IL-6/sIL-6R/SCF combination stimulates cell growth of multiple lineages from human CD34$^+$ cells in suspension culture

When human CD34$^+$ cells purified from umbilical cord blood were incubated with sIL-6R in the presence of SCF and IL-6, the total cell count increased dramatically in line with the proportion of sIL-6R. The addition of sIL-6R in optimal proportion to the combination of IL-6 and SCF increased the total cell count by 5-10 fold in serum-containing suspension culture. In the absence of IL-6, however, sIL-6R failed to increase the cell count. The increase in the total cell count by IL-6/sIL-6R in the absence of SCF was also extremely modest, suggesting the action of IL-6/sIL-6R is synergistically associated with SCF. A more striking synergistic effect between IL-6/sIL-6R and SCF was found in the serum-free culture, in which an approximately 2000-fold increase in the total cell count was observed at day 21 of culture whereas IL-6 and SCF without sIL-6R induced only a minimal increase, clearly indicating that sIL-6R is functional and capable of stimulating dramatic cell generation from human hemopoietic stem/progenitor cells in the presence of IL-6 and SCF (Figure 2).

It is interesting to examine the nature of the cells developed from human CD34$^+$ cells induced by IL-6/sIL-6R in the presence of SCF. Cell morphological and immunological studies with APAAP staining and FACS analysis revealed that the generated cells were heterogeneous and contained various cell lineages. Notably, while most of the cells were blast cells at day 7, a significant proportion were erythroid cells megakaryocytes in addition to blast and myeloid cells at days 14 and 21. Differences in the development stages of various cell lineages such as enucleated erythrocytes were also detectable, indicating that a combination of IL-6/sIL-6R and SCF may play a novel role in the development of various hemopoietic cell lineages (10, 11 and unpublished data).

Effect of sIL-6R, IL-6 and SCF on colony formation from CD34+ cell in serum-containing methylcellulose culture

Observations from the suspension culture suggested the possibility that sIL-6R/IL-6 stimulates proliferation of hemopoietic progenitors including primitive hemopoietic progenitors in the presence of SCF, resulting in the increase in cells in the culture. This possibility was confirmed by methylcellulose clonal culture of CD34+ cells with various combinations of sIL-6R, IL-6 and/or SCF (10, 11). In the serum-containing culture, as shown in Table 1, sIL-6R, IL-6, sIL-6/IL-6 or SCF alone induced only a small amount of colony formation. A combination of IL-6 and SCF enhanced the formation of GM and blast colonies over IL-6 or SCF alone. The most striking generation of colonies was observed in the culture supplemented with sIL-6R, IL-6 and SCF at a plating efficiency as high as > 50%. Interestingly, considerable numbers of large GEMM colonies and Blast colonies were developed in addition to a number of Meg colonies and erythroid bursts in the combination of sIL-6R, IL-6 and SCF. More than 60% of the colonies induced by the three factors were GEMM and Blast colonies, both of which are derived from more immature progenitors, whereas most of the colonies induced by IL-3, GM-CSF and G-CSF were GM colonies.

Effect of sIL-6R, IL-6 and SCF on colony formation from CD34+ cell in serum-free methylcellulose culture.

To exclude any possible influences by unknown factors contained in the serum, a serum-free methylcellulose culture was prepared. No colonies were detectable in the culture with IL-6, sIL-6 or sIL-6/IL-6, and only a few GM colonies developed in the culture with IL-3, GM-CSF, G-CSF and SCF alone or a combination of SCF and IL-6. The most significant colony formation was again observed in the culture with IL-6, sIL-6R and SCF. The addition of sIL-6R to the combination of IL-6 and SCF increased the total colony count 17.5-fold , and stimulated the formation of a large number of GEMM and Blast colonies in addition to Meg colonies and erythroid bursts. These results clearly indicate that sIL-6R/IL-6 potently stimulates the proliferation of immature hemopoietic progenitor cells in the presence of SCF.

When sIL-6R/IL-6 was combined with IL-3, IL-11, LIF, GM-CSF or G-CSF, which were reported to be able to affect primitive progenitor cells(1), a slight synergy was observed in the serum-containing culture. However, no synergy was found between sIL-6R/IL-6 and these factors in the serum-free culture, indicating that sIL-6R/IL-6 specifically synergizes with SCF for the proliferation of CD34$^+$ progenitor cells. The ddition of IL-3 to the combination of sIL-6R, IL-6 and SCF enhances the colony formation in both serum-containing and serum-free methylcellulose cultures. Interestingly, the addition of G-CSF to the combination appears to inhibit the colony formation (P<0.01)(10, 11). Since SCF is a cytokine with tyrosine kinase receptor, the possible synergy of sIL-6R/IL-6 with other cytokines of the tyrosine kinase receptor was also examined. No significant synergy of sIL-6R/IL-6 with EGF, M-CSF, FGF, or PDGF was observed in colony formation from CD34$^+$ cells in the presence or abscence of SCF in both serum-containing and serum-free methylcellulose cultures.

Effects of sIL-6R and IL-6 with SCF on expansion of hemopoietic progenitor cells in serum-containing suspension culture.

gp130 has been shown to be expressed in embryonic stem (ES) cells, and the activation of gp130 by LIF or a combination of IL-6/sIL-6R can sustain the self renewal of the ES cells (12), suggesting that gp130 plays a role in the self-renewal process of stem cells. The dramatic increase in the total cell count in the suspension culture as well as the efficient colony formation observed above also suggest that the combination of SCF, IL-6 and sIL-6R is useful for the expansion of human stem/progenitor cells. Indeed, this was clearly demonstrated by our subsequent expansion studies (10). Total progenitors dramatically increased in accordance with the concentration of sIL-6R. The number of progenitor cells increased approximately 70-fold over the input number by day 14 in the presence of sIL-6R/IL-6/SCF. In the absence of IL-6, however, sIL-6R failed to increase the total progenitor cell count (Figure 3). These results indicate that sIL-6R is functional and capable of transducing proliferative signals in CD34+ cells only in combination with sIL-6R and IL-6 for the expansion of progenitor cells in a suspension culture in the presence of SCF .

Effects of sIL-6R and IL-6 with SCF on expansion of hemopoietic progenitor cells in serum-free suspension culture

To examine the effect of sIL-6R/IL-6 on the expansion of hemopoietic progenitor cells in more detail, a serum-free suspension culture supplemented with sIL-6R and/or IL-6 in combination with other factors was set up over a period of 3 weeks with weekly analysis of the progenitor cells. No progenitors were assayable in the culture with IL-6 or sIL-6. SCF with IL-6 increased the progenitors by 6-fold, 5-fold and 5-fold by days 7, 14 and 21, respectively. A combination of sIL-6R, IL-6 with SCF dramatically increased the expansion of progenitor cells in the serum-free suspension cultures. When compared with the pre-expansion value, the overall increase in progenitors was 30-fold, 45-fold, 25-fold in the serum-free culture by days 7, 14, and 21, respectively. An approximately 80-fold increase in $CD34^+$ cells was also observed by flow cytometric analysis .

A combination of sIL-6R, IL-6 and SCF stimulates expansion of primitive hemopoietic progenitors

Weekly analyses of different subtypes of expanded progenitors in methylcellulose assay showed that all types of progenitors including GM colony-forming units (CFU-GM), erythroid burst-forming unit (BFU-E), CFU-Meg, CFU-Blast and CFU-GEMM continued to be generated throughout the 3 weeks of culture in the presence of sIL-6R, IL-6 and SCF, although Mix colonies were barely detectable in other combinations of factors. The number of CFU-Mix increased 60-fold and 80-fold in the serum-containing culture and 49-fold and 68-fold in the serum-free culture by days 7 and 14, respectively. Of interest, considerable numbers of CFU-Mix remained assayable at day 21 of the serum-free culture, while the CFU-Mix decreased sharply in the serum-containing culture at the same time. These results revealed that sIL-6R/IL-6 acts synergistically with SCF in the expansion of primitive hemopoietic progenitors.

sIL-6R/IL-6/SCF is a more potent combination than IL-6/IL-3/SCF for expansion of primitive hemopoietic progenitors

A combination of IL-6, IL-3 and SCF has been shown to be potent and was extensively used for the expansion study and gene transfer experiments. Thus we next compared the effect of the combination of sIL-6R, IL-6 and SCF with that of the combination of IL-6, IL-3 and SCF on the increase in the total progenitor count as well as the primitive progenitor count. The expansion of total progenitors by the combination of sIL-6R, IL-6 and SCF was 1.5 times that by the combination of IL-6, IL-3 and SCF. A combination of sIL-6R, IL-6 and SCF expanded the CFU-Mix approximately 49-fold and 68-fold in the serum-free culture by days 7 and 14, respectively (Figure 4). Progenitors generated by a combination of IL-

6, IL-3 and SCF were mainly of granulocyte and/or macrophage lineage, and the CFU-Mix were only expanded about 10-fold in the serum-free culture by day 14 of culture. The addition of IL-3 to the combination of sIL-6R, IL-6 and SCF did not increase the expansion of the CFU-Mix, and, intriguingly, the addition of G-CSF to the combination appeared to have negative effects on the expansion. This result revealed that a combination of sIL-6R, IL-6 and SCF is more potent especially on the expansion of primitive progenitors.

Effects of other cytokines on expansion of progenitors induced by a combination of sIL-6/IL-6/SCF

The addition of EGF, M-CSF, IL-1β, IL-10, IL-11, LIF, OSM or CNTF to the combination of sIL-6R/IL-6/SCF was not found to enhance expansion. In contrast, the addition of TNF or TGF-β to the combination significantly inhibited the expansion supplemented with sIL-6R/IL-6/SCF, which is in agreement with previous reports of TNF and TGF-β as negative hemopoietic regulators.

gp130 is the signal transducer for IL-6/sIL-6R and unparalleled expression of gp130 and IL-6R on human CD34+ cells

To verify the involvement of gp130 in the sIL-6R/IL-6 complex mediated expansion of hemopoietic progenitor cells, the effects of mouse anti-human gp130 mAbs and anti-human IL-6R mAb on the expansion of progenitors in suspension culture were examined. The addition of anti-gp130 mAbs or anti-IL-6R mAb dose-dependently inhibited the expansion of total progenitor cells as well as CFU-Mix in the serum-containing suspension culture with a combination of sIL-6R, IL-6 and SCF, whereas the mAbs had no effect on the expansion supplemented with SCF and IL-3 (Figure 5). Similar results were obtained in the serum-free suspension culture.

The significant proliferation and differentiation of human hemopoietic progenitor cells in cultures with sIL-6R in the presence of IL-6 and SCF and the lack of this effect in cultures without sIL-6R suggest that sIL-6R confers IL-6 responsiveness to human CD34+ cells on which gp130 but not IL-6R are expressed. The unparalleled expression pattern of gp130 and IL-6R on human CD34+ was first demonstrated by our recent flow cytometric studies, in which all of the CD34+ cells were found to express gp130 but a majority lack IL-6R expression. In cultures stimulated by a combination of SCF, IL-6 and sIL-6R or a combination of SCF, IL-3, EPO, and G-CSF, CD34+IL-6R- cells generated a large number of cells and colonies of multiple hemopoietic lineages whereas the progenies of CD34+IL-6R+ under the same conditions were mainly myeloid (Tajima et al. unpublished data). Thus CD34+gp130+IL-6R- may be the phenotype for most human hemopoietic progenitors such as CFU-Mix, CFU-Blast, BFU-E, CFU-Mk, and the gp130 activation in these progenitors by a complex of sIL-6R/IL-6, but not by IL-6 alone mediates a novel function in the proliferation and differentiation of human hemopoietic stem/progenitor cells.

Future prospects

Ex vivo expansion of hemopoietic progenitor cells is an attractive way to prepare suitable hemopoietic cells for potential clinical application including blood and marrow stem cell transplantation and gene therapy. Co-activation of gp130 and c-Kit signal pathways by IL-6, sIL-6R and SCF as shown in our study may provide a novel approach for the expansion of human stem/progenitor cells for potential clinical application. It is conceivable that human hemopoietic stem cells express both gp130 and c-Kit, so our finding also raises the possibility that the maintenance of self-renewal of human hemopoietic stem cells occurs through the co-activation of the two signal pathways. Today, such studies are hampered by the heterogeneity of the accessible normal progenitor/stem cell population in vitro.

The ubiquitously expressed gp130 and unparalleled expression of receptors for IL-6 and IL-6 related cytokines on CD34+ cells suggest that gp130 plays an important role in vivo and may function as a signal transducer for unknown cytokines or cytokine receptors. The essential role of gp130 in hemopoiesis in vivo was confirmed in gp130$^{-/-}$ knockout mice (13). The mutant embryos have greatly reduced numbers of pluripotential and committed hemopoietic progenitors such as CFU-S, CFU-GM, BFU-E, and CFU-Mk in the liver, and some show severe anemia due to impaired maturation of erythroid cells. The in vivo role of c-Kit in hemopoiesis has been well-documented in W mutation mice (14). Taken together, our in vitro data suggest that gp130 and c-Kit signalings play a vital role in the proliferation and differentiation of human hemopoieitc stem/progenitor cells in vivo. sIL-6R, IL-6 as well as a functional complex of IL-6/sIL-6R, and SCF are present in human serum (15, 16, 17) and the half-maximal effect of sIL-6R in the serum-free culture was observed at a concentration within the physiologic range of sIL-6R in human serum (Sui et al. unpublished data). Thus IL-6/sIL-6R might be the human physiological stimulator for the ubiquitously expressed gp130 and might play a critical role in the development of human blood cells in vivo. However, we could not exclude other possibilities such as the existence of a new member of the IL-6 family that signals via gp130 and plays a crucial role in human hemopoieis. The striking effects induced by a IL-6/sIL-6R complex in human hemopoiesis may be mimicking the function of such a novel cytokine, yet to be identified.

58

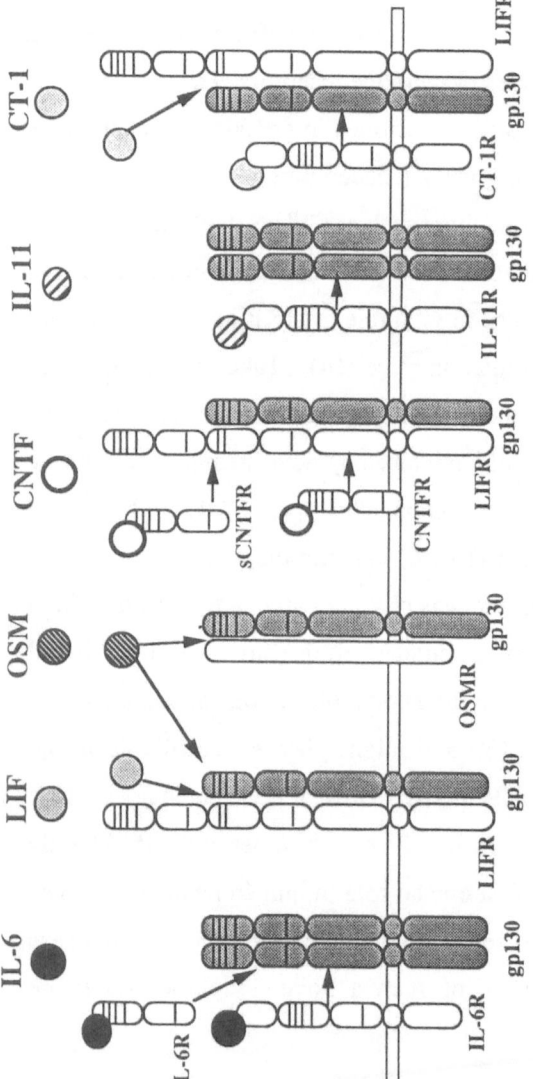

Figure 1.

Cytokine receptor systems sharing gp130 as a signal transducer. In these cytokine receptor complexes, gp130 is utilized in common. Signals are believed to be initiated by the ligand-induced homo- or heterodimerization of receptor components, which leads to the interaction of their cytoplasmic regions, resulting in activation of associated tyrosine kinases.

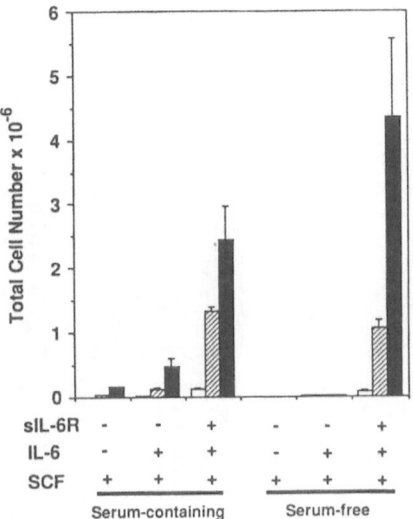

Figure 2.

Proliferative effect of sIL-6R on human CD34+ cells. 2000 CD34+ cells were initiated in the cultures. The progenies of CD34+ cells were examined at weekly intervals. The results are from three separate experiments. Standard deviations are represented by error bars.

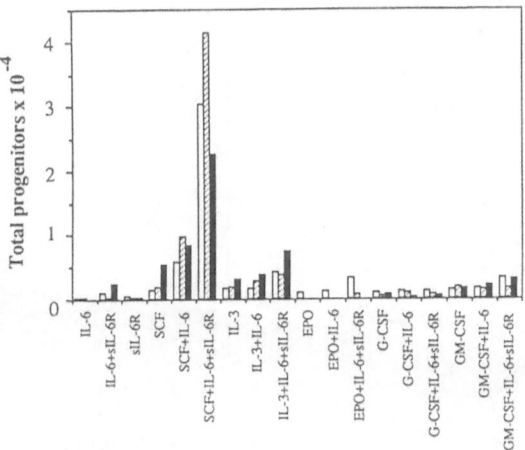

Figure 3.

Generation of total progenitors from 2000 CD34+ cells containing 684 progenitors in serum-containing suspension culture supplemented with single factors or in combinations at day 7(open bars), day 14(oblique bars) and day 21 (filled bars).

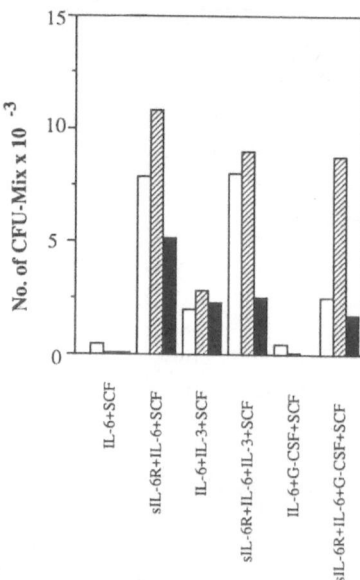

Figure 4.
Generation of CFU-Mix in serum-free suspension culture supplemented with single factors or in combinations at day 7 (open bars), day 14 (oblique bars) and day 21 (filled bars).

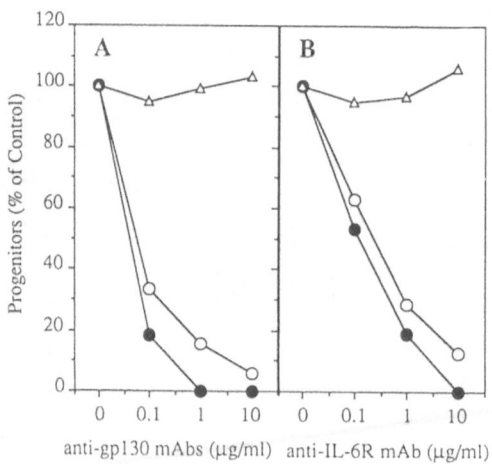

Figure 5.
Effects of various concentrations of anti-human gp130 mAbs (A) and anti-human IL-6R mAb on the expansion of total progenitor cells (open circles) and CFU-Mix (filled circles) with a combination of sIL-6R, IL-6 and SCF or total progenitor cells with a combination of IL-3, IL-6 and SCF (open triangles).

References

1. Ogawa, M. :Differention and proliferation of hematopoietic stem cells. Blood 81, 2844,1993.

2. Kishimoto, T., Taga, T. & Akira, S. :Cytokine signal transduction. Cell 76, 253,1994.

3. Miyajima, A., Kitamura, T., Harada, N., Yokota, T. & Arai, K. : Cytokine receptors and signal transduction. Ann. Rev. Immunol. 10, 295,1992.

4. Stahl, N. & Yancopoulos, G.D.:The alphas, betas, and kinases of cytokine receptor complexes. Cell 74, 587,1993.

5. Metcalf, D.: Hematopoietic regulators: redundancy or subtlety. Blood 82,3515,1993.

6. Taga,T. & Kishimoto, T.: Signaling mechanism through cytokine receptors that share signal transducing receptor components. Current Opinion in Immunology 7, 17,1995.

7. Hibi, M., Murakami, M., Satio, M., Hirano, T., Taga, T., & Kishimoto, T.: Molecular cloning and expression of an IL-6 signal transducer, gp130. Cell 63, 1149,1990.

8. Saito, M., Yoshida, K., Hibi, M., Taga, T. & Kishimoto, T.: Molecular cloning of a murine IL-6 receptor-associated signal transducer, gp130, and its regulated expression in vivo. J. Immuno. 148, 4066,1992.

9. Koike, K., T. Nakahata, T. Takagi, T. Kobayashi, A. Ishiguro, K. Tsuji, K. Naganuma, A. Okano, Y. Akiyama, and T. Akabane.: Synergism of BSF-2/interlukin 6 and interlukin 3 on development of multi-potential hemopoietic progeniotrs in serum-free culture. J. Exp. Med. 168:879,1988.

10. Sui X, Tsuji K, Tanaka R, Tajima S, Muraoka K, Ebihara Y, Ikebuchi K, Yasukawa K, Taga T, Kishimoto T, Nakahata T.: gp130 and c-Kit

signalings synergize for ex vivo expansion of human primitive hemopoietic progenitor cells. Proc. Natl. Acad. Sci. USA 92:2859,1995.

11. Sui X, Tsuji K, Tajima S, Tanaka R, Muraoka K, Ebihara Y, Ikebuchi K, Yasukawa K, Taga T, Kishimoto T, Nakahata T Erythropoietin-independent erythrocyte production: signals through gp130 and c-Kit dramatically promote erythropoiesis from human CD34+ cells. J. Exp. Med. in press.

12. Yoshida K, Chambers I, Nichols J, Smith A, Saito M, Yasukawa K, Shoyab M, Taga T, Kishimoto T.: Maintenance of the pluripotential phenotype of embryonic stem cells through direct activation of gp130 signaling pathways. Mech. Dev. 45:163,1994.

13. Yoshida K, Taga T, Saito M, Suematsu S, Kumanogoh A, Tanaka T, Fujiwara H, Hirata M, Yamagami T, Nakahata T, Hirabayashi T, Yoneda Y, Tanaka K, Wang WZ, Mori C, Shiota K, Yoshida N, and Kishimoto T Targeted disruption of gp130, a common signal transducer for IL-6-family of cytokines, leads to myocardial and hematological disorders. Proc. Natl. Acad. Sci. USA in press.

14. Russell ES: Hereditary anemias of the mouse: a review for genetics. Adv. Genet. 20:357,1979.

15. Honda M, Yamamoto S, Cheng M, Yasukawa K, Suzuki H, Saito T, Osugi Y, Tokunaga T, Kishimoto T.: Human soluble IL-6 receptor, its detection and enhanced release by HIV infection. J. Immunol. 148:2175,1992.

16. Lanley KE, Bennett LG, Wypych J, Yancik SA, Liu XD, Westcott KR, Chang WD, Smith KA, Zsebo KM.: Soluble stem cell factor in human serum. Blood 81:656,1993.

17. Montero-Julian FA, Liautard J, Flavetta S, Romagne F, Gaillard JP, Brochier J, Klein B, Brailly H.: Immunoassay for functional human

soluble interleukin-6 receptor in plasma based on ligand/receptor interactions. J. Immuno. Methods 169:111,1994.

Hemopoietic Stem Cell-stimulating Ingredients in Kampo (Japanese Herbal) Medicine "Juzen-Taiho-To".

Masumi Sakurai[1], Hiroaki Kiyohara[1], Haruki Yamada[1], Hiroko Hisha[2], Yongan Li[2], Norito Takemoto[3], Hideki Kawamura[3], Katunori Yamaura[2], Seiich Shinohara[3], Yasuhiro Komatsu[3], Masaki Aburada[3] and Susumu Ikehara[2].

[1]Oriental Medicine Research Center, the Kitasato Institute, Minato-ku, Tokyo, Japan. [2]1st Dept. Pathology, Kansai Medical University, Moriguchi, Osaka, Japan. [3]Tsumura & Co., Chiyoda-ku, Tokyo, Japan.

SUMMARY

We have previously found that one of the kampo (Japanese herbal) medicines, Juzen-Taiho-To (TJ-48), accelerates recovery from hemopoietic injury induced by radiation and an anti-cancer drug.   n-Hexane-soluble substances from TJ-48 showed significant stimulatory activity on the proliferation of hemopoietic stem cells *in vitro*.   Chromatographic separation and spectrometric identification using NMR and GC-MS revealed that the active fraction of TJ-48, which contained fatty acids such as oleic, linoleic and linolenic acids, accelerated stem cell proliferation.   Oral administration of oleic acid to mitomycin C-treated mice enhanced CFU-S counts on day 14 to twice the control group.   When the fatty acid composition of TJ-48 was compared with other kampo medicines, the same active fatty acids were detected even in other kampo prescriptions which had not been found to accelerate recovery from hemopoietic injury, but in different ratios. Although not all kampo medicines tested showed the stimulatory activity, their fatty acid fractions did.   These results suggest that hemopoietic stimulation by TJ-48 might be the result of the combined effect of the active unsaturated fatty acids and other hydrophilic ingredients.

KEY WORD : hemopoietic stem cells , the kampo (Japanese herbal) medicines, Juzen-Taiho-To (TJ-48), fatty acids

INTRODUCTION

"Juzen-Taiho-To" (TJ-48), which is a kampo (Japanese herbal) medicine, being a decoction of ten herbs, has been used for patients recovering from surgery or suffering from chronic diseases in order to promote improvement of their debilitated condition.   Therefore TJ-48 has traditionally been administered to patients with anemia, anorexia or fatigue. Recently it has also been found to improve the general condition of cancer patients receiving chemotherapy and/or radiation therapy [1].   TJ-48 is known to influence the immune system specifically; it significantly enhances the anti-SRBC response [2], phagocytosis [3] and mitogenic activity against spleen B cells in mice [4]. The peripheral blood cell counts were maintained at a higher level in patients who took TJ-48 orally in combination with the anticancer drug [5]. Recently, Ikehara *et al*. found that TJ-48 facilitates hematopoietic recovery from mitomycin C-induced bone-marrow or radiation injuries by increasing the number of spleen colony-forming units (CFU-S) [6].   Thus, TJ-48 is a unique medicine that acts directly on hematopoietic stem cells. TJ-48 contains several compounds from the component herbs. Yamada *et al* . have found that the pectic polysaccharides in TJ-48 actively promote immunopotentiation [7].   However, the substances that actively promote hematopoietic recovery have not yet been identified.
The present paper deals with the hematopoietic stem cell-stimulating ingredients in TJ-48.

MATERIALS AND METHODS

Juzen-Taiho-To (TJ-48) obtained from Tsumura & Co. (Tokyo, Japan) was prepared as follows: A mixture of crude drugs consisting of Astragali radix (3.0g, root of *Astragalus membranaceus* Bunge), Cinnamomi cortex (3.0g, barke of *Cinnamomum cassia* Blume), Rehmanniae radix (3.0g, root of *Rehmannia glutinosa* Libosch *var*. purpurea Makino), Paeoniae radix (3.0g, rhizome of *Paeonia lactiflora* Pall), Cnidii rhizoma (3.0g, *Cnidium officinale* Makino), Atractylodis lanceae rhizoma (3.0g, rhizome of *Atractylodes lancea* DC.), Angelicae radix (3.0g, root of *Angelica* activity at 0.5 and 1.0μg/ml.   When F-1-1E was further fractionated by silica gel chromatography, F-1-1/E-4 and E-5 showed the more potent activity at 0.5 and 1.0μg/ml.   Because HPLC analysis of E-5 showed 4 peaks (E-5-1 to 4), these fractions were purified, respectively.   As shown in Table 3, E-5-3 showed the most potent stem cell proliferation activity at 0.05 - 0.2μg/ml.

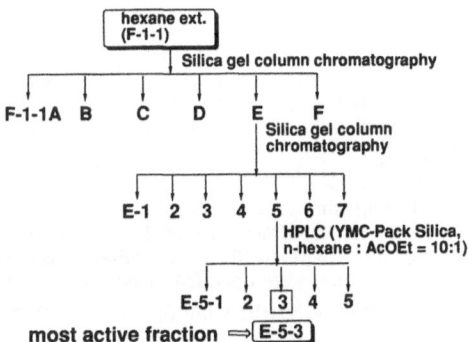

Fig. 1 Purification and identification of active substances from F-1-1

The ^{1}H-NMR spectrum suggested that E-5-3 was a fatty acid containing an unsaturated bond.   GC and GC-EI-MS indicated that E-5-2 and E-5-3 contained at least 4 fatty acids.   GC peaks gave fragment ions at m/z 270 and 298 $[M + H]^+$, suggesting the presence of palmitic acid and stearic acid.   In addition, the peaks which gave $[M + H]^+$ at m/z 296 and 292 were also detected, and these are indicated the presence of C_{18}-monoen and trien acids. Commercially available palmitic acid   and stearic acid had no stem cell proliferation activity, but oleic acid and linolenic acid showed potent activity.

Because C_{18}-unsaturated fatty acid had stem cell proliferation activity, total fatty acids in TJ-48 were reanalysed. TJ-48 was extracted with $CHCl_3$/MeOH (2 : 1) and a free fatty acid fraction obtained by acetone fractionation (F-1A, yield 0.1%). GC-EI-MS indicated that F-1A contained at least 6 fatty acids, which were determined to be palmitic acid, stearic acid, oleic acid, vaccenic acid, linoleic acid and linolenic acid [weight ratios (%) ; 16.2 : 1.6 : 13.5 : 1.6 : 61.7 : 5.4] by comparing retention times and $[M + H]^+$ of standard fatty acids. These results indicate that the active substances in TJ-48 are oleic acid and linolenic acid.   Twenty seven commercially available free fatty acids were tested for stem cell proliferation. Oleic acid $(C_{18 : 1})$, elaidic acid $(C_{18 : 1})$ and linolenic acid $(C_{18 : 3})$ showed potent stem cell proliferation activity at 0.2 - 1.0μg/ml, but the other fatty acids had little or no activity (data not shown).

Oleic acid and linoleic acid seem to be common to many Kampo medicines; both are also found in Ninjin-youei-to (TJ-108) and Shou-seiryu-to (TJ-19).   The former has been reported to stimulate hemopoiesis, but the latter not.   Indeed, we have found that the fatty acids in TJ-48, TJ-108 and TJ-19 were almost identical (Table 1), but the TJ-108 extract had a similar stimulatory effect on HSCs as TJ-48, whereas TJ-19 had no such effect (Table 2).

To confirm the effect of the fatty acids, we demonstrated the stimulation of HSCs in vivo. CFU-S counts were assessed using MMC-treated mice administered various doses of oleic acid: The

Table 1 Component of fatty acids in TJ-48, TJ-108 and TJ-19

Fatty acid	Palmitic acid	Stearic acid	Oleic acid	Vaccenic acid	Linoleic acid	Linolenic acid	yield (%)
			w/w (%)				
TJ-48	16.2	1.6	13.5	1.6	61.7	5.4	0.10
TJ-108	10.8	2.1	23.8	1.0	58.5	3.7	0.23
TJ-19	11.7	15.1	13.7	1.1	57.0	1.1	0.17

acutiloba Kitagawa), Ginseng Radix (3.0g, root of *Panax ginseng* C.A. Meyer), Hoelen (3.0g, fungus of *Poria cocos* Wolf.) and Glycyrrhizae radix (1.5g, root of *Glycyrrhiza uralensis* Fisch. *et* DC.) was added to 285 ml of water and extracted at 100°C for 1h. The extracted solution was filtered and spray-dried to obtain the dry extract powder (TJ-48, 2.3g).   TJ-19 and TJ-108 were also obtained from Tsumura & Co. All fatty acid standards were purchased from Funakoshi Co. (Japan).

Silica gel column chromatography was carried out on Wako gel C-200.   Thin-layer chromatography (TLC) was performed on precoated silica gel 60 F254 (Merck) plates, and spots were visualized by spraying with 10% sulfuric acid solution followed by heating at 110°C. ^{1}H- and ^{13}C-NMR spectra were recorded in CDCl$_3$ on a Varian XL-400 spectrometer operating at 400MHz for ^{1}H-NMR and 100 MHz for ^{13}C-NMR.

E-5-2 and E-5-3 were methylesterified by heating (100°C, 30 min) with 0.5% HCl-MeOH. The products were analyzed by GC-EI-MS on a Hewlett Packard model 5890 gas chromatograph and model 5970B mass-selective detector equipped with an SP-2380 capillary column (0.2-μm film thickness, 0.25 mm i.d. X 30 m, Supelco), which were operated under a temperature program of 60°C for 1 min, 60→140 °C (30°C/min), 140→160°C (0.5°C/min), and 160→250°C (30°C/min).

Bone marrow cells were collected by flushing femurs and tibias, and single cell suspensions were obtained by repeated aspiration through needles.. These cells were then passed through a Sephadex G-10 column to remove adherent cells such as macrophages and stromal cells. They were further purified by discontinuous Percoll density gradient (1.060< p < 1.073). HSC-enriched fractions (low density cells: LD cells) were collected and 10^4 cells per well were then cultured in triplicate in 96-well plates which had become confluent with 20 Gy irradiated MS-5 (a mouse stromal cell line derived from C3H bone marrow cell), with various concentrations of fraction of TJ-48 or standard fatty acid. These substances were dissolved in MeOH/dimethyl sulfoxide (DMSO) (1:1, vol/vol) and were appropriately diluted in culture medium. In all the cultures, the final concentration of the solvent was less than 0.025%, which did not affect the cell proliferation. As a control, LD cells were cultured with MS-5 cells in culture medium containing MeOH/DMSO. The culture was incubated for 4 or 5 days, after which ^{3}H-thymidine was introduced into each well. After 20 to 24 hours, the cells were harvested and the incorporation of ^{3}H-thymidine was measured. The stimulation indices of samples (fractions of TJ-48 or standard fatty acids) were expressed as ratios to the control: ^{3}H-thymidine incorporation on the sample showed a stimulatory activity when the value was more than 1.3.

C58BL/6 (B6) mice were divided into two groups (4 mice/group). One group was administered oleic acid or linolenic acid dissolved in 1% tween 80, p.o. at the dose of 1, 10, 100 or 1000 mg/Kg every day for 3 weeks. The other group (control) was administrated 1% tween alone. MMC (1mg/Kg) was injected i.p. into the mice of both groups every day for the first week. These mice were sacrificed and their bone marrow cells then injected into 8.5 Gy-irradiated syngenic mice. Eight or fourteen days later, the numbers of CFU-S were counted.

RESULTS

Since we have demonstrated that TJ-48 enhances CFU-S counts after hematopoietic suppression induced by radiation and MMC treatment *in vivo*, purification of the active components in TJ-48 was attempted.

TJ-48 was extracted by refluxing with MeOH to give MeOH-soluble (F-1) and MeOH-insoluble fractions, and the latter was further successively fractionated into the four fractions F-2 to F-5 by solubility, dialysis and EtOH precipitation.   The results showed that F-1 (MeOH-soluble fraction), F-3 (dialyzable low-molecular weight fraction) and F-4 (supernatant fraction of EtOH precipitation) enhanced GM-CFC counts at 10μg/ml [6].   Further fractionation revealed that a hexane-soluble fraction (F-1-1) obtained from F-1 had the capacity to enhance GM-CFC counts [6].   Further purification was guided by the proliferation assay of the purified stem cells.

When F-1-1 was further fractionated by silica gel chromatography (Fig. 1), F-1-1E showed the most potent stem cell proliferation activity at 0.1 - 1.0 μg/ml.   F-1-1F also showed significant

Table 2 Stem cell proliferation stimulatory activity of TJ-48, TJ-108 and TJ-19

	0.5 (μg/ml)	1.0 (μg/ml)	5.0 (μg/ml)	10.0 (μg/ml)
TJ-48	N.D.	N.D.	1.49	1.15
TJ-108	N.D.	N.D.	1.49	0.91
TJ-19	N.D.	N.D.	1.08	0.80
Fatty acid fraction				
TJ-48	1.35	1.03	0.86	0.91
TJ-108	1.29	0.85	0.75	1.01
TJ-19	1.26	0.97	0.82	0.91
Oleic Acid	1.39	N.D.	N.D.	N.D.
Linolenic Acid	2.95	N.D.	N.D.	N.D.

administration of MMC significantly decreased day 14 CFU-S counts. An increase in CFU-S counts however, was observed when oleic acid was given to the mice at concentrations of 1 to 1000mg/Kg. The most significant effect was observed at a dose of 10mg/Kg. Similar stimulation was also observed in mice administered linolenic acid (data not shown).

CONCLUSION

The present study suggests that the ingredients in TJ-48 that actively promote hematopoietic recovery are certain C_{18} unsaturated free fatty acids such as oleic acid and linolenic acid. In addition, we have found that C_{18} and C_{22} fatty acids such as elaidic acid and behenic acid can also stimulate the proliferation of HSCs. On the other hand, the stimulatory activity of TJ-48 subfractions on GM-CFC and HSCs was observed not only in the F-1 (methanol-soluble fraction) but also in the F-3 (water-soluble dialyzable fraction) and F-5 (polysaccharide fraction) [6]. TJ-108 extract also had a similar stimulatory effect on HSCs as TJ-48, whereas TJ-19 had no such effect. It is therefore conceivable that the combinations and contents of fatty acids and/or other constituents such as polysaccharides in prescriptions are important for the efficacy of TJ-48. Elucidation of other active ingredients in TJ-48 is now in progress.

Oleic acid and linolenic acid are common constituents of plant and animal cells, and it is known that they play important roles as energy stores or constituents of the cellular membrane. These fatty acids may therefore provide some signal for the proliferation of stem cells or the interaction between stem cells and stromal cells. Based on the present findings, the administration of TJ-48 should be of benefit to patients receiving chemotherapy, radiation therapy or bone marrow transplantation.

REFERENCES

1. Nabeya K, Ri S (1983) Effect of oriental medical herbs on the restoration of the human body before and after operation. Proc Symp Wakan-Yaku 16:201
2. Komatsu Y, Takemoto N, Maruyama H, Tsuchiya H, Aburada M, Hosoya E, Shinohara S, Hamada H (1986) Effect of Juzentaihoto on the anti-SRBC response in mice. Jap J Inflammat 6:405-408
3. Takemoto N, Kawamura H, Maruyama H, Komatsu Y, Aburada M, Hosoya E (1989) Jap J Inflammat 9: 49-52
4. Maruyama H, Kawamura H, Takemoto N, Komatsu Y, Aburada M, Hosoya E (1988) Effect of Kampo medicines on phagocytes. Jap J Inflammat 8: 65-66
5. Takemoto N, Kawamura H, Komatsu Y, Aburada M, Hosoya E (1989) Jap J Inflammat 9: 137-140
6. Ikehara S, Kawamura H, Komatsu Y, Yamada H, Hisha H, Yasumizu R, Ohnishi-Inoue Y, Kiyohara H, Hirano M, Aburada M, Good RA (1992) Effect of Medicinal plants on hemopoietic cells. Microbial Infections H. Fredman et al.(Eds), Plenum press, New York ; pp319-330
7. Kiyohara H, Takemoto N, Komatsu Y, Kawamura H, Hosoya E, Yamada H (1991) Charactarization of mitogenic pectic polysaccharides from Kampo (Japanese Herbal) Medicine "Juzen-Taiho-To" Planta Med 57: 254-259

Hematopoietic Reconstitution after Peripheral Blood Stem Cell Transplantation: Effects of Granulocyte Colony-Stimulating Factor and Progenitor Cell Dose

Chihiro Shimazaki, Hideo Goto, Eishi Ashihara, Noboru Yamagata, Hideyo Hirai, Takehisa Kikuta, Toshiya Sumikuma, Yoshikazu Sudo, Tohru Inaba, Naohisa Fujita, and Masao Nakagawa

Second Department of Medicine, Kyoto Prefectural University of Medicine, 465 Kawaramachi-Hirokoji, Kamigyoku, Kyoto, 602 Japan

SUMMARY

The effect of granulocyte colony-stimulating factor (G-CSF) on accelerating the rate of neutrophil recovery after peripheral blood stem cell transplantation (PBSCT) remains controversial.)\We retrospectively analyzed 37 patients who received high-dose chemotherapy followed by PBSCT. Patients were divided into three groups: those who received no G-CSF (control), a low dose (50 mg/m^2), or a high dose (150 mg/m^2), subcutaneously. Seven patients who received increased numbers of colony forming units-granulocyte macrophage (CFU-GM) (>100x10^4/kg) and either low- or high-dose G-CSF were separately analyzed. Neutrophil recovery (0.5 x10^9/l) was accelerated in the G-CSF-treated patients. It occurred at a median of 10 and 9 days in the low- and high-dose G-CSF groups compared with 14 days in the control group (p< .0001). In patients receiving increased numbers of progenitor cells, the time until recovery was 9 days. No statistically significant differences were observed for platelet and reticulocyte recovery, transfusions, days febrile and parenteral antibiotic requirement. Thus, the administration of low-dose G-CSF is recommended in PBSCT.

KEY WORDS: PBSCT, Hematopoietic recovery, G-CSF, CFU-GM

INTRODUCTION

The administration of granulocyte colony-stimulating factor (G-CSF) accelerates neutrophil recovery after autologous or allogeneic bone marrow transplantation (BMT) [1,2]. However, it remains controversial whether the use of G-CSF in the post-transplantation period further accelerates the rate of neutrophil engraftment in PBSCT. We and other investigators have demonstrated that the use of G-CSF enhances neutrophil recovery in patients undergoing PBSCT [3-6], though another group failed to show this effect [7-9]. Furthermore, the dosage and route of administration of G-CSF in PBSCT varied in each study, and it is also known that the speed of hematopoitic recovery in PBSCT depends on the number of progenitor cells infused [10].

Based on these considerations we retrospectively analyzed hematopoietic reconstitution in 37 patients with various types of malignancies who underwent PBSCT. The patients were divided into three groups: patients who received no G-CSF, a low dose G-CSF or a high dose G-CSF. Patients who received a large number of colony forming units-granulocyte macrophage (CFU-GM) (>100x10^4/kg) were separately analyzed.

MATERIALS AND METHODS

Patients

Thirty seven patients with various malignancies underwent a high-dose chemotherapy followed by PBSCT a total of 39 times. Of these 7 patients were analyzed separately because they received a large number of CFU-GM (>100x10⁴/kg). Therefore, 30 patients underwent PBSCT a total of 32 times. These patients included 6 with acute myelogenous leukemia (AML), 6 with acute lymphoblastic leukemia (ALL), 15 with malignant lymphoma (ML), and 1 with multiple myeloma (MM), Ewing's sarcoma (ES) and small cell lung cancer (SCLC). The patients ranged in age from 18 to 59 years and included 20 males and 17 females.

Transplant protocol and G-CSF administration All patients received high-dose myeloablative chemotherapy followed by PBSCT. Details of procedures for PBSCT have previously been described [11]. The pretransplant conditioning regimen for AML and ALL consisted of busulfan (16 mg/kg) and cyclophosphamide (CY, 120 mg/kg), while for ML it consisted of CY (120 mg/kg), etoposide (ETP, 1500 mg/m^2) and ranimustine (MCNU, 500 mg/m^2). MM patients received melphalan (140 mg/m^2), ETP (750 mg/m^2) and MCNU (250 mg/m^2), ES patients received ETP (1200 mg/m^2) and ifosphamide (12 g/m^2), and SCLC patients received CY (3 g/m^2), ETP (1000 mg/m^2) and carboplatin (1200mg/m^2). PBSC were infused on day 0. Eleven patients received rhG-CSF of 50mg/m^2 and nine patients received rhG-CSF of 150mg/m2. Twelve patients were not given rhG-CSF. Treatment with rhG-CSF started on day 1 using a single daily subcutaneous injection and was discontinued when the neutrophil count exceeded 5x10^9/l. The patients who received rhG-CSF were well matched to the control group with regard to age, disease status and the number of CFU-GM infused (Table 1). All patients received prophylactic oral antibiotics and antifungal therapy. Patients who developed a temperature >38-C received broad-spectrum intravenous antibiotics. Packed red blood cell transfusions were given as required to maintain a hematocrit >20%, and platelets were given to maintain a platelet count >20x10^9/l.

Table 1. Patient Characteristics

	Control n=12	Low-dose G-CSF n=11	High-dose G-CSF n=9	Increased progenitors n=7
Median age in year (range)	38 (17-49)	45 (26-57)	45 (20-59)	28 (18-52)
male/female	9/3	3/8	6/3	3/4
Disease				
AML	3	5	0	1
ALL	1	2	3	0
ML	8	2	5	5
MM	0	1	0	0
Solid Tumor	0	1	1	1
Disease status (CR/NR)	10/2	8/3	5/4	3/4
CFU-GM infused	55.8 ±	52.3 ±	48.6 ±	278.4 ±
(x 10⁴/kg) (mean±SD)	11.8	20.7	12.7	38.5

AML: acute myelogenous leukemia, ALL: acute lymphoblastic leukemia,
ML: malignant lymphoma, MM: multiple myeloma, CFU-GM: colony forming unit-granulocyte macrophage, CR: complete remission, NR: not remission

Statistical analysis

Comparisons of PBSC infused, hematopoietic recovery, use of blood products and parameters of infection were made using the Student's t test for unpaired data.

RESULTS

Neutrophil recovery was significantly enhanced by the administration of rhG-CSF after PBSCT (Table 2). The median time until neutrophil recovery ($0.5 \times 10^9/l$ and $1 \times 10^9/l$) in the low- and high-dose rhG-CSF groups respectively were 10 and 10 days, and 9 and 10 days compared with 14 and 17 days in the control group (low-dose G-CSF vs control group: $p < .0001$, high-dose G-CSF vs control group: $p < .0001$). All patients who received increased numbers of progenitor cells with either low- or high-dose rhG-CSF achieved neutrophil recovery at a median of 9 days. The median time until platelet recovery ($50 \times 10^9/l$) in the control, low- and high-dose rhG-CSF groups and the increased numbers of progenitors group, were 13, 11, 13, and 10 days, respectively. These were no statistically significant differences for platelet recovery between groups. Similarly, no statistically significant differences were demonstrated for reticulocyte recovery. There were no statistically significant differences in red cell or platelet transfusion requirements, the number of days febrile, and parenteral antibiotic requirements between the groups.

Table 2. Hematopoietic recovery

	Control	Low-dose G-CSF	High-dose G-CSF	Increased progenitors
days to recover (median, range)				
ANC>$0.5 \times 10^9/l$	14 (11-17)	10 (7-13)	9 (8-10)	9 (8-10)
ANC>$1 \times 10^9/l$	17 (11-21)	10 (8-14)	10 (9-11)	9 (8-10)
PLT>$50 \times 10^9/l$	13 (9-17)	11 (9-105)	13 (9-20)	10 (10-15)
Ret>1%	16 (14-25)	21 (14-120)	14 (13-22)	14 (13-21)

ANC: absolute neutrophil count, PLT: platelet, Ret: reticulocyte, G-CSF: granulocyte colony-stimulating factor

DISCUSSION

We demonstrated that the administration of G-CSF in the post-transplantation period accelerated neutrophil, but not platelet, recovery after PBSCT as previously described [3]. In addition, we showed that the effect of G-CSF on neutrophil engraftment was the same between doses of 50 mg/m² and 150 mg/m² and that a large number of progenitor cells did not accelerate the rate of neutrophil recovery to less than 9 days.

Thus far, several reports of the effect of G-CSF on neutrophil engraftment after PBSCT have produced conflicting results and recommendations regarding its usefulness [3-9]. These conflicting results might be due to different patient populations, but the number of CD34+ cells and CFU-GM infused and the dosage and route of G-CSF administration should also be considered.

It is noteworthy that the median time until neutrophil recovery ($0.5 \times 10^9/l$) in the G-CSF- treated groups has been similar (10-11days) in all reports except one in which the mean time until recovery was 13.4 days [8]. In these studies the time to recovery in the control groups ranged from 12 to 17 days. In the present study, the patients who received increased numbers of CFU-GM ($278.4 \pm 38.5 \times 10^4/kg$) with either low- or high-dose G-CSF did not accelerate their neutrophil recovery to less than 9 days. These observations suggest that 9 days is the minimum time required for differentiation to mature neutrophils from myeloid-restricted progenitor cells.

Most other studies have used much higher doses of G-CSF (5-10 µg/kg either subcutaneously or intravenously). In this context, we and others have previously demonstrated that the endogenous concentrations of G-CSF increased immediately following graft infusion in PBSCT [12,13]. The peak concentration of endogenous

G-CSF in patients receiving PBSCT was around 2000 pg/ml, while those in patients given low- (50 μg/m2) and high- (150 μg/m2) dose rhG-CSF after PBSCT were approximately 10,000 and 30,000 pg/ml, respectively [14]. These findings suggest that high-dose G-CSF is not always necssary to accelerate neutrophil recovery in PBSCT.

In conclusion, the effect of G-CSF administration in the post-transplantation period on neutrophil recovery is less dramatic in patients receiving PBSCT compared with those undergoing BMT. It does not appear that high-dose G-CSF is necessary in PBSCT, and we therefore recommend the use of low doses, especially in patients with lower numbers of CFU-GM in their infusion.

REFERENCES

1. Sheridan WP, Morstyn G, Wolf M, Dodds A, Lusk J, Maher D, Layton JE, Green MD, Souza L, Fox RM (1989) Granulocyte colony-stimulating factor and neutrophil recovery after high-dose chemotherapy and autologous bone marrow transplantation. Lancet ii:891-895.
2. Schriber JR, Chao NJ, Long GD, Negrin RS, Tieney DK, Kusnierz-Glaz C, Lucas KS, Blume KG (1994) Granulocyte colony-stimulating factor after allogeneic bone marrow transplantation. Blood 84:1680-1684.
3. Shimazaki C, Oku N, Uchiyama H, Yamagata N, Tatsumi T, Hirata T, Ashihara E, Okawa K, Goto H, Inaba T, Fujita N, Haruyama H, Nakagawa M (1994) Effect of granulocyte colony-stimulating factor on hematopoietic recovery after peripheral bloodprogenitor cell transplantation. Bone Marrow Transplant 13:271-275.
4. Spitzer G, Adkins DR, Spencer V, Dunphy FR, Petruska PJ, Velasquez WS, Bower CE, Kronmueller N, Niemeyer R, Mclntyre W (1994) Randomized study of growth factors post-peripheral blood stem cell transplant: neutrophil recovery is improved with modest clinical benefit. J Clin Oncol 12:661-670.
5. Van der Wall E, Richel DJ, Holtkamp MJ, Slaper-Cortenbach ICM, van der Schoot CE, Dalesio O, Nooijen WJ, Schornagel JH, Rodenhuis S (1994) Bone marrow reconstitution after high-dose chemotherapy and autologous peripheral blood progenitor cell transplantation: effect of graft size. Ann Oncol 5:795-802.
6. Klumpp TR, Mangan KF, Goldberg SL, Pearlman ES, Macdonald JS (1995) Granulocyte colony-stimulating factor accelerates neutrophil engraftment following peripheral blood stem cell transplantation: a prospective, randomized trial. J Clin Oncol 13:1323-1327.
7. Dunlop DJ, Fitzsimons EJ, McMurray A, Morrison M, Kyle E, Alcorn MJ, Steward WP (1994) Filgrastim fails to improve haematopoietic reconstitution following myeloablative chemotherapy and peripheral blood stem cell rescue. Br J Cancer 70:943-945.
8. Suzue T, Takaue Y, Watanabe A, Kawano Y, Watanabe T, Abe T, Kuroda Y, Matsushita T, Kikuta A, Iwai J, Shimokawa T, Eguchi H, Murakami T, Kosaka Y, Kudo T, Shimizu H, Koizumi S, Fujimoto T (1994) Effects of rhG-CSF (filgrastim) on the recovery of hematopoiesis after high-dose chemotherapy and autologous peripheral blood stem cell transplantation in children: a report from the Children's Cancer and Leukemia Study Group of Japan. Exp Hematol 22:1197-1202.
9. Cortelazzo S, Viero P, Bellavita P, Rossi A, Buelli M, Borleri M, Marziali S, Bassan R, Commotti B, Rambaldi A, Barbui T (1995) Granulocyte colony-stimulating factor following peripheral-blood progenitor cell transplant in non-Hodgkin's lymphoma. J Clin Oncol 13:935-941.
10. Kawano Y, Takaue Y, Watanabe T, Saito S, Abe T, Hira A, Sato J, Ninomiya T, Suzue T, Koyama T, Shimokawa T, Yokobayashi A, Asano S, Masaoka T, Takaku F, Kuroda Y (1993) Effects of progenitor cell dose and preleukapheresis

use of human recombinant granulocyte colony-stimulating factor on the recovery of hematopoiesis after blood stem cell autografting in children. Exp Hematol 21:103-108.

11. Shimazaki C, Oku N, Ashihara E, Okawa K, Goto H, Inab T, Ito K, Fujita N, Tsuji H, Murakami S, Haruyama H, Nishio A, Nakagawa M (1992) Collection of peripheral blood stem cell mobilized by high-dose Ara-C plus VP-16 or aclarubicin followed by recombinant human granulocyte colony-stimulating factor. Bone Marrow Transplant 10:341-346.

12. Uchiyama H, Shimazaki C, Fujita N, Tatsumi T, Yamagata N, Hirata T, Ashihara E, Oku N, Goto H, Inaba T, Haruyama H, Nakagawa M (1993) Kinetics of serum cytokines in adults undergoing peripheral blood progenitor cell transplantation. Br J Haematol 88:639-642.

13. Kawano Y, Takaue Y, Saito S, Sato J, Shimizu T, Suzue T, Hirao A, Okamoto Y, Abe T, Watanabe T, Kuroda Y, Kimura F, Motoyoshi K, Asano S (1993) Granulocyte colony-stimulating factor (CSF), macrophage-CSF, granulocyte-macrophage CSF, interleukin-3 and interleukin-6 levels in sera fom children undergoing blood stem cell autografts. Blood 81:856-860.

14. Shimazaki C, Uchiyama H, Fujita N, Araki S, Sudo Y, Yamagata N, Ashihara E, Goto H, Inaba T, Haruyama H, Nakagawa M. Serum levels of endogenousand exogenous granulocyte colony-stimulating factor after autologous blood stem cell transplantation. Exp Hematol (in press).

Cord-Placental Blood Banking

Minoko Takanashi, Shinobu Iwai, Masahiro Ueda, Mitsuo Tsubokura, Kazunori Nakajima, Kenji Tadokoro, Takeo Juji

Research Department, The Japanese Red Cross Central Blood Center, 4-1-31 Hiroo, Shibuya-ku, Tokyo, 150 Japan

SUMMARY

Cord-placental blood, a rich source of hemopoietic stem cells, has come to be used clinically for stem cell transplantations. With the cooperation of the obstetrics staff of the Japanese Red Cross Medical Center, cord blood was withdrawn in the 3rd stage of labor with the written consent of the mother. If the mother had a positive viral marker or if the baby had a genetic abnormality, then the cord blood was not withdrawn. The mean volume obtained was 32.5 ml. We used 10 ml of the blood mixed with anticoagulant for the cell count, blood typing, HLA typing and infectious marker screening, keeping the plasma and DNA frozen for future analysis. The samples were processed for RBC reduction with HES, analysed for colony forming ability and CD34$^+$ population, and then frozen in liquid nitrogen. The frozen samples had a mean of 3.7×10^8 nucleated cells, 1.5×10^5 CFU-GM and 2.9×10^5 CD34$^+$ cells. As a source for collecting stem cells, cord blood is the least obtrusive for the donor. A limitation is the volume, with only a small proportion of the samples giving an adequate number of stem cells. While the cord blood samples with more than 5×10^8 cells are few in number, they are ready to be used for transplantation, and the project is proceeding.

KEY WORDS: cord-placental blood, hemopoietic stem cells, banking, transplantation

INTRODUCTION

Cord-placental blood contains a high level of hemopoietic stem cells [1] and has been used for stem cell transplantations in clinical practice [2]. It has been proven to be able to reconstitute hemopoiesis in children, causes less severe GVHD, and needs less strict HLA matching. When a banking system was planned [3], the blood center was well positioned with an established system for donor screening, HLA typing and blood product handling. We analysed techniques for hemopoietic stem cell counting and freezing, and last spring we began the banking system. The cord blood stem cell banking system is now ready for use in transplantations.

MATERIALS AND METHODS

With the cooperation of the obstetrics staff of the Japanese Red Cross Medical Center, cord blood was withdrawn in the 3rd stage of labor with the written consent of the mother. The cord blood was not withdrawn if the mother had a positive viral marker nor if the baby had a genetic abnormality (ex. Down's syndrome). The blood was collected by gravity into a bag containing CPD solution (a mixture of sodium citrate, citric acid, dextrose, and sodium dihydroxyphosphate), and was kept at room temperature until separated.

The separation was performed under sterile conditions. The cord blood bag was weighed, and a 10 ml test sample was withdrawn. Then a small separation bag, containing 12% hydroxyethyl starch

(HES) at a volume of one quarter of the cord blood, was connected to the cord blood bag. The HES was transferred from the separation bag to the cord blood bag and mixed with the blood. After settling at room temperature for 90 minutes with a clamp between the two bags, the sedimented RBC were dispensed into the separation bag. The nucleated cell fraction of less than 4% hematocrit was processed for a cell count, colony assay, CD34+ count, and preservation. The cryopreservation was done with between 4 to 8 x 10^7 cells /ml using 5% dimethylsulfoxide, 6% HES and 4% human albumin, in a -80°C freezer overnight and then in liquid nitrogen [4]. The RBC fraction was used to test for bacteria and fungi with the Signal blood culture system (Oxoid, Hampshire, England).

Cell count by a Sysmex microcell counter, ABO/Rh blood typing and STS were done using 0.5 ml of test sample, and the rest of the 10 ml was separated by centrifugation on Ficoll-Paque. The plasma fraction was processed for screening tests for viral infection, i.e. HBsAg, anti-HBcAb, anti HCVAb, anti-HTLV-I, anti-HIV-1 and anti-HIV-2, leaving 2 tubes for cryopreservation. The mononuclear cells were processed for class I and class II HLA typing, and leftover DNA was kept for future tests. The bottom RBC with nucleated WBC were frozen for future DNA extraction.

For the clonogenic assay, 2 x 10^4 cells/ml were suspended in α-MEM containing 30% fetal calf serum, 1% bovine serum albumin, 5 x 10^{-5} M 2-mercaptoethanol, 5 u/ml IL-3, 10 ng/ml G-CSF, 2 u/ml Epo, and 1.2% methylcellulose. Cells were incubated in 5% CO_2 at 37°C for 14 days. Colonies were counted with an inverted microscope as CFU-GM, BFU-E, CFU-Eo, CFU-EoGM, CFU-Emix, and CFU-Mϕ.

CD34+ cells were counted using anti-CD34 antibody conjugated with FITC and a flowcytometer, Cytoron (Ortho Diagnostics, Tokyo, Japan). The gate was set in the lymphocyte area, and cells positive for CD34 were counted in the two-colour program, with red fluorescence of propidium iodide for dead cells.

RESULTS

Efficiency of blood collection

Table 1. Amounts of cord blood and stem cells for 57 samples.

	mean ± SD	range	median
blood volume	32.5 ± 21.9 ml	1 ~ 101 ml	29.9 ml
nucleated cells	3.7 ± 2.7 x 10^8	0.4 ~ 14.4 x 10^8	3.3 x 10^8
CFU-GM	1.49 ± 1.81 x 10^5	0 ~ 9.09 x 10^5	0.96 x 10^5
Total CFU	5.79 ± 6.36 x 10^5	0.08 ~ 31.22 x 10^5	3.92 x 10^5
CD34+ cells	2.91 ± 8.32 x 10^5	0.01 ~ 58.65 x 10^5	0.95 x 10^5

A total of 57 samples were analysed (Table 1). The mean blood volume withdrawn was 29.9 ml, which was less than we expected, as a previous study in which blood was collected after placental delivery gave a mean of 48.6 ml [5]. Eight of the samples (14.0%) contained more than 50 ml of blood. For 15 samples (26.3%), more than 5×10^8 cells were cryopreserved. More than 10^5 CFU-GM were cryopreserved in 28 samples (49.1%) and more than 10^5 CD34$^+$ cells were cryopreserved in 27 of 56 samples (48.2%).

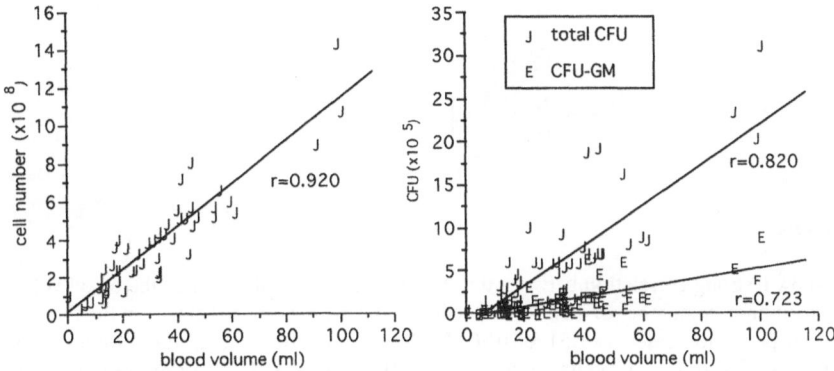

Fig.1 Correlation between the parameters.
The correlation between: blood volume and cell number (left), blood volume and total CFU or CFU-GM (right) were significant.

There was a strong correlation between CFU-GM and total CFU (r=0.955), blood volume and cell number (r=0.920), blood volume and total CFU (r=0.820), and blood volume and CFU-GM (r=0.723) (Fig.1). The correlation was lower between blood volume and CD34$^+$ cells (r=0.622), CD34$^+$ cells and total CFU (r=0.670), and CD34$^+$ cells and CFU-GM (r=0.601).

Laboratory tests

There were 9 samples in which the HLA typing was unsuccessful, mostly in samples having a small volume or kept too long in excess anticoagulant. The smaller the volume collected, the more diluted the sample became, and the more acidic the condition was that the cells stayed in.

There was one sample with bacterial contamination, and Propionibacterium acnes, a gram positive anaerobic rod, was isolated.

No sample was positive for the screening tests for viral markers.

Effect of freezing and thawing

Eight samples kept frozen in liquid nitrogen for more than a year were thawed and their colony forming ability was analysed. The mean cell number recovered was 56.2% of pre-freezing (Fig.2). In spite of the overall low recovery of viable cells, recovery of the colony forming cells was good. The morphological differentiation of WBC showed that the segmented cell fraction decreased from 54.8% to 29.5%, in 5 of the samples. That is, the mononuclear cells had a higher survival rate.

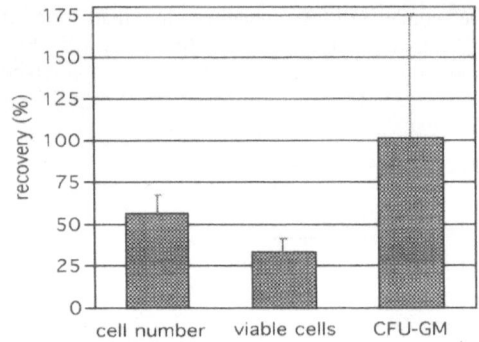

Fig.2 Effect of freezing procedure:
recovery of cells and CFU-GM

DISCUSSION

The results show a strong correlation between the stem cell number collected and the blood volume collected. The minimum number of stem cells needed to reconstitute hemopoiesis, in the reports of cord blood transplantation cases, is 1.51×10^4 CFU-GM or 0.4×10^8 cells/kg body weight. So at least 3×10^5 CFU-GM or 8×10^8 cells are needed for 20kg children. Only 12.3% of our samples meet the CFU-GM limitation and 7.0% satisfy the total cell number minimum. Thus a present target must be to increase the efficiency of blood collection, which is now done by obstetrics staff. Giving more information and improving communication with the pregnant women as well as further education of the medical staff would help this project. At present we use a syringe to withdraw blood from the umbilical cord in the 3rd stage of labor, and we use only the samples with more than 40ml of blood for conducting all of the procedures. In the future we will analyse the possibility of expanding the stem cell fraction without differentiation.

From the clinical point of view, samples for transplantation must be safe and reliable to use. Therefore our samples must be infection free and have at least a minimum number of hematopoietic stem cells. As allogeneic cord blood stem cell transplantation is quite new, it is reasonable to use those samples as a rescue for cases with unsuccessful transplantation or severe myelosuppression after chemotherapy.

REFERENCES

[1] Broxmeyer HE, Douglas GW, Hangoc G, Cooper S, Bard J, English D, Army M, Thomas L, Boyse EA (1989) Human umbilical cord blood as a potential source of transplantable hematopoietic stem/progenitor cells. Pro Natl Acad Sci USA 86:3828-3832
[2] Wagner JE (1994) Umbilical cord blood transplantation: overview of the clinincal experience. Blood Cells 20:227-234
[3] Harris DT, Schumacher MJ, Rychlik S, Booth A, Acevedo A, Rubinstein P, Bard J, Boyse EA (1994) Collection, separation and cryopreservation of umbilical cord blood for use in transplantation. Bone Marrow Transplant 13:135-143
[4] Stiff PJ, Koester AR, Weidner MK, Dvorak K, Fisher RI (1987) Autologous bone marrow transplantation using unfractionated cells cryopreserved in dimethylsulfoxide and hydroxyethylstarch without controlled-rate freezing. Blood 70:974-978
[5] Iwai S, Takanashi M, Tsukui K, Ueda M, Nakajima K, Tadokoro K, Juji T (1996) Trials and analysis of umbilical cord blood collection, separation and cryopreservation methods for transplantation. (submitted)

Eosinophilic Precursors in the Fibroreticular Network of Human Thymus

Inchul Lee[1], Eunsil Yu[1], Robert A. Good[2] and Susumu Ikehara[3]

[1] Department of Diagnostic Pathology, Asan Medical Center, Ulsan University, Seoul,
[2] Department of Pediatrics, All Children's Hospital, University of South Florida, St. Petersburg, Florida USA; [3] First Department of Pathology, Kansai Medical University, Osaka, Japan

SUMMARY

The distribution of myeloid cells in the human thymus was investigated using a series of seventy four thymic samples from newborn to 37 year-old patients. By light microscopy, eosinophilic precursors (promyelocyte, myelocytes and metamyelocytes) were readily identified. These immature granular cells were present in all pre-involutional thymi; they made up 30-50% of the total eosinophilic population and were frequently observed as a group of cells at various stages of differentiation, suggesting that they differentiate from existing precursors in the thymus. These eosinophilic precursors were mostly located in the intralobular septa and fibroreticular network at the corticomedullary junction, while mature eosinophils were scattered throughout the thymus. Flow cytometric analyses using stem cell-enriched preparations showed cells expressing CD33 or CD34 to constitute on average 2.55% and 3.33% (0.09% and 0.12% of the total cells) respectively. $CD33^+/CD34^+$ coexpressors were also identified, and they constituted 0.36% of the analyzed cells (0.01% of the total cells). No statistical difference in the proportions of $CD33^+$ and/or 34^+ cells was noted between any age groups. It is concluded that eosinophilic precursors present in the thymus differentiate into cells in eosinophilic lineage in particular areas such as intralobular septa and the fibroreticular network of the outer medulla in pre-involutional human thymi.

KEY WORDS : human thymus, eosinophilic precursor, fibroreticular network

INTRODUCTION

Thymocytes differentiate and mature in the complex thymic microenvironment [1-8]. However, it is not clear whether thymocyte precursors or truly pluripotent hemopoietic stem cells (HSCs) migrate into the thymus and undergo terminal differentiation (reviewed in 9). To understand the dynamics of cellular migration into the thymus, several fundamental questions should be answered: 1) whether HSCs exist in the thymus at all, 2) if they exist in the thymus, whether they are pluripotent HSCs or hematopoietic stem cells already committed, 3) how their frequency and localization in the thymus change with age, and 4) wherther there is any direct evidence of in situ differentiation into other hematopoietic lineage.

In an attempt to answer these questions, we carried out histological and immunocytochemical studies using an extensive series of samples of human thymic samples.

MATERIALS AND METHODS

Thymic Samples

Seventy four human thymic samples were investigated by light and electron microscopy, immunohistochemistry, and/or flow cytometry (Table 1). Postnatal thymic samples were freshly obtained during open heart surgery from newborn babies to patients up to 37 years old. The subjects suffered from various congenital cardiovascular diseases without any known immunologic or other systemic disorders. Samples were routinely processed for histologic and electron microscopic examination. Reticulin and Masson's trichrome stainings were also carried out routinely.

Immunohistochemistry

For immunohistochemistry, 4μ-thick frozen sections were used. Sections were air-dried, fixed in cold acetone for 10 minutes, and then immunostained using the ABC method; the monoclonal anti-cytokeratin antibody CK-217, monoclonal anti-CD33 and anti-CD34 antibodies (Becton-Dickinson Immunocyto-Chemistry Systems, San Jose, CA), polyclonal rabbit antisera against fibronectin and laminin (Chemicon Co.) were used.

Flow cytometry

Cells from forty five fresh thymic samples were examined using flow cytometry. To enrich HSCs, low-density cells were prepared as previously described [10], but with a few modifications. Briefly, single cell suspensions were prepared from fresh thymic samples by gently mincing over a steel mesh in RPMI-1640 medium with 5% fetal calf serum. After washing twice, the viability, which was greater than 95% in each preparation, was determined by trypan blue staining. The suspension in RPMI with 10% fetal calf serum was incubated overnight on Sephadex G-10 column in 5% CO_2. The cells were then pelleted, overlaid by 3 step-discontinuous Percoll gradients (r=1.075, 1.065, and 1.055 respectively), and incubated on ice for 10 minutes. After centrifugation for 30 minutes at 2000g, a low density fraction (1.055 < r < 1.065) was harvested.

The harvested cells were 3.68% of the total starting cells in average (0.71-10.34%). Double-immunostaining was carried out using monoclonal anti-CD33 (phycoerythrin-labeled) and anti-CD34 (FITC-labeled) antibodies (Becton-Dickinson Immunocyto Systems, San Jose, CA). Samples were also analyzed using anti-CD4, anti-CD8, anti-CD5, anti-CD36 and anti-CD13 antibodies (Becton-Dickinson Immunocytometry Systems). Flow cytometric analyses were performed on a FACScan (Becton-Dickinson Immunocytometry Systems, CA.).

RESULTS

Fibroreticular network

It is well known that the thymic lobules (the functional units of thymus) consist of cortex and medulla, and that they are circumscribed by interlobular septa. Multiple loose intralobular septa branch into the medulla from the interlobular septa (Fig. 1). The interlobular septa mostly consist of dense connective tissue and occasional blood vessels. The intralobular septa, however, were found to be composed of relatively loose connective tissue, small vessels, and numerous mononuclear cells, particularly in the inner area close to the medulla. As the intralobular septa reach the corticomedullary junction, they expand to form the fibroreticular network, which occupies most of the corticomedullary junction of the thymic lobules.

The intralobular septa were demarcated by an intact layer of epithelial cells and a basement membrane. They were identified by immunocytochemical staining for cytokeratin and laminin respectively. The fibroreticular network, a distinct structure from the medulla or cortex, was also delineated by the epithelial cells and basement membrane. However, the lining was incomplete, and the fibroreticular network merged directly with medulla or cortex at multiple sites. Thus, the fibroreticular network was not just a pure connective tissue compartment but a specific intrathymic parenchymal structure.

Eosinophilic precursors In the fibroreticular network and intralobular sepa, we noted heterogenous cells such as eosinophils, mast cells, macrophages, plasma cells, lymphoid cells, and primitive mononuclear cells. The primitive mononuclear cells were similar to HSCs in terms of certain morphological criteria such as their nuclear shape and chromatin pattern and high nuclear/cytoplasmic ratio. However, they could not be readily identified on the morphological basis. In contrasts eosinophilic precursors could be identified without difficulty, since the precursors had abundant eosinophilic granules in the cytoplasm (Fig. 2). The precursors had large, premature nuclei which were round, ovoid, or band-form depending on their stage of differentiation. The nuclear/cytoplasmic ratio was high, and the chromatin was diffusely dispersed. Eosinophilic cells undergoing mitosis were occasionally noted. Electron microscopic studies revealed eosinophilic promyelocytes and myelocytes with characteristic cytoplasmic granules that contained crystalline inclusions. The eosinophilic promyelocytes, myelocytes, metamyelocytes, and mature eosinophils were frequently observed as close aggregates. The presence of aggregates of eosinophilic cells in various differentiational stages strongly suggests that eosinophilic cells differentiate from precursors within the thymus.

Table 1. Distribution of eosinophils and their precursors in human thymi.

Group	Case number	Eosinophilic precursors	Mature eosinophils	Locations of eosinophilic precursors				
				Intelobular septum	Intralobular septum	FRN	Cortex	Medulla
Postnatal (< 1 Mo)	18	++/+++	+/++	+	+++	+++	+	+
1 Mo < 1 Yr	29	++/+++	+/++	−	++	+++	−/+	−/+
1 Yr < 5 Yr	14	+/+++	+/++	−	+	++	−	−/+
5 Yr < involution	8	+/++	+	−	+	++	−	−
Involuted (18-37 Yr)	5	−/+	−/+	−	−	−	−	−

− : absent   + : focally scattered
++ : seen in less than 1/2 of lobules   +++ : seen in more than 1/2 of lobules

Eosinophilic precursors were present in all thymi examined (before thymic involution) (Table 1). They made up 30-50% of the total eosinophilic population. They tended to decrease with age, although considerable numbers still existed in the thymi of adolescents. The eosinophilic precursors were mostly confined to the fibroreticular network and intralobular septa. In the newborn thymi, they were occasionally present also in the interlobular septa. With age, however, there was a tendency for only mature eosinophils to be present in the interlobular septa (Table 1). In involuted thymi, the distinction between fibroreticular network and medulla became ambiguous, and eosinophils as well as the precursors had mostly disappeared. By immunohistochemistry using anti-CD34 and anti-CD33 antibodies, the immunostaining was largely confined to the mononuclear cells in the septa and fibroreticular network, while the cortex and medulla did not immunostain.

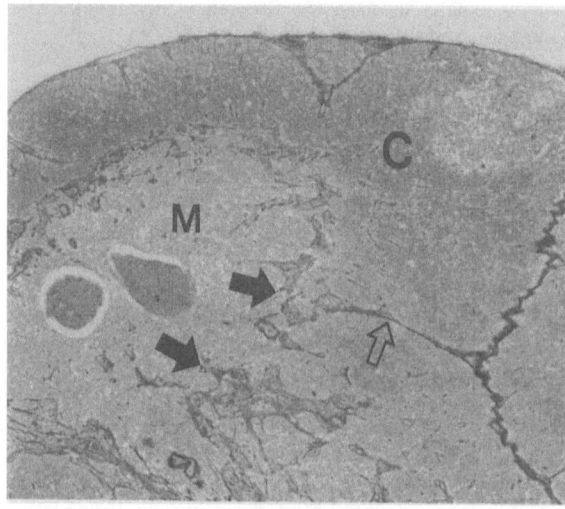

Fig. 1 : Thymus from 2 year-old: At the corticomedullary junction, the intralobular septa (empty arrow) expand and disperse to form the fibroreticular network (arrow). It occupies most of the corticomedullary junction, while the medulla (M) and cortex (C) are largely devoid of connective tissue fibers. Note the two Hassall's corpuscles in the middle of the medulla. (Reticulin staining X 60)

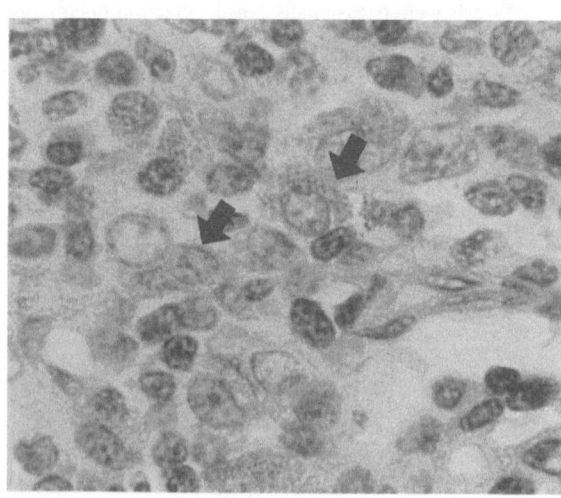

Fig. 2 : Same thymus as figure 1. Note eosinophilic myelocytes with large, round nuclei in the fibroreticular network (arrows) (H & E staining, X 950).

Intrathymic myeloid stem cells

The HSC-enriched preparations from 45 fresh thymic samples were analyzed using flow cytometry. The percentage of CD4$^+$ cells varied from 45 to 67% (mean 59%), and that of CD8$^+$ cells were from 16 to 29% (mean 24%). The percentage of CD5$^+$ cells varied from 81 to 93% (mean 89%). The CD36$^+$ or CD13$^+$ cells were under the detectable level.

The expression of myeloid and/or stem cell markers (i.e. CD33 and CD34) was also examined. In all samples, considerable CD33$^+$ or CD34$^+$ cells were identified with wide individual variation. The percentage of CD34$^+$ cells varied from 0.19 to 14.28% (mean 3.33%) of the analyzed cells; 0.01-0.46% of the total starting cells (mean 0.12%). The CD33$^+$ cells were from 0.15 to 9.44% (mean 2.55%); 0.01-0.34% of the total starting cells (mean 0.09%). No statistically significant difference was seen between any age-groups; samples included those from newborn babies to those from 10 year-old patients.

In all thymi, there were significant $CD33^+/34^+$ coexpressors which apparently represented myeloid stem cells. They varied from 0.10 to 2.45% (mean 0.36%) of the analyzed cells; 0.04-0.08% of the total starting cells (mean 0.01%). As with single positive cells, no statistical difference was seen between any age-groups.

CONCLUSION

Hemopoietic stem cells as well as eosinophilic precursors are normally present in pre-involutional human thymi. Eosinophilic precursors are mostly in the fibroreticular network as clusters of various differentiational stages. It is suggested that the eosinophilic lineage may represent an intrathymic myeloid differentiation.

REFERENCES

1. Haynes BF. (1984) The human thymic microenvironment. Advances Immunol. 36: 87-142
2. Weiss L. (1988) The thymus. In : Weiss L, ed cell and tissue biology. Urban & Schwarzenberg, Baltimore pp481-495
3. Kendall MD. (1989) The morphology of perivascular space in the thymus. Thymus 13: 157-164
4. Goldstein G. (1966) Plasma cells in the human thymus. Austr. J. Exp. Biol. Med. Sci. 44: 695-8
5. Hayward AR. (1972) Myoid cells in the human fetal thymus. J. Pathol. 106: 45-8
6. Kaiserling E, Stein H, Müller-Hermelink HK. (1974) Interdigitating reticulum cells in the human thymus. Cell Tissue Res. 155: 754-5
7. Ikehara S, Tanaka H, Nakamura T, Furukawa F, Inoue S, Sekita K, Shimizu J, Hamashima Y and Good RA. (1985) The influence of thymic abnormalities on the development of autoimmune diseases. Thymus 7: 25-36
8. Bhatal PS and Campbell PE. (1965) Eosinophil leucocytes in the child's thymus. Aust. Ann. Med. 14: 210-213
9. Adkins B, Müller C, Okada CY, Reichert RA, Weissman IL, and Spangrude GJ. (1987) Early events in T cell maturation. Ann. Rev. Immunol. 5: 325-65
10. Kumamoto T, Inaba M, Imamura H, Nango K, Adachi Y, Soe Than, Inaba K, Kagawa T, Ikehara S. (1991) Characterization of B cells in human thymus. Immunobiol. 183: 88-93

Growth Factors
and Their Receptors

Biology of Flt3 Ligand, a Novel Regulator of Hematopoietic Stem and Progenitor Cells

Hilary J. McKenna and Stewart D. Lyman

Immunex Corporation, 51 University St., Seattle, WA 98101

SUMMARY

Flt3 Ligand (Flt3L) is a protein that plays a key role in the regulation of early events in the development of multiple hematopoietic lineages. Flt3L stimulates the development of primitive multipotent precursors, as well as more committed or restricted myeloid precursors. Flt3L has an effect on early B cell development as well as on T cell development, at least in the embryo. These effects of Flt3L on hematopoietic precursors are similar to those observed with Steel factor (SLF), and both of these proteins synergize with a variety of cytokines to stimulate the proliferation of these cells. However, there are a number of differences between the biological effects of these two hematopoietic factors, the most notable being the lack of effect of Flt3L on mast cells. Mice lacking the Flt3 receptor have a mild defect in early B cell development, and stem cells isolated from these mice have an impaired ability to reconstitute lethally irradiated recipients. Serum levels of Flt3L are normally quite low in healthy humans (< 100 pg/ml), but are highly elevated in individuals afflicted with anemias with a stem cell component, such as Fanconi or acquired aplastic anemia, but not in single lineage anemias, such as Diamond-Blackfan. These data suggest that Flt3L may be a key physiological regulator of stem cells in vivo. Flt3L may find clinical utility in the treatment of hematopoietic disorders, especially those involving multiple lineages.

KEY WORDS: Flt3 ligand, stem cells, hematopoiesis, tyrosine kinase receptors

INTRODUCTION

The growth, differentiation, and survival of hematopoietic cells is primarily regulated by proteins that interact with specific receptors on the surfaces of these cells. Among these proteins are the colony stimulating factors (CSFs) and the interleukins, which bind to different families of receptors. The discovery of the Flt3 tyrosine kinase receptor [1, 2] (also referred to as flk-2 [3]or STK-1[4]) led to the discovery of the ligand for this receptor, known as the Flt3 ligand (Flt3L)[5-7]. This protein is structurally related to the CSF-1 and SLF proteins in that all three proteins share conserved cysteine residues, are transmembrane proteins that give rise to soluble, biologically active proteins, and have a similar intron/exon structure [8]. Space constraints limit the focus of this article to a review of the biological activities of Flt3L and suggestions for some of its potential uses in the clinic. Information on discovery of the Flt3L and its receptor, expression of these proteins, structure and chromosomal locations of the genes, identification of isoforms of the protein, and signaling through the Flt3 receptor have been covered in other articles [8, 9].

HEMATOPOIETIC ACTIVITIES OF FLT3L

As mentioned in the introduction, Flt3L, SLF, and CSF-1 are structurally-related hematopoietic growth factors. SLF has multiple effects on lymphoid and myeloid development, as well as on primitive hematopoietic cells [10]. In contrast, CSF-1 functions primarily within the monocyte-macrophage lineage [11]. Prior to the cloning of Flt3L, indirect evidence that Flt3L affected hematopoietic cell development was obtained by Small and coworkers [4]. Antisense oligonucleotides directed against human Flt3R inhibited colony formation of Granulocytic-Monocytic (GM) colonies, Burst Forming Unit-Erythroid (BFU-E) colonies, and Granulocytic-Erythroid-Monocytic-Megakaryocytic (GEMM) colonies from human CD34$^+$ bone marrow cells. Perhaps surprisingly, however, it was later shown that antisense oligonucleotides directed against Flt3L alone did not inhibit hematopoiesis in vitro, although when combined with antisense oligonucleotides against SLF inhibition was observed [12].

The initial reports describing the cloning of Flt3L showed that Flt3L stimulated a low level of proliferation of enriched hematopoietic precursors from different sources: purified c-kit^+ mouse bone marrow cells [5], murine AA4.1$^+$ Sca-1$^+$ lin^{lo} fetal liver cells [5], and human CD34$^+$ bone marrow cells [6]. By itself, Flt3L had only weak proliferative effects, but it synergized with IL-3, IL-7 and SLF [5] to give enhanced proliferation. Flt3L alone stimulated the formation of a small number of colonies from murine Thy^{lo} Sca-1$^+$ Lin$^-$ bone marrow cells [7], human CD34$^+$ CD33$^+$ Lin$^-$ fetal liver cells [7] and human CD34$^+$ bone marrow cells [6]. Flt3L synergized with IL-6 [7], IL-3, GM-CSF, [6, 7] and Pixy321 [6] (a fusion protein of IL-3 and GM-CSF [13]), to increase the number of colonies. Since these initial reports, a number of papers have been published outlining the effects of flt3L on primitive and more committed myeloid and lymphoid progenitor cells. These observations have been summarized in the following sections.

THE EFFECT OF FLT3L ON MYELOID PRECURSORS

The effects of Flt3L on primitive myeloid precursors have been examined in clonal assays. High-proliferative-potential (HPP) colonies represent myeloid precursors with considerable proliferative capacity along the granulocytic and monocytic lineages. Murine Thy-1^{lo} Sca-1$^+$ bone marrow-derived cells did not form HPP colonies in response to Flt3L alone, but Flt3L synergized with GM-CSF, G-CSF, IL-3 and IL-6, though not with SLF [14]. The level of synergy was less than that observed when SLF was added to these factors. The exception was flt3L + IL-6, where levels of synergy were equivalent to that seen with SLF + IL-6. Similarly, human fetal liver-derived CD34^{++} CD38$^+$ Lin$^-$ and CD34^{++} CD38$^-$ Lin$^-$ cells [15] or bone marrow-derived CD34$^+$ cells [16] did not form HPP colonies in response to Flt3L alone. Flt3L synergized with IL-3 and GM-CSF [15] or Pixy321 [16] but not SLF [15, 16]. Both Flt3L and SLF synergized with a cocktail of factors to induce HPP colony formation from human progenitor cells, but interestingly, HPP colonies grown with Flt3L had greater potential in secondary recloning assays [17].

Lin$^-$ Sca-1$^+$ bone marrow cells cultured with Flt3L plus G-CSF, IL-11 or IL-12, resulted in a high proportion of cells with a primitive blast cell phenotype [18]. Similarly, Flt3L added to either IL-6, IL-11, or G-CSF resulted in the formation of undifferentiated blast cell colonies from murine Lin$^-$ Sca-1$^+$ precursors from post 5-Fluorouracil bone marrow [19]. A similar effect was noted by Hudak and coworkers [14]. Flt3L combined with IL-3, IL-6, G-CSF or SLF, but not GM-CSF, resulted in colonies comprising large numbers of undifferentiated blast cells from Thy-1^{lo} Sca-1$^+$ bone marrow cells [14]. Flt3L combined with IL-3 + IL-6 + βFGF induced the formation of blast cell colonies from human hematopoietic progenitors to a similar degree as the addition of SLF [17].

GEMM colonies form from a primitive precursor with multilineage potential. When Flt3L was added to Pixy321 plus erythropoietin, multipotent GEMM colonies formed from CD34$^+$ bone marrow-derived cells [16]. A similar effect was noted by Broxmeyer and coworkers who found that Flt3L combined with IL-3 + EPO induced the formation of GEMM colonies from cord blood cells, though not to the same extent as SLF + IL-3 + EPO [20].

Effects of Flt3L on less primitive myeloid progenitors (as judged by low proliferative potential [LPP] or lineage restriction) have also been observed. Using purified Lin$^-$ Sca-1$^+$ murine bone marrow cells as a source of progenitor cells, Flt3L alone had little effect on colony formation, but synergized with GM-CSF, G-CSF, CSF-1, IL-3, IL-6, IL-11, IL-12, and SLF [18]. In contrast, no synergy of Flt3L with several of these factors was seen on the more committed Lin$^-$ Sca-1$^-$ cells. The effects of Flt3L appeared to be direct since these effects could be observed on single cells. Synergistic effects of Flt3L with SLF, G-CSF, IL-6 or IL-11 were noted on the development of GM colonies from Thy-1^{lo} Sca-1$^+$ murine bone marrow-derived progenitors [14]. A study of murine Lin$^-$ Sca-1$^+$ cells isolated from post 5-Fluorouracil marrow showed that Flt3L synergized with IL-6, IL-11, or G-CSF, but not with IL-3 or SLF, to promote colony formation, and that the colonies formed by Flt3L in combination with other factors were not as large as those formed by combinations of factors plus SLF [19].

Hematopoietic progenitors purified from human fetal liver (CD34^{++} CD38$^+$ Lin$^-$, CD34^{++} CD38$^+$ Lin$^-$) formed LPP colonies in response to Flt3L plus IL-3, GM-CSF, or SLF [15]. When SLF was used in place of Flt3L, the level of synergy observed was somewhat higher. Conversely, CD34$^+$ human bone marrow-derived cells formed similar numbers of GM colonies in response to either Flt3L + Pixy321 or SLF + Pixy321 [16]. Similarly, both Flt3L and SLF synergized with GM-CSF, G-CSF, IL-3, or CSF-1 to induce CFU-GM formation from cord blood progenitors [20].

The addition of Flt3L to human myeloid Dexter cultures augmented the production of both mature cells and colony-forming cells (CFC) [16]. Agonistic antibodies directed against Flt3 receptor also stimulated the growth of cells in a murine Dexter type culture system beyond that seen with the feeder layer alone [21].

ERYTHROID PRECURSORS

Though Flt3L has been shown to have an effect on CFU-GM, CFU-GEMM and HPP-CFC, no effects have been reported on erythroid committed progenitors (BFU-E). This is a lineage in which obvious differences in the response to either Flt3L or SLF are seen. SLF has potent synergistic effects with EPO and IL-3 on erythroid progenitors [10], but Flt3L has no effect on colony formation of these cells from either human fetal liver [7], human bone marrow [16], or murine bone marrow [14, 18]. However, it was recently reported that Flt3L synergized with EPO and EPO + IL-3 to induce BFU-E formation from cord blood cells, while SLF did not [20].

MAST CELLS AND THEIR PRECURSORS

Another lineage in which there is a major difference between Flt3L and SLF activity is the mast cell lineage. SLF stimulates the development, proliferation and activation of mast cells [reviewed in 10], whereas Flt3L does not appear to have this activity [22]. SLF induces proliferation of murine mast cell lines (MC-6, H7, R+SV40), while Flt3L does not [22]. Flt3L had no effect on the formation of mast cell colonies in the presence of IL-4 + IL-10, unlike SLF, which synergized with these two factors to induce colonies [14]. Intravenous administration of SLF in mice results in a respiratory distress syndrome characterized by breathing difficulties; the syndrome is believed to result from degranulation of mast cells in the lungs [23]. Flt3L did not induce respiratory distress in mice following the injection of a large intravenous dose [22].

OTHER MYELOID LINEAGES

Flt3L in the presence of IL-3 had no effect on the development of megakaryocytic colonies, and in the presence of IL-5 or GM-CSF had no effect on the formation of eosinophil colonies [14].

EFFECT OF FLT3L ON LYMPHOID PROGENITOR CELLS

T Cell Precursors

The role of Flt3L in T cell development is unclear. Expression of the Flt3 receptor has been described in the murine fetal thymus (day 13 and 16) and the adult thymus where it was restricted to populations enriched for primitive intra-thymic cells (Thy-1^{lo}, CD4$^-$, CD8$^-$ cells) [3]. This is in contrast to a recent report in which Flt3 receptor expression in the thymus was studied by in situ hybridization [24]. Flt3 receptor was not detected in the fetal thymus until day 16.5 of gestation, and was also seen in the newborn and adult thymus. Expression of the receptor was restricted to the medullary area of the thymus, and not the cortex where the more primitive thymocytes are found [24]. The type of cell expressing Flt3 receptor was not identified, though it was postulated that it may be a cell type comprising the thymic stroma. There has been only one report of an effect of Flt3L on T cell progenitors. Flt3L alone or in combination with IL-7 stimulated the proliferation of day 14 murine fetal thymocytes [7].

B Cell Precursors

There is growing evidence that Flt3L has an important role in B cell development. The most conclusive evidence comes from studies of mice in which the Flt3 receptor was disrupted [25]. The phenotype of the homozygous knock-out mice showed a defect in B cell development, specifically a decrease in the number of pro- and pre-B cells in the bone marrow. In a study where Flt3 receptor expression was examined on highly enriched subsets of immature B cells, the highest level of Flt3 receptor expression was detected in the primitive pre-pro-B cells, and as B cell development progressed to the pre-B stage, Flt3 receptor was down-regulated [26].

Flt3L when combined with IL-6, IL-11 or G-CSF supported the proliferation of purified murine hematopoietic progenitors that were able to give rise to B cell colonies in methylcellulose culture. Flt3L alone induced the proliferation of purified B-cell progenitors and synergized with IL-7 and SLF [19].

CAN FLT3 RECEPTOR EXPRESSION BE USED TO DELINEATE STEM CELL POPULATIONS?

Cell surface expression of the c-*kit* tyrosine kinase receptor has proven to be a useful marker for the enrichment of primitive progenitors from human and murine hematopoietic tissue. Similarly, Flt3 receptor expression has also been looked at as a marker of stem cells. Enriched populations of murine progenitor cells have been sub-divided on the basis of Flt3 receptor expression. Bone marrow cells highly enriched for both pluripotent hematopoietic stem cells (PHSC) and colony forming unit-spleen cells (CFU-S_{12}), or CFU-S_{12} alone were found to express Flt3 receptor, while the cells in the most primitive population, enriched solely for PHSC, did not express Flt3 receptor [27]. The authors hypothesized that Flt3 receptor was expressed on stem cells in cell cycle, but not quiescent pluripotent stem cells. A similar conclusion was drawn by Zeigler and coworkers [21]. Stem cell populations from bone marrow and fetal liver were fractionated on the basis of Flt3 receptor expression. Both the Flt3 receptor^{high} and Flt3 receptor^{low} cell fractions were shown to contain primitive stem cells on the basis of competitive repopulation experiments. Cell cycle analysis showed that Flt3 receptor^{low} cells have a greater percentage of cells in G_0 than Flt3 receptor^{high} cells. From these results it was suggested that the most quiescent stem cells are Flt3 receptor^{low}, and that the Flt3 receptor is expressed on a subset of hematopoietic stem cells that are destined to differentiate into more committed progenitor cells.

Cell surface Flt3 receptor has been detected on enriched CD34$^+$ cells from human bone marrow, but not on CD34$^-$ cells [16]. The murine myeloid M1 cell line expresses cell surface Flt3 receptor when cultured in an undifferentiated state. Although these cells do not proliferate in Flt3L, addition of the growth factor does stimulate phosphorylation of the Flt3 receptor. Upon exposure to leukemia inhibitory factor (LIF), the M1 cells are induced to terminally differentiate to macrophage-like cells. Differentiation is accompanied by a down-regulation of Flt3 receptor and concomitant up-regulation of Flt3L [28].

ARE FLT3L AND SLF FUNCTIONALLY REDUNDANT IN THE HEMATOPOIETIC SYSTEM?

The issue of functional redundancy was elegantly addressed in a recent report describing the production of mice homozygous for a disrupted Flt3 receptor [25]. In general these mice were quite healthy, which is in marked contrast to the lethality observed in mice homozygous for the deletion of the c-*kit* receptor [29]. The loss of a functional Flt3 receptor resulted in a reduction in the number of B cell precursors and a defect in primitive stem cells as assayed in a long-term competitive repopulation assay. Upon adoptive transfer to irradiated secondary recipients, stem cells from Flt3 receptor$^{-/-}$ mice had an impaired ability to repopulate myeloid and T and B lymphoid lineages compared to stem cells from wild type marrow.

The Flt3 receptor$^{-/-}$ mice were crossed with mice (*W/W^v*) that carry a partial deletion of the c-*kit* gene on one chromosome and a mutated form of this receptor on the other [30]. *W/W^v* mice are severely anemic, but this anemia is not lethal. Offspring were obtained from this cross, but they had severely reduced numbers of hematopoietic cells and died between 20 and 50 days of age [25]. These experiments demonstrated a requirement for both Flt3 and c-*kit* receptors in the development of a normal, functional hematopoietic system.

THE ROLE OF FLT3L IN NORMAL AND ABNORMAL HUMAN HEMATOPOIESIS

Although the Flt3 receptor has been shown to be expressed on a wide range of leukemic cell lines and on primary leukemic cells [28, 31-34], the role, if any, that Flt3L or Flt3 receptor plays in the leukemic process is unclear. What is clear from studies of Flt3L serum levels in humans is that this protein appears to be a key physiological regulator of stem cells in vivo [35]. Normal healthy individuals have low serum levels of circulating Flt3L (53 out of 60 had levels below 100 pg/ml, the level of detection). Serum levels of Flt3L in patients with a variety of hematological disorders were determined. Patients with pure red blood cell anemia, polycythemia, α–thalassemia, Diamond-Blackfan anemia, anemias of undetermined origin, or idiopathic thrombocytopenia purpura did not show elevated serum Flt3L levels. In contrast, patients with stem cell based disorders had greatly elevated levels of Flt3L in their serum. Fanconi anemia and acquired aplastic anemia patients had Flt3L serum levels that were elevated approximately 100- and 33-fold, respectively. One of the Fanconi anemia patients was successfully treated with a cord blood transplant, and hematopoietic recovery was accompanied by a return to normal Flt3L serum levels. Levels of Flt3L in serum appear to be inversely correlated with the level of functional stem cells in the patients [35].

POTENTIAL USES OF FLT3L IN THE CLINIC

Ex vivo expansion of stem cells is an area receiving intense clinical study at present, and Flt3L would be an excellent candidate for this setting. Incubation of Thy-1^{lo} Sca-1$^+$ murine bone marrow cells in liquid culture with Flt3L + IL-3 or Flt3L + SLF generated large numbers of mature myeloid cells [18]. Culture of these same cells in the presence of Flt3L + G-CSF or IL-11 resulted in the generation of cells with an immature blast cell phenotype, and clonogenic progenitors were expanded over 40-fold after 14 days in culture [18]. Ex vivo expansion of progenitors was also noted with the combination of Flt3L with IL-3, SLF, IL-6 or G-CSF [14]. Flt3L was more potent than SLF in combination with IL-6 or G-CSF at generating CFU in liquid culture. The combination of Flt3L + IL-6 was the most potent at generating CFU-S$_{12}$ cells in vitro, demonstrating that primitive cells could be expanded with Flt3L +.IL-6 and still retain functional potential [14].

Flt3L as a single factor was able to maintain human bone marrow-derived CFU-GM and HPP ex vivo for 3-4 weeks, and when combined with IL-1 + IL-3 + IL-6 + EPO resulted in a similar level of CFU-GM expansion as was seen when SLF was added to this combination of factors [16].

Flt3L may be of some utility in gene therapy. Infection of stem cells with retroviruses requires that the cells be cycling, and therefore Flt3L may be used to induce cycling of candidate stem populations to facilitate this process.

Flt3L may also be useful for mobilizing bone marrow stem cells to the peripheral blood for transplantation. Preliminary data in both mice and primates indicate that Flt3L is capable of increasing the number of colony forming cells (CFU-GM, CFU-GEMM, and BFU-E) in peripheral blood [36]. As no toxic effects of Flt3L in vivo have been reported to date, the clinical potential of this molecule appears to be bright.

REFERENCES

1. Rosnet O, Schiff C, Pebusque MJ, Marchetto S, Tonnelle C, Toiron Y, Birg F, Birnbaum D (1993) Human FLT3/FLK2 gene: cDNA cloning and expression in hematopoietic cells. Blood 82:1110-1119
2. Rosnet O, Marchetto S, de Lapeyriere O, Birnbaum D (1991) Murine Flt3, a gene encoding a novel tyrosine kinase receptor of the PDGFR/CSF1R family. Oncogene 6:1641-1650
3. Matthews W, Jordan CT, Wiegand GW, Pardoll D, Lemischka IR (1991) A receptor tyrosine kinase specific to hematopoietic stem and progenitor cell-enriched populations. Cell 65:1143-1152
4. Small D, Levenstein M, Kim E, Carow C, Amin S, Rockwell P, Witte L, Burrow C, Ratajczak MZ, Gewirtz AM, Civin CI (1994) STK-1, the human homolog of Flk-2/Flt-3, is selectively expressed in CD34+ human bone marrow cells and is involved in the proliferation of early progenitor/stem cells. Proc Natl Acad Sci U S A 91:459-463
5. Lyman SD, James L, Vanden Bos T, de Vries P, Brasel K, Gliniak B, Hollingsworth LT, Picha KS, McKenna HJ, Splett RR, Fletcher FF, Maraskovsky E, Farrah T, Foxworthe D, Williams DE, Beckmann MP (1993) Molecular cloning of a ligand for the flt3/flk-2 tyrosine kinase receptor: a proliferative factor for primitive hematopoietic cells. Cell 75:1157-1167
6. Lyman SD, James L, Johnson L, Brasel K, de Vries P, Escobar SS, Downey H, Splett RR, Beckmann MP, McKenna HJ (1994) Cloning of the human homologue of the murine flt3 ligand: a growth factor for early hematopoietic progenitor cells. Blood 83:2795-2801
7. Hannum C, Culpepper J, Campbell D, McClanahan T, Zurawski S, Bazan JF, Kastelein R, Hudak S, Wagner J, Mattson J, Luh J, Duda G, Martina N, Peterson D, Menon S, Shanafelt A, Muench M, Kelner G, Namikawa R, Rennick D, Roncarlo M-G, Zlotnick A, Rosnet O, Dubreuil P, Birnbaum D, Lee F (1994) Ligand for FLT3/FLK2 receptor tyrosine kinase regulates growth of haematopoietic stem cells and is encoded by variant RNAs. Nature 368:643-648
8. Lyman SD, Stocking K, Davison B, Fletcher F, Johnson L, Escobar S (1995) Structural analysis of human and murine flt3 ligand genomic loci. Oncogene 11: in press
9. Lyman SD (1995) Biology of flt3 ligand and receptor. Int. J. Hematol.
10. Galli SJ, Zsebo KM, Geissler EN (1994) The kit ligand, stem cell factor. Adv Immunol 55:1-96
11. Roth P, Stanley ER (1992) The biology of CSF-1 and its receptor. Curr Top Microbiol Immunol 181:141-67
12. Ratajczak MZ, Kuczynski WI, Sokol DL, Moore JS, Pletcher Jr. CH, Gewirtz AM (1995) Expression and physiologic significance of *kit* ligand and stem cell tyrosine kinase-1 receptor ligand in normal human CD34$^+$, c-*kit*$^+$ marrow cells. Blood 86:2161-2167
13. Curtis BM, Williams DE, Broxmeyer HE, Dunn J, Farrah T, Jeffery E, Clevenger W, deRoos P, Martin U, Friend D, Craig V, Gayle R, Price V, Cosman D, March CJ, Park LS (1991) Enhanced hematopoietic activity of a human granulocyte/macrophage colony-stimulating factor-interleukin 3 fusion protein. Proc. Natl. Acad. Sci. USA 88:5809-5813
14. Hudak S, Hunte B, Culpepper J, Menon S, Hannum C, Thompson-Snipes L, Rennick D (1995) FLT3/FLK2 ligand promotes the growth of murine stem cells and the expansion of colony-forming cells and spleen colony-forming units. Blood 85:2747-2755
15. Muench MO, Roncarolo MG, Menon S, Xu Y, Kastelein R, Zurawski S, Hannum CH, Culpepper J, Lee F, Namikawa R (1995) FLK-2/FLT-3 ligand regulates the growth of early myeloid progenitors isolated from human fetal liver. Blood 85:963-972
16. McKenna HJ, de Vries P, Brasel K, Lyman SD, Williams DE (1995) The effect of flt3 ligand on the ex vivo expansion of human CD34$^+$ hematopoietic progenitor cells. Blood

86: in press

17. Gabbianelli M, Pelosi E, Montesoro E, Valtieri M, Luchetti L, Samoggia P, Vitelli L, Barberi T, Testa U, Lyman S, Peschle C (1995) Multi-level effects of flt3 ligand on human hematopoiesis: Expansion of putative stem cells and proliferation of granulomonocytic progenitors/monocytic precursors. Blood 86:1661-1670

18. Jacobsen SE, Okkenhaug C, Myklebust J, Veiby OP, Lyman SD (1995) The FLT3 ligand potently and directly stimulates the growth and expansion of primitive murine bone marrow progenitor cells in vitro: synergistic interactions with interleukin (IL) 11, IL-12, and other hematopoietic growth factors. J Exp Med 181:1357-63

19. Hirayama F, Lyman SD, Clark SC, Ogawa M (1995) The flt3 ligand supports proliferation of lymphohematopoietic progenitors and early B-lymphoid progenitors. Blood 85:1762-8

20. Broxmeyer HE, Lu L, Cooper S, Ruggieri L, Li Z-H, Lyman SD (1995) Flt3 ligand stimulates/costimulates the growth of myeloid stem/progenitor cells. Exp. Hematol. 23:1121-1129

21. Zeigler FC, Bennett BD, Jordan CT, Spencer SD, Baumhueter S, Carroll KJ, Hooley J, Bauer K, Matthews W (1994) Cellular and molecular characterization of the role of the flk-2/flt-3 receptor tyrosine kinase in hematopoietic stem cells. Blood 84:2422-2430

22. Lyman SD, Brasel K, Rousseau AM, Williams DE (1994) The flt3 ligand: a hematopoietic stem cell factor whose activities are distinct from steel factor. Stem Cells 12:99-107

23. Lynch DH, Jacobs C, DuPont D, Eisenman J, Foxworthe D, Martin U, Miller RE, Roux E, Liggitt D, Williams DE (1992) Pharmacokinetic parameters of recombinant mast cell growth factor (rMGF). Lymphokine Cytokine Res. 11:233-243

24. deLapeyriere O, Naquet P, Planche J, Marchetto S, Rottapel R, Gambarelli D, Rosnet O, Birnbaum D (1995) Expression of Flt3 tyrosine kinase receptor gene in mouse hematopoietic and nervous tissues. Differentiation 58:351-359

25. Mackarehschian K, Hardin JD, Moore KA, Boast S, Goff SP, Lemischka IR (1995) Targeted disruption of the flk2/flt3 gene leads to deficiencies in primitive hematopoietic progenitors. Immunity 3:147-161

26. Wasserman R, Li Y-S, Hardy RR (1995) Differential expression of the blk and ret tyrosine kinases during B lineage development is dependent on Ig rearrangement. J. Immunol. 155:644-651

27. Orlic D, Fischer R, Nishikawa S, Nienhuis AW, Bodine DM (1993) Purification and characterization of heterogeneous pluripotent hematopoietic stem cell populations expressing high levels of c-kit receptor. Blood 82:762-770

28. Brasel K, Escobar S, Anderberg R, de Vries P, Gruss H-J, Lyman SD (1995) Expression of the flt3 receptor and its ligand on hematopoietic cells. Leukemia 9:1212-1218

29. Bernstein A, Forrester L, Reith AD, Dubreuil P, Rottapel R (1991) The murine W/c-kit and Steel loci and the control of hematopoiesis. Semin Hematol 28:138-142

30. Nocka K, Tan JC, Chiu E, Chu TY, Ray P, Traktman P, Besmer P (1990) Molecular bases of dominant negative and loss of function mutations at the murine c-kit/white spotting locus: W^{37}, W^v, W^{41} and W. Embo J 9:1805-1813

31. Birg F, Courcoul M, Rosnet O, Bardin F, Pebusque MJ, Marchetto S, Tabilio A, Mannoni P, Birnbaum D (1992) Expression of the FMS/KIT-like gene FLT3 in human acute leukemias of the myeloid and lymphoid lineages. Blood 80:2584-2593

32. Da Silva N, Hu ZB, Ma W, Rosnet O, Birnbaum D, Drexler HG (1994) Expression of the FLT3 gene in human leukemia-lymphoma cell lines. Leukemia 8:885-888

33. Birg F, Rosnet O, Carbuccia N, Birnbaum D (1994) The expression of FMS, KIT and FLT3 in hematopoietic malignancies. Leuk Lymphoma 13:223-227

34. Meierhoff G, Dehmel U, Gruss H-J, Rosnet O, Birnbaum D, Quentmeier H, Dirks W, Drexler HG (1995) Expression of flt3 receptor and flt3 ligand in human leukemia-lymphoma cell lines. Leukemia 9:1368-1372

35. Lyman SD, Seaberg M, Hanna R, Zappone J, Brasel K, Abkowitz JL, Prchal JT, Schultz JC, Shahidi NT (1995) Flt3 ligand plasma/serum levels are low in normal individuals and are highly elevated in patients with Fanconi anemia and acquired aplastic anemia. Blood 86: in press
36. Lyman SD (1995) Biological activities of flt3 ligand and its role in hematopoiesis. Exp. Hematol. 23:798 (abstract)

Effects of Recombinant Human Thrombopoietin (rhTPO) on Thrombopoiesis in Bone Marrow-Transplanted Mice.

Koji Kabaya, Kazunori Shibuya, Yoshifumi Torii, Hiromichi Akahori, Yuko Nitta, Masumi Ida, Takashi Kato, and Hiroshi Miyazaki[1]

[1]Pharmaceutical Research Laboratory, Kirin Brewery Co., Ltd., 3 Miyahara-cho, Takasaki, Gunma 370-12, Japan.

SUMMARY

We examined whether recombinant human thrombopoietin (rhTPO) is capable of preventing thrombocytopenia and promoting thrombopoietic reconstitution following bone marrow transplantation (BMT) in mice. Immediately after receiving 10Gy whole-body irradiation, 7-week-old male C3H/HeN mice were inoculated with 10^6 bone marrow cells obtained from syngeneic mice (day 0). In control mice undergoing BMT, platelet counts decreased below 5% of the normal counts with a nadir on day 10, and then returned to the normal level on day 28. Consecutive treatment with rhTPO at daily doses of 3 to 300µg/kg s.c. from day 1 significantly prevented thrombocytopenia on day 10, and promoted the recovery on day 14 in a dose-dependent manner. A plateau was achieved by consecutive subcutaneous injections of 30µg/kg. Variations in white blood cell counts and hemoglobin concentration following BMT were not influenced by the rhTPO-treatment. We, then, investigated the administration schedule of rhTPO in this model. rhTPO-injection starting from day 5 did not prevent thrombocytopenia on days 10 and 12 after BMT, but enhanced the recovery on day 14. Furthermore, administration with rhTPO on alternate days at 55.7µg/kg/day for 7 days or at an interval of two days at 78µg/kg/day for 4 days was less effective than consecutive administration at 30µg/kg/day for 13 days. These findings suggest the usefulness of consecutive treatment with rhTPO from day 1 after BMT.

KEY WORDS: recombinant human thrombopoietin (rhTPO), bone marrow transplantation (BMT), thrombopoiesis, platelet, mice

INTRODUCTION

Bone marrow transplantation (BMT) has been performed on patients with leukemia or aplastic anemia and the cure rate has been increasing in recent years [1-3]. However, thrombocytopenia, anemia, and/or neutropenia before hematopoietic reconstitution are major problems influencing the success of BMT. Recent studies have demonstrated the clinical benefit of recombinant human granulocyte colony-stimulating factor (rhG-CSF) on the granulocytic recovery [4, 6] and recombinant human erythropoietin (rHuEPO) on the anemia [7, 8] following BMT. On the other hand, platelet transfusion has been the only supportive care for thrombocytopenia. However, platelet transfusions were usually accompanied by complications, such as infection and alloimmunization [9, 10].

We recently purified the rat thrombopoietin (TPO), which has been thought to be the major regulator of platelet production for a long time, from the plasma of irradiated rats, and determined the partial amino acid sequence of the rat TPO and isolated the cDNA for rat TPO. Further, we cloned the cDNA for human TPO from human liver cDNA library [11, 12].

In the present study, we examine the effects of recombinant human TPO (rhTPO) on hematopoiesis in normal mice and the efficacy on thrombocytopenia and thrombopoietic reconstitution following BMT in mice.

MATERIALS AND METHODS

Mice. Male Balb/c mice, 8-weeks old (Japan SLC Inc., Shizuoka, Japan), and C3H/HeN mice, 7-weeks old (Charles River Japan, Kanagawa, Japan) were used. They were housed in autoclaved cages and maintained in an air-conditioned, specific pathogen-free animal room regulated at a temperature of 21-23°C and relative humidity of 50-60%. The lighting cycle was 12/12 hours beginning from 8:00 a.m. The mice were given sterilized commercial rodent chow and *water ad libitum*. All experiments were approved by the Institutional Animal Care and Use Committee.

BMT model mice.   Immediately after receiving 10Gy whole body X-ray irradiation (MBR-1520R, Hitachi, Tokyo, Japan, dose rate; 1.8Gy/min at 150kV and 20mA with 0.5mm Al + 0.5mm Cu filters, focus and sample distance [FSD]; 45 cm), mice were inoculated with 10^6 syngeneic bone marrow cells (day 0).

Collection of blood and measurement of peripheral blood cell counts.   Mice were injected with rhTPO at various doses and approximately 250μl of blood was collected daily at 9 a.m. with heparinized capillary tubes (75 mm, Funakoshi Pharmaceuticals Inc., Tokyo, Japan) from the retro-orbital plexus. Platelet counts, hemoglobin concentration and white blood cell (WBC) counts were measured by the use of microcell counter (E-2500, Towa Medical Electronics Inc., Kobe, Japan). The smears of blood cells stained with Brecher's New Methylene Blue (Muto Pure Chemicals. Ltd., Tokyo, Japan) were used for the determination of reticulocyte count.

Measurements of the size and number of megakaryocytes in the femur.   Formalin-fixed paraffin-embedded decalcified femurs were sectioned longitudinally and stained with hematoxylin-eosin. To measure the megakaryocyte size, morphometric analysis was performed with a VIDAS image analyzer composed of a light microscope (Kontron-Zeiss, Germany). The number of megakaryocytes per six randomly chosen 400x fields in the femur section was counted using a light microscope.

Measurements of colony forming-units of megakaryocyte (CFU-Mk).   Culture   was performed according to the method previously described by Miyazaki [13] with minor modifications. Briefly, approximately 2 x10^5 bone marrow cells were cultured in 1 ml of 0.3% Noble agar (Difco, Detroit, Michigan) containing Iscove's modified Dulbecco's medium (IMDM, Sigma) supplemented 10% FCS, 2mM glutamine, 1mM sodium pyruvate, 50μM 2-mercaptoethanol (MERCK, Germany) in the presence of 50ng recombinant mouse interleukin-3 (mIL-3) in a 35ml tissue culture dish (Nunc, Naperville, Illinois). After 7 days of culture, agar disks were detached from the culture disks and placed onto glass slides and stained with acetylcholine esterase (AchE) according to the method described by Jackson [14]. Megakaryocyte colonies comprising four or more cells were counted as CFU-Mk-derived colonies.

RESULTS

Effects of rhTPO on normal mice.

Firstly, the effects of rhTPO on thrombopoiesis in normal Balb/c mice were investigated.

Five consecutive injections with rhTPO into normal mice (day 1 through 5) induced a dose-dependent thrombocytosis with a peak on day 8 (Fig.1).

No change in reticulocyte and white blood cell counts, but a dose-related decrease in hemoglobin concentration were observed with rhTPO (data not shown).

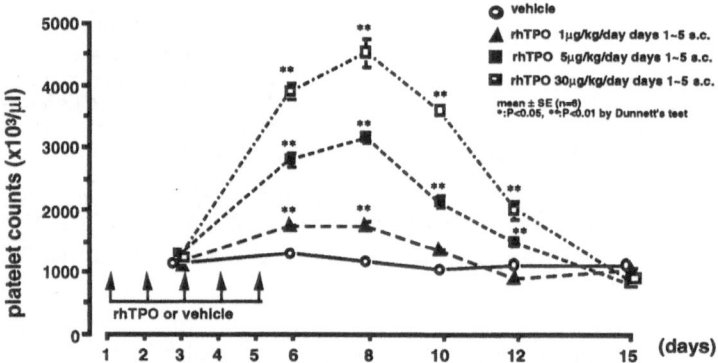

Fig. 1. Effects of rhTPO on platelet counts in normal mice.

Marrow megakaryocyte size significantly enlarged to 1.5-fold by day 3 with rhTPO injections, and gradually decreased thereafter (Fig.2A). Furthermore, the number of megakaryocytes rose to 6-fold with a peak on day 6 (Fig.3B), indicating that rhTPO increased the marrow megakaryocyte size prior to a promotion of proliferation of megakaryocyte precursors. Recent *in vitro* studies have shown TPO stimulated a marked increase in the ploidy of megakaryocytes [15, 16]. Significant increase in marrow megakaryocyte size observed in the present study suggests that rhTPO administration induced the polyploidization *in vivo* as well as *in vitro*.

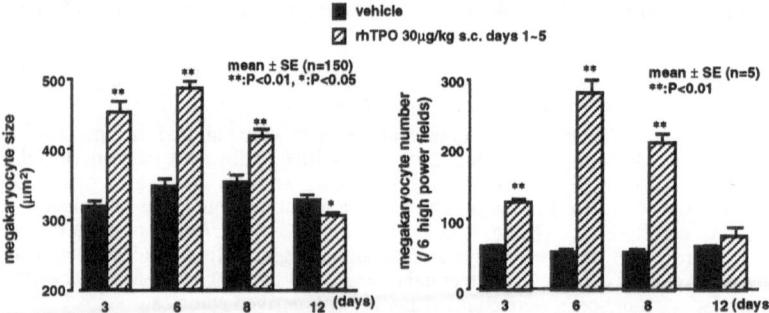

Fig. 2. Effects of rhTPO on megakaryocyte size and number in the femur of normal mice.

Administration of rhTPO also increased the number of CFU-Mk to around 2-fold on day 8 (Fig.3). Since a peak level of megakaryocyte size and number was observed on day 6 in rhTPO-treated mice, rhTPO increases megakaryocyte size and number prior to an increase in early stages of megakaryocytic progenitors.

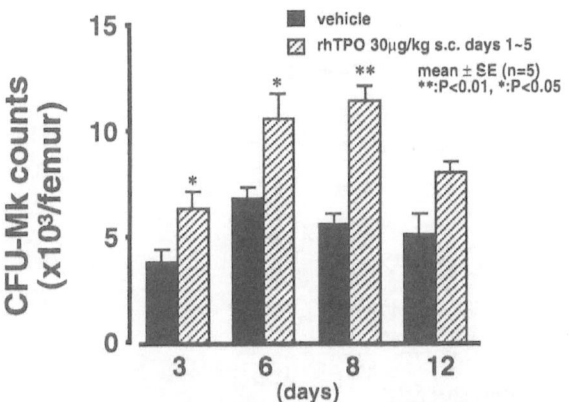

Fig. 3. Effects of rhTPO on CFU-Mk in the femur of normal mice.

Effects of rhTPO on thrombocytopenia after BMT in mice.

Administration of rhTPO at daily doses of 3 to 300µg/kg from the next day after BMT for 13 consecutive days improved the thrombocytopenia on days 10 and 14. A dose dependent effect was noted with the 3 and 30µg/kg dosages but the 100 and 300µg/kg dosages were not more potent than 30µg/kg dosage (Fig. 4). Therefore, the optimum dose of rhTPO in this model may be 30µg/kg.

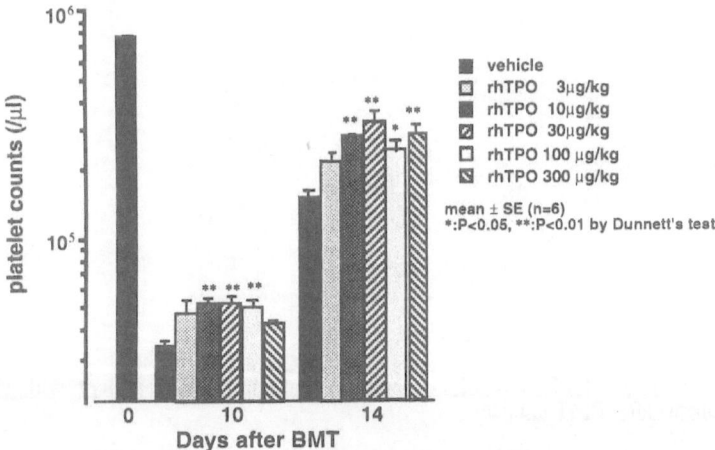

Fig. 4. Effects of rhTPO on platelet counts following BMT in mice.
Next, we investigated the effects of rhTPO-treatment from 5 days after BMT, when platelet counts began to decrease. As shown in Fig. 5, this treatment was less effective than that starting from the next day after BMT.

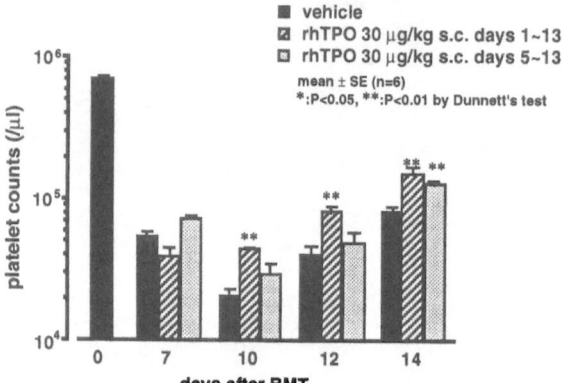

Fig. 5 Less potent effect of rhTPO-treatment starting from 5 days after BMT in mice.

Furthermore, we compared the therapeutic efficacy of rhTPO on thrombocytopenia after BMT on consecutive days, alternate days, or at an interval of three days for 2 weeks. The total injection dosage of rhTPO in the three groups was the same. Treatment schedule and dosages are shown in Fig. 6. rhTPO-treatment of alternate days or at an interval of trhee days showed a significant efficacy but was less effective than consecutive treatment. These results indicate that the optimum treatment schedule of rhTPO is consecutive treatment from the next day after BMT.

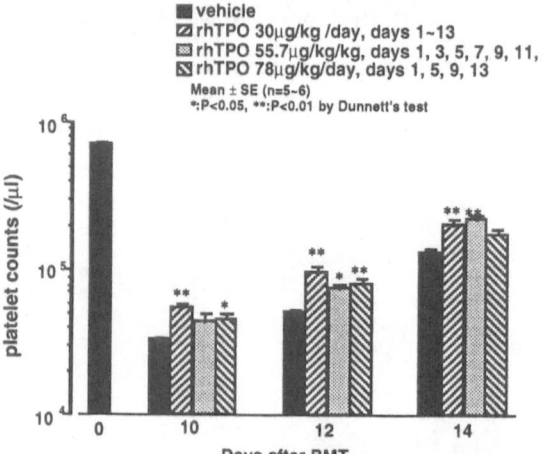

Fig. 6 Comparison of efficacy of consecutive and alternate treatment with rhTPO on thrombocytopenia after BMT in mice.

Concecutive treatment with rhTPO at a daily dose of 30µg/kg induced an increase in CFU-Mk counts in the femur in BMT mice (Fig. 7).

CONCLUSION

1. rhTPO induces a dose-dependent thrombocytosis.

2. rhTPO increases the size and number of marrow megakaryocytes.

99

3. rhTPO significantly reduces the platelet nadir and enhances the platelet recovery following BMT.

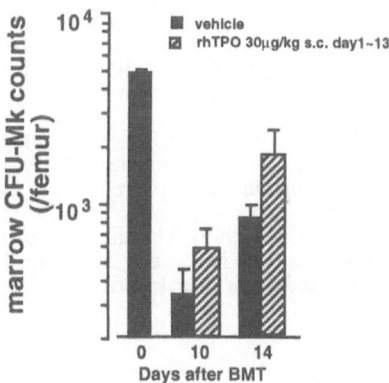

Fig. 7 Effects of rhTPO on marrow CFU-Mk counts following BMT in mice.

REFERENCES

[1] Chaplin, C ,RP Gale (1987) Bone marrow transplantation for acute leukemia: recent advances and comparison with alternative therapies. Semin Hematol 24: 55
[2] Bortin, MM (1983) Bone marrow transplantation registry. Exp Hematol 12: 205
[3] Bortin, MM, RP Gale ,AA Rim (1981) Allogeneic bone marrow transplantation for 144 patients with severe aplastic anemia. J A M A 245: 1132
[4] Masaoka, T, F Takaku, S Kato, Y Moriyama ,Y Kodera (1989) Recombinant human granulocyte colony-stimulating factor in allogeneic bone marrow transplantation. Exp Hematol 17: 1047-1050
[5] Takahashi, S, S Okamoto, N Shirafuji, M Shimane, T Inoue, E Matsushi, K Tajima, T Turuta, K Kozai, T Iwahori, H Ogura, S Irie, K Watari, H Uemura, H Ogura, A Tojo, K Ikebuchi, K Tani, N Sato, K Ozawa ,S Asano (1991) Possible benefit of rhG-CSF combined conditioning regimen for allogeneic/syngeneic BMT in patients with relapsed acute myeloid leukemia (AML) -preliminary report-. Int J Hematol 54: [suppl.1] 308 (Abstr)
[6] Takahashi, S ,H Kodo (1990) Clinical application of recombinant human colony-stimulating factor (rhG-CSF) in bone marrow transplantation. Jpn J Clin Hematol 31: 589-596
[7] Locastelli, F, M Zecca, P Pedrazzoli, L Prete, S Quaglini, P Comoli, P De Stefano, Y Beguin, G Robustelli della Cuna, F Severi ,M Cazzola (1994) Use of recombinant human erythropoietin after bone marrow transplantation in pediatric patients with acute leukemia: effect on erythroid repopulation in autologous versus allogeneic transplants. Bone Marrow Transplant 13: 403-410
[8] Klaesson, S, O Ringden, P Ljungman, B Lonnqvist ,L Wennberg (1994) Reduced blood transfusions requirements after allogeneic bone marrow transplantation: results of randomised, double-blind study with high-dose erythropoietin. Bone Marrow Transplant 13: 397-402
[9] Godeau, B, P Fromont, T Seror, N Duedari ,P Bierling (1992) Platelet alloimmunization after multiple transfusions: a prospective study of 50 patients. Br J Hematol 81: 395-400
[10] Schiffer, CA (1989) Prevention of alloimmunization in platelet transfusion recipients. In: T. J. Kunichi and J. N. George, ed. Platelet immunobiology:molecular and clinical aspects., Philadelphia, Lippincott, pp 454-470
[11] Souma, Y, H Akahori, N Seki, T Hori, K Ogami, T Kato, Y Shimada, K Kawamura ,H Miyazaki (1994) Molecular cloning and chromosomal localization of the human thrombopoietin gene. FEBS Lett 353: 57-61

[12] Kato, T, K Ogami, Y Shimada, A Iwamatsu, Y Sohma, H Akahori, K Horie, A Kokubo, Y Kudo, E Maeda, K Kobayaashi, H Ohashi, T Ozawa, H Inoue, K Kawamura ,H Miyazaki (1995) Purification and characterization of thrombopoietin. J Biochem 118: 229-236

[13] Miyazaki, H, H Inoue, M Yanagida, K Horie, T Mikayama, H Ohashi, M Nishikawa, T Suzuki ,T Sudo (1992) Purification of rat megakaryocyte colony-forming cells using a monoclonal antibody aganst rat platelet glycoprotein IIb/IIIa. Exp Hematol 20: 855-861

[14] Jackson, CW (1973) Cholinesterase as a possible marker for early cells of the megakaryocytic series. Blood 42: 413-421

[15] Kaushansky, K, S Lok, RD Holly, VC Broudy, N Lin, MC Bailey, JW Forstron, MM Buddle, PJ Oort, FS Hagen, GJ Roth, T Papayannopoulou ,DC Foster (1994) Promotion of megakaryocyte progenitor expansion and differentiation by the c-Mpl ligand thrombopoietin. Nature 369: 568-571

[16] Broudy, VC, ML Lin, K Kaushansky (1995) Thrombopoietin (c-mpl ligand) acts synergistically with erythropoietin, stem cell factor, and interleukin-11 to enhance murine megakaryocyte colony growth and increases megakaryocyte ploidy in vitro. Blood 85: 1719-1726

Physiological and pathological role of gp130, a common signal transducer for IL-6-family of cytokines

Tetsuya Taga[1], Kanji Yoshida[1], Hisao Hirota[1,2], and Tadamitsu Kishimoto[2]

[1]Institute for Molecular and Cellular Biology, Osaka University, 1-3 Yamada-oka, Suita, Osaka 565, Japan
[2]Department of Medicine III, Osaka University Medical School, 2-2 Yamada-oka, Suita, Osaka 565, Japan

SUMMARY

Receptor complexes for interleukin-6 (IL-6), IL-11, leukemia inhibitory factor (LIF), oncostatin M (OM), ciliary neurotrophic factor (CNTF) and cardiotrophin-1 (CT-1) utilize membrane glycoprotein gp130 as a common signal-transducing component. In order to investigate detailed physiological roles of gp130 and to determine pathological consequences of complete lack or abnormal activation of gp130, mice deficient for gp130 protein or expressing continuously activated gp130 protein have been made. A gp130 null mutation is lethal, and embryos deficient for gp130 protein progressively die between 12.5 days post coitum (dpc) and term. They show, at 16.5 dpc, hypoplastic development of the ventricular myocardium. They have greatly reduced numbers of pluripotential and committed hematopoietic progenitors in the liver, as measured on 13.5 dpc. gp130-/- placentas on and after 14.5 dpc are smaller than controls and exhibit impaired maternofetal transport. Continuous activation of gp130 *in vivo* by overexpressing both IL-6 and IL-6R leads to hypertrophy of ventricular myocardium and thickened ventricular walls of the heart in adulthood. These results indicate crucial roles of gp130 in cardiomyocyte regulation, hematopoiesis, and placental development.

KEY WORDS: cytokine, signal transduction, gp130, interleukin-6

INTRODUCTION

Cytokine signals are mediated through specific receptor complexes expressed on target cells. Most of the cytokine receptor components, in particular those involved in hematopoietic cell regulation, belong to a large group of proteins called the cytokine receptor family [1]. Receptor complexes from this family are usually composed of a ligand-specific receptor chain and a signal transducer common to multiple cytokines [2, 3]. gp130 is a ubiquitously expressed signal-transducing receptor component shared by several cytokines including interleukin-6 (IL-6), IL-11, leukemia inhibitory factor (LIF), oncostatin M (OM), ciliary neurotrophic factor (CNTF) and cardiotrophin-1 (CT-1) [4-9]. This membrane glycoprotein was initially identified as a signaling component which associates with the IL-6 receptor (IL-6R) when the receptor binds with IL-6 [10, 11]. The discovery of this shared signal transducer, gp130, helps to explain how these different cytokines can mediate overlapping biological functions [12]. The first step in the process of signaling by the receptor complexes sharing gp130 is the ligand-induced dimerization of receptor components: IL-6-binding to IL-6R induces homodimerization of gp130 [13], whereas stimulation by LIF, OM, CNTF, and CT-1 leads to heterodimerization of gp130 with a closely related protein, LIFR [6, 9, 14]. OM is suggested to signal also through a different type of heterodimer composed of OM-specific receptor and gp130 [15]. From the close structural similarity of IL-6R and IL-11R, the gp130 homodimer could be a candidate complex for IL-11 signaling [16]. Ligand-induced homo- or heterodimerization of gp130 triggers the activation of associated cytoplasmic tyrosine kinases, JAK1, JAK2 and TYK2, which are in the JAK family [17-19]. This leads to tyrosine-phosphorylation of a latent cytoplasmic transcription factor, APRF/STAT3 (for acute phase response factor or signal transducer and activator of transcription 3) [20-22]. Phosphorylation of a serine residue in STAT3 (presumably by MAPK) has recently been shown to be important for the full activation of STAT3 [23-25]. The Ras/MAPK cascade is known to be activated following gp130-stimulation [26-28]. One of the targets of MAPK is NF-IL6, which was demonstrated to be activated upon threonine phosphorylation by MAPK [29]. A precise mechanism which links the gp130-dimerization and MAPK activation remains to be elucidated.

gp130 is expressed in almost all organs examined, including heart, spleen, kidney, lung, liver, placenta and brain [11, 30]. In contrast, expression of the ligand-binding receptor chains for the IL-6-family of cytokines shows somewhat restricted distribution and does not necessarily parallel that of gp130. Since the biological functions of gp130 have been studied in most cases *in vitro*, physiological functions of gp130 are not considered to have been fully elucidated. In addition, despite its pleiotropic functions demonstrated by *in vitro* studies, no disease for which an abnormality in gp130-signaling is responsible has yet been reported. To examine the physiological roles of gp130 and to understand the pathological consequences resulting from the lack of this common signal transducer or its continuous activation, we have created two types of model mice, one deficient for gp130 and the other having constitutively activated gp130.

MICE DEFICIENT FOR GP130

Null mutation of the gp130 gene is lethal

Targeted disruption of the gp130 gene was carried out in embryonic stem (ES) cells (from the 129 strain) as described elsewhere [31]. The targeted ES clones were injected into C57BL/6 blastocysts and the resultant chimeric mice were crossed with normal C57BL/6 mice. Three lines of mice from independent ES cell clones were found to transmit the mutation through the germ line (Yoshida et al., in press). Heterozygous mutant (gp130+/-) mice did not show any apparent phenotype. In order to obtain mice homozygous for the gp130 gene mutation (gp130-/-), heterozygotes were intercrossed. Out of 203 offspring from the heterozygous matings, no gp130-/- mice were observed when genotyped at 4-6 weeks of age. Among these offspring, gp130+/- mice appeared at a frequency of 64%, which is close to the theoretical value, 67%, based on Mendelian laws, indicating the lethal phenotype of the null mutation.

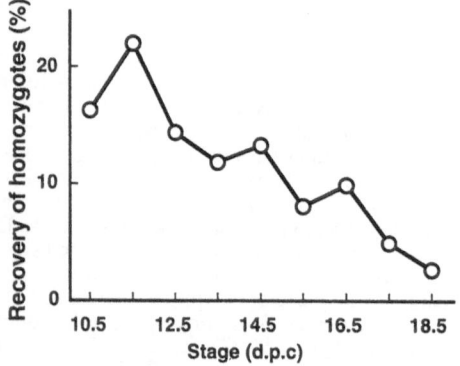

Fig. 1 <u>Recovery of embryos homozygous for the gp130 mutation, from the heterozygous matings.</u>
Genotypes of embryos obtained from intercrossings of gp130+/- mice were determined at the indicated stages (in dpc) by Southern blotting. The number of live gp130-null mutant fetuses was divided by the total number of live fetuses. n (total live fetuses) = 106, 209, 254, 211, 112, 192, 140 and 112 on each day from 11.5 and 18.5 dpc.

To determine the time of death, embryos in utero at 11.5-18.5 days postcoitum (dpc) and newborn pups derived from the heterozygous intercrosses were analyzed for their gp130 genotypes. As summarized in Fig. 1, gp130-/- embryos on 11.5 dpc were found at a frequency of nearly 25%, which follows the Mendelian distribution. Thereafter recovery of live homozygous mutant embryos decreased. At 18.5 dpc, live homozygous mutant embryos were observed at a frequency of only 2.7% of the total live embryos, and eventually in the newborns, no live null-mutants were found. Among the live gp130-/- embryos in particular after 13.5 dpc, approximately half were smaller in size (mostly by about 10%; in a few severe cases by up to 20%) than their wild type and heterozygous littermates. gp130-/- embryos displayed no obvious malformation in surface appearance at any stage examined.

Hypoplastic development of ventricular myocardium in the gp130-/- heart

Histological analysis revealed an extreme hypoplastic development of the myocardium in gp130-/- embryos, apparent at 16.5 dpc and later. As shown in Fig. 2, the ventricular walls of the gp130-/- heart at 16.5 dpc were abnormally thin, showing a minimum thickness of one cell layer. This type of extreme abnormality in the myocardium was observed in all the 16.5 dpc (n=5) and 17.5 dpc (n=1) gp130-/- embryos examined histologically. Although a compact layer of the ventricle was extremely thin, trabeculation inside the ventricle chamber occurred normally in the homozygous mutant hearts. In all the above-mentioned six gp130-/- cases at 16.5 dpc and 17.5 dpc, no ventricular septal defect was detected by examination of serial sections encompassing the entire ventricle. On the contrary, the ventricular thickness of the gp130 null embryos on 14.5 dpc appeared normal relative to the control littermates at 14.5 dpc.

control   gp130-/-

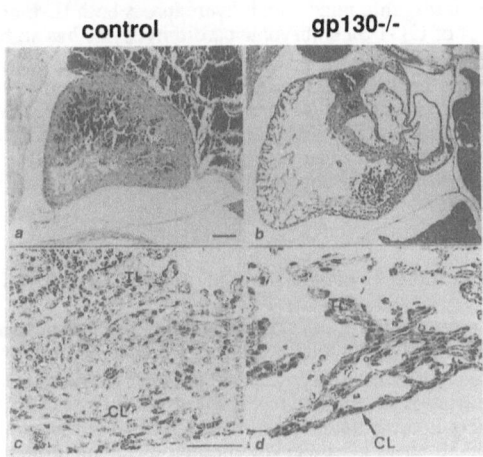

Fig. 2 <u>Histological analysis of the control and gp130 null mutant embryonic hearts.</u> Sagittal sections from control and gp130-/- littermates at 16.5 dpc were stained by hematoxylin and eosin. CL, compact layer; TL, trabecular. Bars, 200 μm (for a and b) and 50 μm (for c and d).

It should be noted that at 17.5 dpc, when the extreme thinning of the compact layer in the gp130-/- heart was observed, the presence and shape of subcellular structures such as nuclei, mitochondria, myofibrils, sarcomeric Z bands, and intercalated discs in the cardiomyocytes of the gp130-/- compact layer were indistinguishable from those of the control. In normal mouse embryos, it has been reported that the compact layer cells of the 14.5 dpc heart are less differentiated and possessed poorly organized myofibrils [32]. They become more differentiated, having well-organized myofibrils with clear Z bands at 16.5 dpc and later. In contrast, trabecular cells are already well differentiated at 14.5 dpc, as reported previously. We considered that if precocious differentiation of the compact layer cells occurred in the gp130-/- heart, this could possibly lead to abolishment of the maintenance of normal compact layer cells. We thus examined the ultrastructures of the gp130-/- heart at 14.5 dpc. The presence and shape of subcellular structures in the cells of the 14.5 dpc gp130-/- compact layer and trabeculae showed no difference from those in the wild type controls. The scarce appearance of organized myofibrils in the compact layer cells (in both control and gp130-deficient hearts) is consistent with a previous report showing that cells at this stage are normally less differentiated than trabecular cells. Trabecular cells of both genotypes showed well-organized myofibrils as expected. Our data thus indicate that the differentiation status of the myocardium in terms of ultrastructural organization was not altered in the gp130-/- heart.

We then examined whether the hypoplastic development of myocardium in the gp130-/- heart was due to the lack of proliferative signals transmitted from gp130 in cardiomyocytes. Since a combination of IL-6 and an extracellular soluble form of IL-6 receptor (sIL-6R) is known to interact with gp130 and induce its homodimerization to trigger cytoplasmic signaling [10, 33], this combination was added to the cultured cardiomyocytes derived from 16.5 dpc normal ICR embryos. Stimulation of gp130 by the IL-6/sIL-6R complex led to an approximately 2.5-fold increase in DNA synthesis in comparison with the medium control. Either IL-6 or sIL-6R alone showed no effect.

The number of cardiomyocytes in the thin-walled compact layer of the gp130$^{-/-}$ ventricle appeared to be very much reduced at 16.5 dpc or later. These cells, however, possessed normal ultrastructural components and expressed ventricle-specific markers comparable to the wild type cardiomyocytes. Taken together with the result that stimulation of gp130 by the IL-6/sIL-6R complex induced proliferation of 16.5 dpc cardiomyocytes, this suggests that, while gp130 signaling plays a role in the growth of cardiomyocytes, it does not influence their differentiation, at least at around 16.5 dpc. Our findings suggest the possible existence of a new member of the IL-6-family which regulates heart muscle cell growth. Myocardial proliferation caused by IL-6/sIL-6R-complex stimulation may be mimicking the function of such a cytokine. A novel cytokine called cardiotrophin-1 (CT-1) has recently been cloned; it acts on neonatal cardiomyocytes to cause hypertrophy, and its structure is closely related to, for example, LIF and CNTF [34]. CT-1 is suggested to act through the LIFR/gp130 heterodimer, since CT-1 and LIF cross-compete for binding to their target cells and CT-1-binding to these cells can be inhibited by anti-gp130 antibody [9]. A role of gp130 in inducing myocardial hypertrophy has also been shown by transgenic mice which overexpress both IL-6 and IL-6R [35] as will be described below. The effect of CT-1 on embryonic cardiomyocytes has so far not been examined. Because the size of each cardiomyocyte in the gp130$^{-/-}$ embryonic heart appeared to be comparable to that observed in the wild type heart, the function of CT-1, assuming it to be mediated during embryogenesis by gp130, might be to maintain (or increase) the cell number rather than to cause hypertrophy. If the lack of CT-1 signaling is responsible for the extreme thinning of the compact layer of the gp130 deficiency, LIFR may not be the exclusive dimerizing partner of gp130 in the functional receptor for CT-1. This is because the severe phenotype in the cardiac development in gp130 deficient mice was not observed in LIFR deficient mice [31, 36].

Extreme reduction in the number of hematopoietic progenitors in gp130$^{-/-}$ embryos

The total number of mononuclear cells in the 13.5 dpc fetal liver was dramatically reduced in the null mutant embryos. The colony forming unit in spleen (CFU-S; a total count per liver), as measured by injecting the fetal liver mononuclear cells into lethally irradiated mice (2 x 10^5 cells per recipient), was also greatly reduced in the homozygous mutant embryos as compared with wild type littermates (Fig. 3a). CFU-S counts in the heterozygous livers were intermediate between those in the wild type and homozygous livers. The result indicated that gp130 plays a critical role in the development of the pluripotent stem cell pool in the fetal liver.

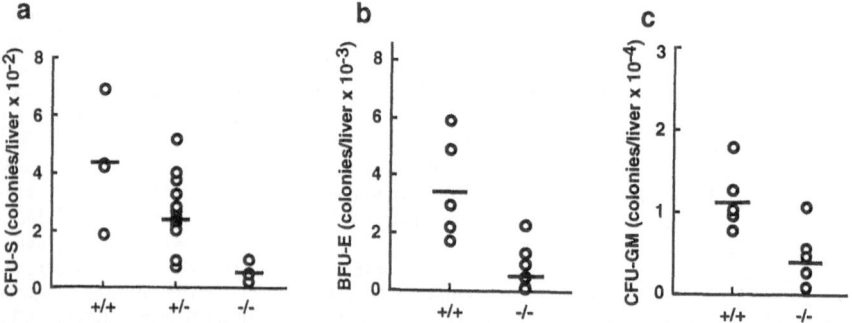

Fig. 3 <u>Reduction of hematopoietic progenitors in 13.5 dpc gp130-deficient fetal livers.</u>
(a) The number of spleen colonies (CFU-S). Colonies formed in the recipient spleen 11 days after inoculation of 2x10^5 mononuclear cells from gp130$^{+/+}$ (n=4), gp130$^{+/-}$ (n=18) and gp130$^{-/-}$ (n=4) fetal livers were counted. (b) The number of erythroid progenitors (BFU-E). gp130$^{+/+}$ (n=5) and gp130$^{-/-}$ (n=6) fetal liver mononuclear cells were subjected to semi-solid in vitro colony assay. (c) The number of granulocyte-macrophage progenitors (CFU-GM). gp130$^{+/+}$ (n=6) and gp130$^{-/-}$ (n=5) fetal liver mononuclear cells were analyzed as in (b). In all these assays, each dot represents the value derived from an individual fetal liver, and horizontal bars represent the mean of each group.

We then examined whether erythroid progenitors (burst-forming unit for erythroid, BFU-E) and granulocyte-macrophage progenitors (CFU-GM) detectable in semi-solid *in vitro* assays were affected by the lack of gp130. As shown in Fig. 3 (b, c), although both types of committed progenitors were present in the gp130 deficient fetal livers, their numbers were very much reduced.

About 20% of gp130$^{-/-}$ embryos at 15.5 through 18.5 dpc exhibited anemic paleness. In these anemic mutant embryos, there were no signs of hemorrhage. Liver sections from a 16.5 dpc wild type embryo and an obviously anemic littermate (gp130$^{-/-}$) were stained with hematoxylin and eosin, and peripherally existing red blood cells found in the blood vessels were inspected microscopically. A larger number of nucleated erythrocytes (and thus a smaller number of enucleated erythrocytes) were found in the blood vessels of the gp130$^{-/-}$ embryo than in the wild type littermate. These results suggested that gp130 deficiency led to impaired proliferation and maturation of erythroid lineage cells.

It may be worth noting that gp130$^{+/-}$ embryos showed intermediate phenotypes in terms of the numbers of total mononuclear cells and CFU-S in the liver. This suggests that the generation of the hematopoietic progenitor pool responds to the dose of gp130 signaling provided. This is not the case in cardiomyocyte development, since gp130$^{+/-}$ embryos did not exhibit any of the defects in the ventricular myocardium observed in gp130$^{-/-}$ embryos. There was variation in the numbers of fetal liver mononuclear cells and CFU-S among differentiated fetuses of the same genotype (see Fig. 3). In addition, among the gp130$^{-/-}$ embryos, the severity of anemic paleness varied considerably (only 20% showed significant anemia). One explanation for these fluctuations might be that the genetic background of the embryos was not uniform, but rather a mixture of 129 and C57BL/6. To clarify this point, we are in the process of generating congenic gp130 mutant mice by repetitive crossing to an inbred strain.

Abnormality in the gp130$^{-/-}$ placenta

The external appearance and histologically examined structures of gp130$^{-/-}$ placentas on and before 12.5 dpc looked normal with regard to the number and shape of trophoblast giant cells, spongiotrophoblasts and labyrinthine trophoblasts. However, at 14.5 dpc, obviously smaller-sized placentas were found (approximately 25% reduction in size). The average thickness of the placentas of gp130$^{-/-}$ embryos measured in the sagittal section under the microscope, was 76.2 ± 8.7% of that of the wild type littermate at 14.5 dpc. Histological examination revealed that this reduction was largely due to a thinner spongiotrophoblast layer and labyrinthine zone in the gp130$^{-/-}$ placentas. Hematoxylin-eosin-stained histological specimens did not reveal any dramatic changes in the cell populations composing these thinned compartments. At 17.5 dpc, however, dilatation and congestion of maternal blood vessels were obvious, and the formation of thrombus of maternal blood was observed in approximately one fifth of the total number of examined placentas from the gp130$^{-/-}$ embryos. In order to investigate potential functional changes in the gp130$^{-/-}$ placenta, the maternofetal transport rate was examined at 13.0 - 13.5 dpc by administrating radio-labeled immunoglobulin into the pregnant mother. As shown in Fig. 4, the transfer of the labeled immunoglobulin to the gp130$^{-/-}$ fetus was significantly lower than that to the wild type fetus. These results suggest an important role of gp130 in the development of the placenta at stages later than 12.5 dpc.

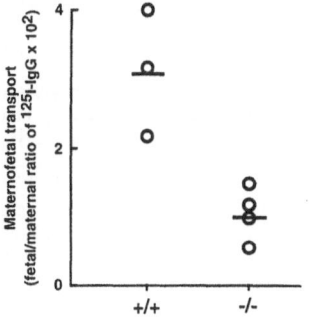

Fig. 4 <u>Functional changes in 13.0 - 13.5 dpc gp130-deficient placentas.</u>
Maternofetal transport of radio-labeled IgG was measured. ^{125}I-IgG was intravenously injected into a pregnant mother from a heterozygous intercrossing (at 13.0 dpc). Radioactivities of ^{125}I-IgG transferred to the fetuses were measured 12 hr later (at 13.5 dpc). Each dot represents the ratio of TCA precipitable ^{125}I-IgG detected in each fetus to that in maternal serum. The value was normalized by the body weight of each fetus.

From studies with LIF-deficient mice, LIF has been shown to be critical for blastocyst implantation [37, 38]: Adult female mice deficient for LIF are infertile as a result of a failure of the embryo to implant. This phenotype arises as a consequence of the lack of LIF production in the maternal host, rather than in the embryo, since LIF$^{-/-}$ embryos develop normally in a wild-type host mother but LIF$^{+/+}$ embryos do not in a LIF$^{-/-}$ mother. Whether LIF acts on the blastocysts or on the endometrium of the uterus in a paracrine manner was not clarified in that LIF knockout study. Since embryos deficient for gp130, the critical component of functional LIF receptor, survived and developed through the implantation stage, LIF is believed to promote implantation via a paracrine effect on the endometrium and not on the blastocyst. After placentation, placental abnormality in gp130$^{-/-}$ fetuses became apparent after 12.5 cpc. The placenta expresses a relatively high level of gp130, and several reports have demonstrated that stimulation of gp130 in placental trophoblasts regulates the expression and/or secretion of placental hormones such as human chorionic gonadtropin [39] and mouse placental lactogen-II [40]. It would be of interest to examine whether production and secretion of these hormones are affected by the lack of gp130. At this moment, it is not clear how the gp130 deficiency caused the thinning of the spongiotrophoblast layer and labyrinthine zone, and led to impairment of maternofetal transport.

MYOCARDIAL HYPERTROPHY IN MICE HAVING CONTINUOUSLY ACTIVATED GP130

Continuous activation of gp130 *in vivo* has been carried out by mating mice from IL-6 and IL-6R transgenic lines, since the IL-6/IL-6R complex is known to induce homodimerization of gp130 and consequent activation of gp130-associated tyrosine kinases. Offspring overexpressing both IL-6 and IL-6R show constitutive tyrosine phosphorylation of gp130 and a downstream signaling molecule, STAT3 [35]. The most notable finding in such mice having constitutively active gp130 is hypertrophy of ventricular myocardium and thickened ventricular walls of the heart in adulthood. The ventricular walls in the IL-6+/IL-6R+ transgenic mice at 5 months old were thicker than those in control mice by approximately 44%. As shown in Figure 5, each cardiomyocyte in the IL-6+/IL-6R+ transgenic heart was thicker than that of the control (on an average, by approximately 48%).

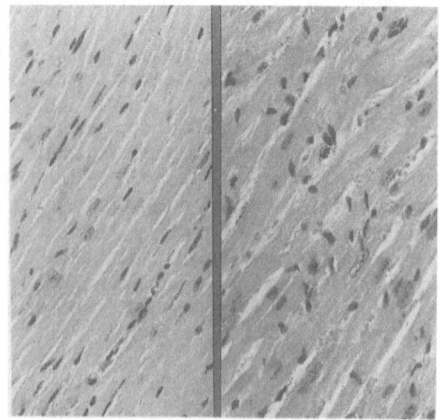

Fig. 5 <u>Myocardial hypertrophy transgenic mice constitutively expressing both IL-6 and IL-6R</u>
Heart sections from nontransgenic (left) and IL-6+/IL-6R+ transgenic (right) mice were shown. Note the thickened cardiomyocytes in the latter.

Transgenic mice overexpressing either IL-6 or IL-6R alone did not show detectable myocardial abnormalities. Neonatal cardiac muscle cells, when cultured *in vitro*, become enlarged in response to a combination of IL-6 and soluble IL-6, a complex which is known to associate with, and activate, gp130.

Since the renin-angiotensin system is considered to be one of the most important regulatory systems in the development of cardiac hypertrophy, we have examined whether this system is involved in myocardial hypertrophy in double-transgenic mice. There were no significant differences in the serum levels of renin, angiotensin II, and cathecholamines among our trangenic mice of the four genotypes.

In the double-transgenic mice, no medial thickness of coronary arteries and arterioles was found, which was in contrast to the transgenic rats expressing renin. Based on these data, the involvement of the renin-angiotensin system in the myocardial hypertrophy occurring in the IL-6+/IL-6R+ transgenic mice may be negligible.

Taken together with the *in vitro* hypertorphic effect of the IL-6/sIL-6R complex [35], our findings with the IL-6+/IL-6R+ transgenic mice strongly suggest that the gp130-mediated signals have a physiological role in cardiomyocyte regulation and, when overstimulated, lead to cardiac hypertorphy as a pathological consequence.

CONCLUSIVE REMARKS

The gp130 deficiency was lethal and affected ventricular myocardial development, hematopoiesis and placental development. Since gp130 is expressed in many organs, it is possible that even the apparently normally developed organs in the gp130-/- fetuses would exhibit abnormalities if the fetuses were to continue to develop. Tissue-specific targeting of the gp130 gene, for instance in the neuronal system, would clarify the role of gp130 in various organs in more detail.

REFERENCES

1. Bazan JF(1990) Structural design and molecular evolution of a cytokine receptor superfamily. Proc Natl Acad Sci USA 87:6934-6938
2. Taga T, and Kishimoto T (1992) Cytokine receptors and signal transduction. FASEB J 6:3387-3396
3. Kishimoto T, Taga T, and Akira S (1994) Cytokine signal transduction. Cell 76:253-262
4. Taga T, Narazaki M, Yasukawa K, Saito T, Miki D, Hamaguchi M, Davis S, Shoyab M, Yancopoulos GD, and Kishimoto T (1992) Functional inhibition of hematopoietic and neurotrophic cytokines by blocking the interleukin 6 signal transducer gp130. Proc Natl Acad Sci USA 89:10998-11001
5. Ip NY, Nye SH, Boulton TG, Davis S, Taga T, Li Y, Birren J, Yasukawa K, Kishimoto T, Anderson DJ, Stahl N, and Yancopoulos GD (1992) CNTF and LIF act on neuronal cells via shared signaling pathways that involve the IL-6 signal transducing receptor component gp130. Cell 69:1121-1132
6. Gearing DP, Comeau MR, Friend DJ, Gimpel SD, Thut CJ, McGourty J, Brasher KK, King JA, Gillis S, Mosley B, Ziegler SF, and Cosman D (1992) The IL-6 signal transducer, gp130: an oncostatin M receptor and affinity converter for the LIF receptor. Science 255:1434-1437
7. Liu J, Modrell B, Aruffo A, Marken JS, Taga T, Yasukawa K, Murakami M, Kishimoto T, and Shoyab M (1992) Interleukin-6 signal transducer gp130 mediates oncostatin M signaling. J BiolChem 267:16763-16766
8. Yin T, Taga T, Tsang ML-S, Yasukawa K, Kishimoto T, Yang Y-C (1993) Involvement of interleukin-6 signal transducer gp130 in interleukin-11-mediated signal transduction. J Immunol 151:2555-2561
9. Pennica D, Shaw KJ, Swanson TA, Moore MW, Sheliton DL, Zioncheck KA, Rosenthal A, Taga T, Paoni NF, and Wood WI (1995) Cardiotropin-1: Biological activities and binding to the leukemia inhibitory factor receptor/gp130 signaling complex. J BiolChem 270:10915-10922
10. Taga T, Hibi M, Hirata Y, Yamasaki K, Yasukawa K, Matsuda T, Hirano T, and Kishimoto T (1989) Interleukin-6 triggers the association of its receptor with a possible signal transducer, gp130. Cell 58: 573-581
11. Hibi M, Murakami M, Saito M, Hirano T, Taga T, and Kishimoto T (1990) Molecular cloning and expression of an IL-6 signal transducer, gp130. Cell 63:1149-1157
12. Kishimoto T, Akira S, and Taga T (1992) Interleukin-6 and its receptor: A paradigm for cytokines. Science 258:593-597
13. Murakami M, Hibi M, Nakagawa N, Nakagawa T, Yasukawa K, Yamanishi K, Taga T, and Kishimoto T (1993) IL-6-induced homodimerization of gp130 and associated activation of a tyrosine kinase. Science 260:1808-1810
14. Davis S, Aldrich TH, Stahl N, Pan L, Taga T, Kishimoto T, Ip NY, and Yancopoulos GD (1993) LIFRß and gp130 as heterodimerizing signal transducers of the tripartite CNTF receptor. Science 260:1805-1808

15. Murakami-Mori K, Taga T, Kishimoto T, and Nakamura S (1995) AIDS-associated Kaposi's sarcoma (KS) cells express oncostatin M (OM)-specific receptor but not leukemia inhibitory facotr/OM receptor or interleukin-6 receptor. J Clin Invest 96:1319-1327
16. Hilton DJ, Hilton AA, Raicevic A, Rakar S, Harrison-Smith M, Gough NM, Begley CG, Metcalf D, Nicola NA, and Willson TA (1994) Cloning of a murine IL-11 receptor α chain; requirement for gp130 high affinity binding and signal transduction. EMBO J 13:4765-4775
17. Narazaki M, Witthuhn BA, Yoshida K, Silvennoinen O, Yasukawa K, Ihle JN, Kishimoto T, and Taga T (1994) Activation of JAK2 kinase mediated by the interleukin 6 signal transducer gp130. Proc Natl Acad Sci USA 91:2285-2289
18. Stahl N, Boulton TG, Farruggella T, Ip NY, Davis S, Witthuhn BA, Quelle FW, Silvennoinen O, Barbieri G, Pellegrini S, Ihle JN, Yancopoulos GD (1994) Association and activation of Jak-Tyk kinases by CNTF-LIF-OSM-IL-6 b receptor components. Science 263:92-95
19. Stahl N, Farruggella J, Boulton T, G Zhong, Z Darnel, JE Yancopoulos, GD (1995) Choice of STATs and other substrates specified by modular tyrosine-based motifs in cytokine receptors. Science 267:1349-1353
20. Akira S, Nishio Y, Inoue M, Wang X-J, Wei S, Matsusaka T, Yoshida K, Sudo T, Naruto M, and Kishimoto T (1994) Molecular cloning of APRF, a novel IFN-stimulated gene factor 3 p91-related transcription factor involved in the gp130-mediated signaling pathway. Cell 77:63-71
21. Lütticken C, Wegenka UM, Yuan J, Buschmann J, Schindler C, Ziemiecki A, Harpur AG, Wilks AF, Yasukawa K, Taga T, Kishimoto T, Barbieri G, Pellegrini S, Sendtner M, Heinrich PC, Horn F (1994) Association of transcription factor APRF and protein kinase Jak1 with the interleukin-6 signal transducer gp130. Science 263:89-92
22. Wegenka UM, Lütticken C, Buschmann J, Yuan J, Lottspeich F, Müller-Esterl W, Schindler C, Roeb E, Heinrich PC, Horn F (1994) The interleukin-6-activated acute-phase response factor is antigenically and functionally related to members of the signal transducer and activator of transcription (STAT) family. Mol Cell Biol 14: 3186-3196
23. Zhang X, Blenis J, Li H-C, Schindler C, Chen-Kiang S (1995) Requirement of serine phosphorylation for formation of STAT-promoter complexes. Science 267:1990-1994
24. Boulton TG, Zhong Z, Wen Z, Darnell JEJr, Stahl N, and Yancopoulos GD (1995) STAT3 activation by cytokines utilizing gp130 and related transducers involves a secondary modification requiring an H7-sensitive kinase. Proc Natl Acad Sci USA 92: 6915-6919
25. Wen Z, Zhong Z, and Darnell JEJr (1995) Maximal activation of transcription by Stat1 and Stat3 requires both tyrosine and serine phosphorylation. Cell 82:241-250
26. Satoh T, Nakafuku M, and Kajiro Y (1992) Function of Ras as a molecular switch in signal transduction. J Biol Chem 267:24149-24153
27. Boulton TG, Stahl N, and Yancopoulos GD (1994) Ciliary neurotrophic factor/ leukemia inhibitory factor/ interleukin 6/ oncostatin M family of cytokines induces tyrosine phosphorylation of a common set of proteins overlapping those induced by other cytokines and growth factors. J Biol Chem 269:11648-11655
28. Daeipour M, Kumar G, and Amaral MC (1993) Recombinant IL-6 activates p42 and p44 mitogen-activated protein kinases in the IL-6 responsive B cell line, AF-10. J Immunol 150:4743-4753
29. Nakajima T, Kinoshita S, Sasagawa T, Sasaki K, Naruto M, Kishimoto T, and Akira S (1993) Phosphorylation at threonine-235 by a ras-dependent mitogen-activated protein kinase cascade is essential for transcription factor NF-IL-6. Proc Natl Acad Sci USA 90: 2207-2211
30. Saito M, Yoshida K, Hibi M, Taga T, and Kishimoto T (1992) Molecular cloning of a murine IL-6 receptor-associated signal transducer, gp130, and its regulated expression in vivo. J Immunol 148:4066-4071
31. Yoshida K, Taga T, Saito M, Suematsu S, Kumanogoh A, Tanaka T, Fujiwara H, Hirata M, Yamagami T, Nakahata T, Hirabayashi T, Yoneda Y, Tanaka K, Wang W-Z, Mori C, Shiota K, Yoshida N, and Kishimoto T (in press) Targeted disruption of gp130, a common signal transducer for IL-6-family of cytokines, leads to myocardial and hematological disorders. Proc Natl Acad Sci USA
32. Rumyantsev PP (1977) Interaction of proliferation and differentiation processes during cardiac myogenesis and regulation. Int Rev Cytol 91:187-273
33. Yasukawa K, Saito T, Fukunaga T, Sekimori Y, Koishikawa T, Fukui H, Ohsugi Y, Matsuda T, Yawata H, Hirano T, Taga T, and Kishimoto T (1990) Purification and characterization of soluble human IL-6 receptor expressed in CHO cell. J Biochem 108:673-676
34. Pennica D, King K, Shaw KJ, Luis E, Rullamas J, Luoh S-M, Darbonne WC, Knutzon DS, Yen R, Chien KR, Baker JB, and Wood W (1995) Expression cloning of cardiotrophin 1, a cytokine that induces cardiac myocyte hypertrophy. Proc Natl Acad Sci USA 92:1142-1146

35. Hirota H, Yoshida K, Kishimoto T, and Taga T (1995) Continuous activation of gp130, a signal transducing receptor component for interleukin6-related cytokines, causes myocardial hypertrophy in mice. Proc Natl Acad Sci USA 92:4862-4866
36. Ware CB, Horowitz MC, Renshaw BR, Hunt JS, Liggitt D, Koblar SA, Gliniak BC, McKenna HJ, Papayannopoulos T, Thoma B, Cheng L, Donovan PJ, Peschon JJ, Bartlett PF, Willis CR, Wright BD, Carpenter MK, Davison BL, and Gearing DP (1995) Targeted disruption of the low-affinity leukemia inhibitory factor receptor gene causes placental, skeletal, neural and metabolic defects and results in perinatal death. Development 121:1283-1299
37. Stewart CL, Kaspar P, Brunet LJ, Bhatt H, Gadi I, Köntgen F and Abbondanzo, JS (1992) Blastocyst implantation depends on maternal expression of leukaemia inhibitory factor. Nature 359:76-79
38. Escary J, Perreau J, Duménil D, Ezine S, and Brûlet P (1993) Leukaemia inhibitory factor is necessary for maintenance of haematopoietic stem cells and thymocyte stimulation. Nature 363:361-364
39. Nishino E, Matsuzaki N, Masuhiro K, Kameda T, Taniguchi T, Takagi T, Sagi F, and Tanizawa O (1989) Trophoblast-derived Interleukin-6 (IL-6) regulates human chorionic gonadotropin release through IL-6 receptor on human trophoblasts. J Clin Endocrinol Metabol 71:536-541
40. Yamaguchi M, Ogren L, Endo H, Thordarson G, Kensinger R, and Talamantes F (1993) Interleukin-6 inhibits mouse placental lactogen-II but not mouse placental lactogen-I secretion in vitro. Proc Natl Acad Sci USA 90:11905-11909

ROLES OF JAK KINASES   IN HUMAN GM-CSF RECEPTOR

Sumiko Watanabe[1], Akihiko Muto[1], Tohru Itoh[1], Tatsutoshi Nakahata[2], Ken-ichi Arai[1]

[1]Department of Molecular and Developmental Biology, [2]Department of Clinical Oncology, Institute of Medical Science, University of Tokyo, 4-6-1, Shirokane-dai, Minato-ku, Tokyo 108, JAPAN

Abstract

The IL-3 and GM-CSF (hGMR) receptors consist of two subunits, α and β, both of which are members of the cytokine receptor superfamily.   Chemical cross-linking and immunoprecipitation revealed that the α and β subunits associate following stimulation with GM-CSF, but the β subunit forms a homodimer even in the absence of the ligand.   We analyzed the mechanism of c-*fos* mRNA activation by GM-CSF using several hGMRβ subunit mutants.   In addition to box1 region, a membrane distal region (a.a. 544-589) of hGMRβ is required for c-*fos* activation. Only one tyrosine residue (Tyr577) exists within the region 544-589, and substitution of Tyr577 to phenylalanine in GMRβ 589 resulted in the loss of c-*fos* activation.   In contrast, the same substitution in a wild type receptor did not affect GM-CSF-induced activities such as c-*fos* mRNA induction and proliferation but abolished Shc phosphorylation. These results suggest that the activation of Shc is not essential for c-*fos* activation and several tyrosine residues coordinate to activate c-*fos* activation.
It is well documented that IL-3 or GM-CSF   activates JAK in various cells. However the role of JAK2 in IL-3/GM-CSF   functions is largely unknown.   We examined the role of JAK2 in GM-CSF-induced signaling pathways.   Dominant negative JAK2 (ΔJAK2) lacking the C-terminus   kinase domain, suppressed IL-3/GM-CSF induced c-*fos* activation, c-*myc* activation and proliferation, suggesting that JAK2 is involved in both signaling pathways.   Several tyrosine residues are known to be phosphorylated by GM-CSF within this region and JAK2 expressed transiently in COS7 cells phosphorylated certain tyrosine residues within hGMRβ. JAK2 also phosphorylated PTP1D in COS7 cells.   PTP1D and Shc are phosphorylated by IL-3/GM-CSF in BA/F3 cells, but these phosphorylation events were inhibited by expression of ΔJAK2.   Taken together, these results indicate that JAK2 is a primary kinase regulating all the known activities of GM-CSF. JAK2 mediates GM-CSF induced c-*fos* activation through receptor phosphorylation and Shc/PTP1D activation.

Introduction

GM-CSF is a cytokine which regulates the differentiation and proliferation of various hemopoietic cells (1).   The receptor of hGM-CSF is composed of two subunits, α and β, both of which are members of the cytokine receptor family (2, 3). In both mice and humans, GM-CSF, IL-3 and IL-5 receptors share a common β subunit. These receptors are composed of a common β subunit and an α subunit specific to each cytokine. In addition to the common β subunit (AIC2B), in the mouse system, an additional β subunit (AIC2A) specific to IL-3 exists. We previously showed that distinct hGMR signaling pathways are involved in c-*myc* mRNA induction/cell proliferation and in the induction of c-*fos*/c-*jun* mRNAs, which is dependent upon a membrane proximal region (a.a. 455-544) and a more cytoplasmic region (a.a. 544-589) of the β subunit respectively (4). To analyze the signals for the activation of c-*myc* and proliferation, we established protocols to monitor the activities of the c-*myc* promoter and DNA replication using a polyoma-replicon (5, 6). Experiments using these systems revealed that E2F/p107 complexes play an important role in the regulation of c-*myc* induction. Further analyses to clarify signaling molecules involved in c-*myc* activation and the initiation of DNA replication are necessary. Although GMR has no intrinsic tyrosine kinase activity, phosphorylation of tyrosine residues in GMR β and several cellular proteins are observed with GM-CSF stimulation. The involvement of JAK family kinases in cytokine signaling has been wel documented. The JAK family of kinase consists of JAK1, JAK2, JAK3 and Tyk2 in mammalian species (7) but their roles in hematopoiesis remain to be determined. Interestingly, a dominant mutation of Drosophila homolog,*hop* gene (*hop*scotch[Tumorous-lethal]) resulted in hemat-opoietic defects (8). Much attention has been directed to JAK family kinases since their roles in interferon (IFN) signals were recognized (9). Studies with IFN receptor signals revealed that JAK family kinases are involved in IFN-specific gene expression in cooperation with STAT proteins (10, 11, 12). Subsequent studies of IL-6 and MGF signaling revealed that the JAK-STAT system plays a role in cytokine-specific gene expression (13, 14). However, it is unclear whether or not JAK family kinase is involved in activities shared by many cytokines such as the induction of cell proliferation or activation of immediate response genes. JAK2 is phosphorylated or activated by many cytokines including IL-3 and GM-CSF (15, 16, 17) and association of JAK2 with the common β subunit of IL-3R and GMR was reported (18). In the present work, we attempted using BA/F3 and COS7 cells to determine whether or not JAK2 is involved in hGMR signals. We found that JAK2, which is activated through the box1 region of hGMRβ, plays essential roles in both c-*myc*/proliferation activation and c-*fos*/c-*jun* activation signaling pathways.

The roles of GM-CSF assessed by loss or gain of function experiments

GM-CSF was initially identified as a factor stimulating the formation of GM colonies. Using gene targeting technology, we re-evaluated the functions of the GM-CSF receptor both in vivo and in vitro. Disruption of genes encoding the IL-3 specific β subunit, AIC2A, elicits no significant phenotype different from normal mouse (19). In contrast, targeting of the gene encoding the common β subunit of IL-3, GM-CSF and IL-5 (AIC2B), no colony was formed *in vitro* in response to GM-CSF or IL-5 using bone marrow cells, though colonies were induced by the addition of IL-3. These results suggest that the GM-CSF or IL-5 signal transduction pathways were defective in this mouse and that AIC2A functioned as a β subunit of IL-3. As expected, this mouse shows a decreased number of eosinophils but, unexpectedly, shows normal peripheral leukocyte counts and differential counts. A previous report indicated that targeting of the gene encoding GM-CSF showed a phenotype similar to a human disease termed alveolar proteinosis (20). The mouse carrying the AIC2B knockout shows a phenotype similar to alveolar proteinosis, probably due to a defect in the macrophages. Taken together, these results indicate that GM-CSF plays a role in proliferation and is involved in the function of alveolar macrophages. Beside GM-CSF, other factor(s) may play roles in the generation of granulocyte and macrophage cell lineages. Essentially, the same results were obtained with a mouse carrying the disrupted genes for the common β subunit and IL-3 (Nishinakamura et al. unpublished results).

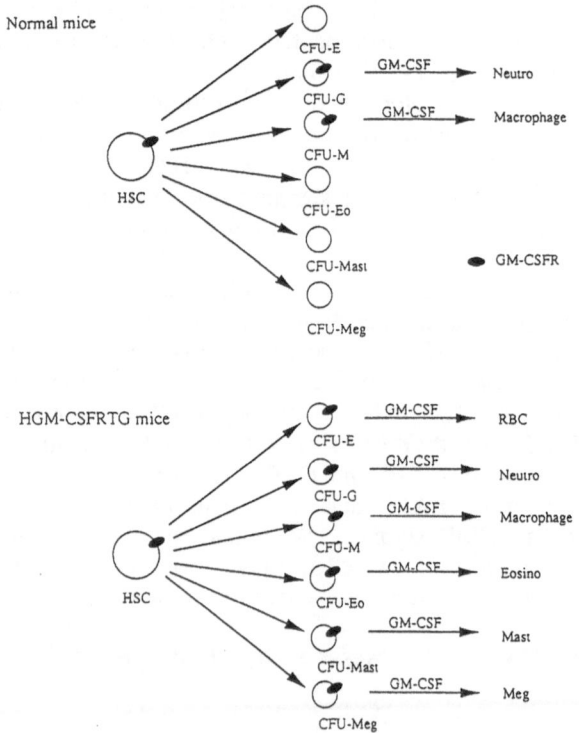

Figure 1   GM-CSF promotes growth in various cells as long as the receptor is expressed.

In normal hematopoiesis, GM-CSF induces GM colonies, suggesting that GM-CSF is a differentiation factor inducing these lineages. In contrast, as long as the receptor is expressed, GM-CSF can stimulate proliferation of almost all lineages.

We have previously shown that reconstituted hGMR in fibroblasts can transduce signals for the activation of immediate early genes and their proliferation (21). This suggests that GM-CSF can transduce signals in non-hemopoietic cells. To test whether reconstituted hGMR in various cells can transduce signals and whether hGMR induces GM-lineage cells when reconstituted in early stage hematopoietic cells, we produced a transgenic mouse (Tg mouse) expressing both hGM-CSF receptor α and β subunits (22). Mouse GM-CSF induces GM colonies predominantly. In contrast, the addition of hGM-CSF to a culture of bone marrow cells from the Tg mouse led to colony formation of all lineages. In addition, hGM-CSF stimulated the formation of erythroid colonies even in the absence of erythropoietin in both serum-containing and serum-free cultures. These results suggest that GM-CSF can function as a potent growth promoting factor rather than differentiation factor specific to G or to M lineages. As long as the receptor and signaling system inside the cells is available, GM-CSF promotes the growth of many different cell types (Fig. 1).

The role of tyrosine residues in the hGMRβ subunit and c-*fos* activation

Similar to other growth factors such as EGF and PDGF, GM-CSF induces cell proliferation and transcription of immediate early genes such as c-*fos*, c-*jun* and c-*myc* (4, 21). In addition, GM-CSF induces ID1, cln and egr genes. Using a series of deletion mutants of the β subunit and tyrosine kinase inhibitors, we examined the signaling mechanism inducing these events (4). There are at least two hGMR signaling pathways (Fig.2).

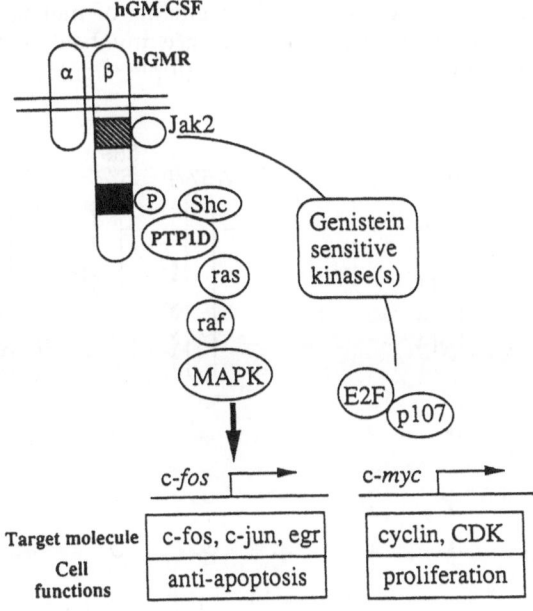

Figure 2　Two distinct signaling pathways of hGMR signals.

One pathway, involving the membrane proximal region (AA 455-517) containing box1 of the receptor β subunit, is required for the activation of c-*myc* transcription and proliferation. This pathway is sensitive to genistein, indicating that a tyrosine kinase sensitive to genistein plays an essential role to activate c-*myc* and proliferation. The other pathway, involving a more membrane-distal region (AA 544-589) in addition to the membrane-proximal region, leads to the activation of c-*fos* and c-*jun* transcription. In contrast to the former pathway, this pathway is not suppressed by genistein, and c-*fos* activation is, rather, augmented by genistein.

Because there are several tyrosine residues within the C-terminus region of the β subunit, we next examined the roles of tyrosine residues in hGMRβ and the involvement of tyrosine kinase in GM-CSF signals. To analyze the requirement of tyrosine residues, we constructed several hGMRβ mutants and analyzed signals through these mutants in BA/F3 cells. Figure 3 is a summary of the various analyses with these mutants. Deletion up to 589 did not affect any of the activities. Further deletion to 544 resulted in the loss of c-*fos* activation and phosphorylation of tyrosine residues of hGMR and cellular proteins. Activation of proliferation is not affected because the box1 region is sufficient for activity. These results suggest that the region between 589 to 544 is essential for activation of the c-*fos* promoter. We next examined the role of tyrosine residues. There are 6 tyrosine residues in the C-terminus region of hGMRβ. Because there is only one tyrosine residue, 577 in the region covering 589 to 544, we first substituted tyrosine residue 577 to phenylalanine of mutant 589. As expected, this mutant did not activate the tyrosine phosphorylation of cellular proteins or the GMRβ, nor did it activate the c-*fos* promoter. On the other hand, the same substitution in the wild type hGMRβ did not affect these activities. This means that tyrosine 577 plays an essential role in the signaling of mutant 588, but in the wild type receptor, multiple tyrosine residues are involved in the c-*fos* gene activation. It is tempting to speculate that multiple signals arise from each tyrosine residue.

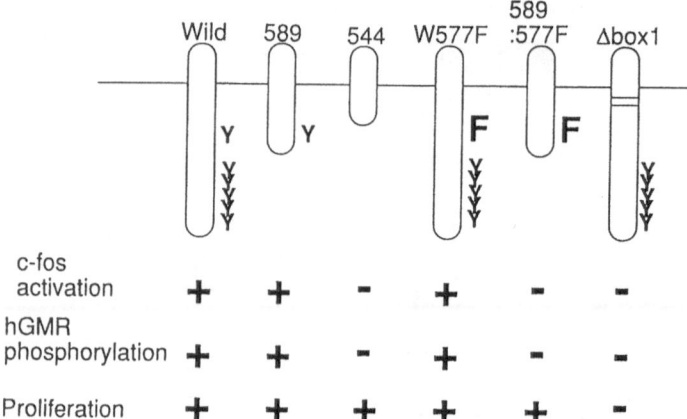

Figure 3   Summary of several mutants of hGMRβ in c-*fos* activation, tyrosine phosphorylation, and cell proliferation in BA/F3 cells.

To test this hypothesis we next determined the involvement of tyrosine 577 in Shc and PTP 1D activation. Shc (23) and PTP1D (24) are known to be phosphorylated by IL-3/GM-CSF (25) and their positive roles in the MAPK cascade have been discussed (26). We analyzed the hGM-CSF induced phosphorylation of these molecules by immunoprecipitation followed by western blotting using anti-phosphotyrosine antibody 4G10 (α PTyr). BA/FGMR cells were depleted of mIL-3 for 5 hr, and stimulated with 5 ng/ml of hGM-CSF for 5 min. Cells were harvested and lysed with lysis buffer. Immunoprecipitations were done with anti Shc or PTP 1D proteins and western blotting was performed with either α PTyr, anti Shc or PTP 1D antibodies.

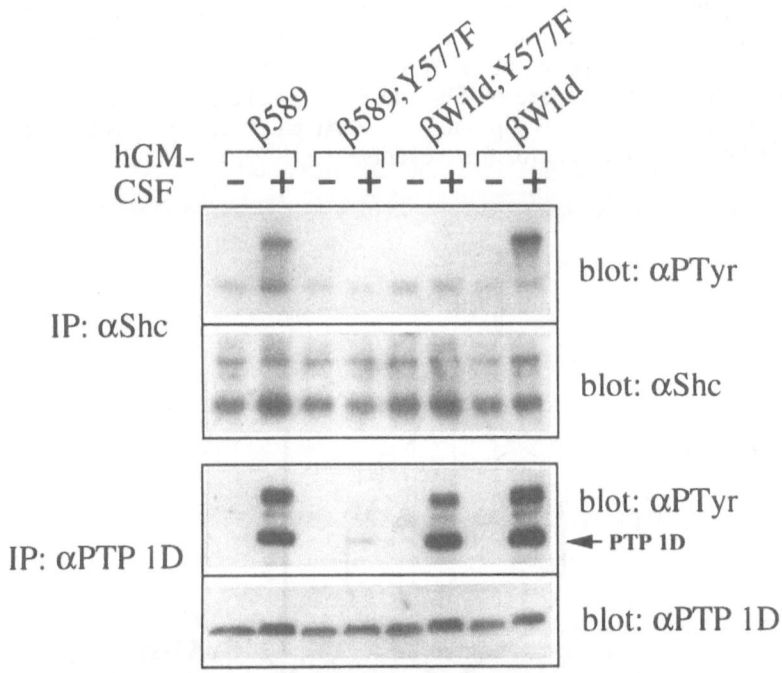

Figure 4   Effects of tyrosine residue substitution in hGMRβ on Shc and PTP 1D phosphorylation.
BA/F3 cells expressing hGMRa and various mutants of hGMRb were depleted of mIL-3 for 5hr and restimulated with hGM-CSF for 5 min. Cells were lysed and proteins were immunoprecipitated and analyzed by western blotting with either anti Shc (A) or anti PTP 1D (B) antibodies.

As shown in Fig. 4A, Shc is phosphorylated with hGM-CSF stimulation in BA/FGMR cells. The phosphorylation of Shc is abolished with a phenylalanine substitution of tyrosine 577 in GMRβ mutant 588. For the same substitution in the wild type receptor, phosphorylation of Shc cannot be observed even though this mutant can activate c-*fos* activation. These results suggest that tyrosine 577 of hGMRβ is essential for Shc activation, and activation of Shc is not essential for activation of the c-*fos* promoter. PTP 1D is also phosphorylated following hGM-CSF stimulation, and substitution of tyrosine 577 to phenylalanin in the 589 mutant abolished GM-CSF induced PTP 1D phosphorylation (Fig. 4B). In contrast to Shc activation, the wild type receptor containing phenylalanine 577 can phosphorylate PTP 1D. These results suggest that tyrosine 577 is not essential for PTP 1D activation. The RAS protein is also known to be involved in the MAP kinase cascade (27). We examined the role of Ras protein using a dominant negative type of mutant ras, ras N17. Co-expression of dominant negative Ras completely suppressed GM-CSF induced c-*fos* activation (data not shown). Taken together, we proposed a model of hGMRβ and signaling molecules as illustrated in Fig. 5. Shc may be activated through tyrosine 577 of the β subunit and PTP 1D can activate either tyrosine 577 or other C-terminal tyrosine residues. Signals transduced by Shc and PTP 1D are integrated at Ras and lead to activation of c-*fos* transcription. We next analyzed the involvement of the tyrosine kinase responsible for these events.

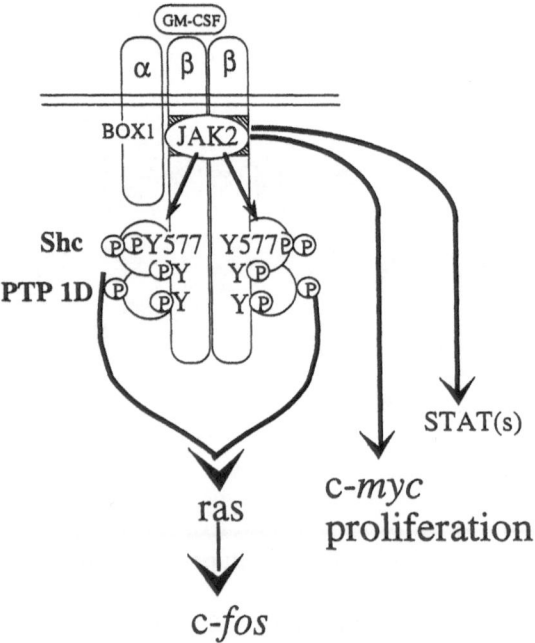

Figure 5   Schematic illustration of signals from hGMR to activate c-*fos* promoter.

Role of JAK2 in GM-CSF signals

Several tyrosine kinases such as the src family tyrosine kinases or Tec kinase were reported to be activated by GM-CSF stimulation (15, 16, 28). JAK2 is activated by IL-3 or GM-CSF and it was reported that the membrane-proximal region, box1 of hGMRβ, is required for phosphorylation of JAK2 (Watanabe et al. submitted). Because the membrane proximal region is essential for all the known activities of hGM-CSF, we analyzed the roles of JAK2 in hGMR signals. We analyzed the involvement of JAK2 in GMR signals with dominant negative JAK2. As schematically shown in Fig. 6, JAK2 lacking the C-terminal kinase domainwas constructed. This mutant dominant negatively inhibited auto-phosphorylation of JAK2 but not JAK1 or JAK3 in COS7 cells (data not shown). We first analyzed the involvement of JAK2 in the pathway to activate the c-*myc* gene and cell proliferati on activation in BA/F3 cells.

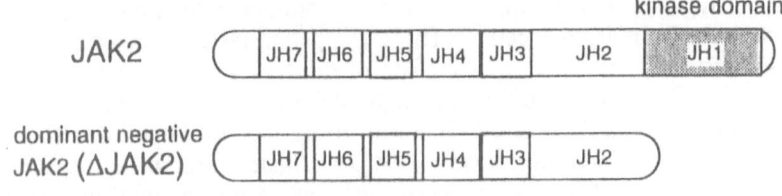

Figure 6   Schematic representation of wild type and kinase-negative JAK2.

We previously established a c-*myc* promoter transient assay (6) using the CAT gene as a reporter gene. As shown in Fig. 7, c-*myc* CAT activity induced by IL-3 or GM-CSF was completely suppressed by co-expression of dominant negative JAK2. DNA replication was monitored using the polyoma replication origin (5) and was also abolished by dominant negative JAK2 (data not shown). These results suggest that JAK2 plays an essential role for signals regulating c-*myc* promoter activation and cell proliferation.

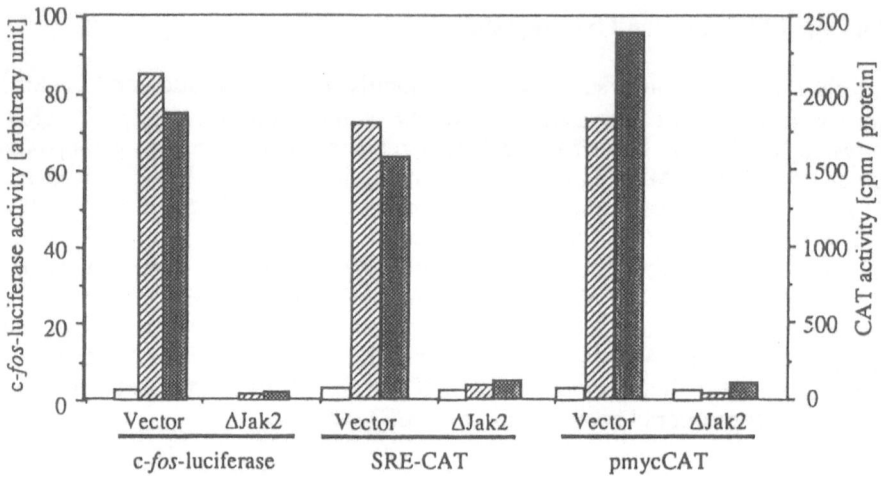

Figure 7   Effect of dominant negative JAK2 in various promoter activities.

The signaling pathway regulating c-*fos* activation by GM-CSF is resistant to the tyrosine kinase inhibitor genistein (4).   Because genistein does not affect GM-CSF induced JAK2 phosphorylation, we tested the possibility that JAK2 is involved in c-*fos* activation.   For this purpose, we used a luciferase plasmid fused with a 0.4 kb fragment of the c-*fos* promoter.   As shown in Fig. 7, dominant negative JAK2 suppressed c-*fos* promoter activation by IL-3 or GM-CSF completely in BA/F3 cells.   The c-*fos* promoter carries an SIE site which contains the GAS sequence, a target site of the STAT protein (29).   To examine whether JAK2 exerts its effect through SIE or SRE, we tested the effect of dominant negative JAK2 on the SRE site using tandem repeats of the SRE site fused to the CAT coding region (30).   Again, dominant negative JAK2 suppressed IL-3 or GM-CSF induced SRE activation suggesting that JAK2 is involved in the STAT independent signaling pathway to the c-*fos* promoter.   To analyze the role of JAK2 in the activation of SRE or c-*fos*, we next examined the effect of dominant negative JAK2 on the signal transducing molecules Shc and PTP1D, which are known to be involved in the activation of the c-*fos* promoter. hGMRα and β were transiently transfected into BA/F3 cells and immunoprecipitation was done with either anti Shc or PTP 1D antibodies. Phosphorylation of Shc or PTP 1D through transiently expressed hGMR was observed and this phosphorylation was completely abolished by co-expression of dominant negative JAK2.   It appears that dominant negative JAK2 interferes with signaling event(s) upstream of Shc or PTP 1D activation, thereby indicating that JAK2 plays an essential role in the activation of both signaling molecules (data not shown).

The hGMR β subunit and PTP 1D are phosphorylated in COS7 cells by either JAK1, JAK2 or JAK3

We next asked whether or not PTP 1D could be phosphorylated in COS7 cells by JAK2. PTP 1D, when expressed alone, was not phosphorylated whereas it was heavily phosphorylated when JAK2 and PTP 1D were co-expressed. PTP 1D is known to be activated by various mitogens such as insulin and insulin-like growth factor-1. We examined the specificity of the JAK family kinases with regard to their potential to phosphorylate PTP 1D. Interestingly, co-expression of either JAK1 or JAK3 resulted in PTP 1D phosphorylation. We then examined whether or not JAK1 or JAK3 is also capable of phosphorylating hGMRβ in COS7 cells. Indeed we found they could phosphorylate hGMRβ (Fig. 8). These results indicate that in COS7 cells there is no target sequence specificity among JAK family members. However, it should be noted that, in BA/F3 cells, mIL-3 or hGM-CSF preferentially activates JAK2 but not JAK1 or JAK3, suggesting that JAK1 and JAK3 do not play a major role in mIL-3 or hGM-CSF signaling.

Conclusion and future aspect

In summary, we conclude that JAK2 is the primary kinase regulating all the known GM-CSF signals such as the activation of proliferation, c-*myc* promoter and c-*fos* promoter. Activation of JAK2 is dependent on the GMR box1 region essential for both signaling pathways and JAK2 phosphorylation. JAK2 may be responsible for hGMRβ phosphorylation and activates a signaling pathway including the phosphorylation of PTP 1D leading to the expression of c-*fos* promoter. These results indicate that JAK2 is involved in multiple pathways of hGMR signals in addition to the STAT dependent pathway. How is JAK2 activated by GM-CSF and its receptor? Because it has been reported that JAK2 is constitutively bound to the hGMRβ subunit, a possible mechanism involves ligand-induced dimerization of the β subunit leading to the phosphorylation and activation of JAK2 kinase followed by phosphorylation of the β subunit. To test this possibility we examined the organization of hGMR subunits using a chemical cross linker. BA/FGMR cells were treated with the chemical cross linker, BS3, and immunoprecipitation was done with the anti β subunit. Figure 9 shows blotting pattern of the immunoprecipitant with anti β subunit antibody and the upper band corresponds to the molecular weight of the β subunit dimer, which is formed even in the absence of hGM-CSF stimulation. We found that the α subunit is associated with the β subunit only when the receptor was stimulated (data not shown).

A

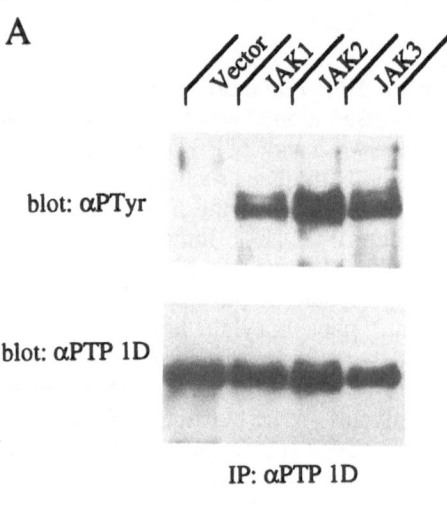

blot: αPTyr

blot: αPTP 1D

IP: αPTP 1D

B

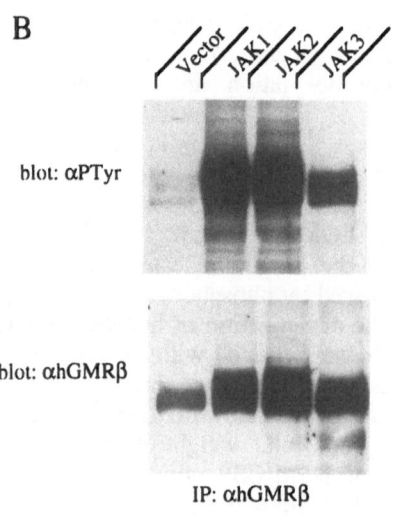

blot: αPTyr

blot: αhGMRβ

IP: αhGMRβ

Figure 8   Phosphorylation of hGMRβ and PTP 1D by JAK family kinases in COS7 cells.

A, B: Plasmid encoding hGMRβ (A) or PTP 1D (B) and control vector, JAK1, JAK2 or JAK3 were co-transfected to COS7 cells.   Immunoprecipitations were done with either anti hGMRβ (A) or PTP 1D (B) followed by western blotting.

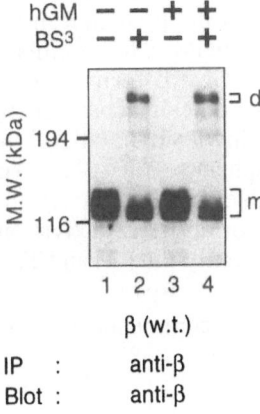

Figure 9 hGMRβ forms a homodimer even in the absence of hGM-CSF in BA/F3 cells.
BA/FGMR cells were stimulated with hGM-CSF (lanes 3 and 4) or without (lanes 1 and 2) and their surface proteins were cross-linked with 0.3 mM BS3 (lanes 2 and 4) or without (lanes 1 and 3).   Proteins were immunoprecipitated and analyzed by western blotting with anti hGMRβ antibody

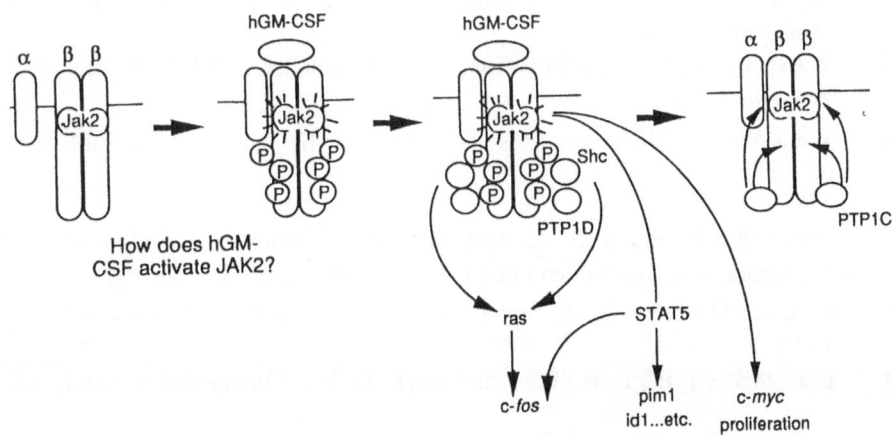

Figure 10   Schematic representation of GM-CSF receptor signals.

In summary, we wish to propose a model of activation of hGMR as shown in Fig. 10. JAK2 forms a homo dimer with the β subunit in the absence of hGM-CSF, and its activation is triggered by hGM-CSF stimulation. Because JAK2 is constitutively bound to hGMRβ and GMRβ forms a homodimer, the mechanism of JAK2 activation seems to involve other mechanisms than simply dimerization induced by hGM-CSF. JAK2 is involved in all of the known activities and signals were extinguished by phosphatase PTP 1C. We obtained evidence that the C-terminal region is responsible for the activation of PTP 1D. We are currently working on the mechanism of JAK2 activation and the roles of other tyrosine kinases such as JAK1, Src family kinases and Tec in GM-CSF signals.

The authors with to thank M. Dahl for comments on the manuscript.

References

1. Arai, K., Lee, F., Miyajima, A., Miyatake, S., Arai, N. and Yokota, T. (1990) Ann. Rev. Biochem. **59**, 783-836
2. Miyajima, A., Kitamura, T., Harada, N., Yokota, T. and Arai, K. (1992) Ann. Rev. Immunol. **10**, 295-331
3. Miyajima, A., Mui, A. L.-F., Ogorochi, T. and Sakamaki, K. (1993) Blood **82**, 1960-1974

4. Watanabe, S., Muto, A., Yokota, T., Miyajima, A. and Arai, K. (1993) Mol. Biol. Cell **4**, 983-992
5. Watanabe, S., Ito, Y., Miyajima, A. and Arai, K. (1995) J. Biol. Chem. **270**, 9615-9621
6. Watanabe, S., Ishida, S., Koike, K. and Arai, K. (1995) Mol. Biol. Cell **6**, 627-636

7. Ihle, J. N., Witthuhn, B. A., Quelle, F. W., Yamamoto, K., Thierfelder, W. E., Kreider, B. and Silvennoinen, O. (1994) TIBS **19**, 222-227
8. Luo, H., Hanratty, W. P. and Dearolf, C. R. (1995) EMBO J. **14**, 1412-1420
9. Darnell Jr., J. E., Kerr, I. M. and Stark, G. R. (1994) Science **264**, 1415-1421
10. Muller, M., Briscoe, J., Laxton, C., Guschin, D., Ziemiecki, A., Silvennoinen, O., Harpur, A. G., Barbieri, G., Witthuhn, B. A., Schindler, C., Pellegrini, S., Wilks, A. F., Ihle, J. N., Stark, G. R. and Kerr, I. M. (1993) Nature **366**, 129-135
11. Watling, D., Guschin, D., Muller, M., Silvennoinen, O., Witthuhn, B. A., Quelle, F. W., Rogers, N. C., Schindler, C., Stark, G. R. and Ihle, J. N. (1993) Nature **366**, 166-170

12. Velazquez, L., Fellous, M., Stark, G. R. and Pellegrini, S. (1992) Cell **70**, 313-322
13. Wegenka, U. M., Lutticken, C., Buschmann, J., Yuan, J., Lottspeich, F., Muller-Esterl, W., Schindler, C., Roeb, E., Heinrich, P. C. and Horn, F. (1994) Mol. Cell. Biol. **14**, 3186-3196
14. Wakao, H., Gouilleux, F. and Groner, B. (1994) EMBO J. **13**, 2182-2191
15. Silvennoinen, O., Witthuhn, B. A., Quelle, F. W., Cleveland, J. L., Yi, T. and Ihle, J. N. (1993) Proc. Natl. Acad. Sci. USA **90**, 8429-8433
16. Quelle, F. W., Sato, N., Witthuhn, B. A., Inhorn, R. C., Eder, M., Miyajima, A., Griffin, J. and Ihle, J. N. (1994) Mol. Cell. Biol. **14**, 4335-4341
17. Taniguchi, T. (1995) Science **268**, 251-255
18. Brizzi, M. F., Zini, M. G., Aronica, M. G., Blechman, J. M., Yarden, Y. and Pegoraro, L. (1994) J. Biol. Chem. **269**, 31680-31684
19. Nishinakamura, R., Nakayama, N., Hirabayashi, Y., Inoue, T., Aud, D., McNeil, T., Azuma, S., Yoshida, S., Toyoda, Y., Arai, K., Miyajima, A. and Murray, R. (1995) Immunity **2**, 211-222
20. Dranoff, G., Grawford, A. D., Sadelain, M., Ream, B., Rashid, A., Bronson, R. T., Dickersin, G. R., Bachurski, C. J., Mark, E. L., Whitsett, J. A. and Mulligan, R. C. (1994) Science **264**, 713-716
21. Watanabe, S., Mui, A. L.-F., Muto, A., Chen, J. X., Hayashida, K., Miyajima, A. and Arai, K. (1993) Mol. Cell. Biol. **13**, 1440-1448

22. Nishijima, I., Nakahata, T., Hirabayashi, Y., Inoue, T., Kurata, H., Miyajima, A., Hayashi, N., Iwakura, Y., Arai, K. and Yokota, T. (1995) Mol. Biol. Cell **6**, 497-508
23. Pelicci, G., Lanfrancone, L., Grignani, F., McGlade, J., Cavallo, F., Forni, G., Nicoletti, I., Grignani, F., Pawson, T. and Pelicci, P. G. (1992) Cell **70**, 93-104
24. Vogel, W., Lammers, R., Huang, J. and Ullrich, A. (1993) Science **259**, 1611-1614
25. Welham, M. J., Dechert, U., Leslie, K. B., Jirik, F. and Schrader, J. W. (1994) J. Biol. Chem. **269**, 23764-23768
26. Li, W., Nishimura, R., Kashishian, A., Batzer, A. G., Kim, W. J. H., Cooper, J. A. and Schlessinger, J. (1994) Mol. Cell. Biol. **14**, 509-517
27. Kaziro, Y., Itoh, H., Kozasa, T., Nakafuku, M. and Satoh, T. (1991) Annu. Rev. Biochem. **60**, 349-400
28. Torigoe, T., O'Connor, R., Santoli, D. and Reed, J. C. (1992) Blood **80**, 617-624
29. Fu, X.-Y. and Zhang, J.-J. (1993) Cell **74**, 1135-1145
30. Fukumoto, Y., Kaibuchi, K., Oku, N., Hori, Y. and Takai, Y. (1990) J. Biol. Chem. **265**, 774-780

TGF-β Receptors and Signal Transduction

Kohei Miyazono

Department of Biochemistry, The Cancer Institute, Tokyo, Japanese Foundation for Cancer Research, 1-37-1 Kami-ikebukuro, Toshima-ku, Tokyo 170, Japan

SUMMARY

Transforming growth factor-β (TGF-β) is a family of 25-kDa dimeric proteins that regulate the cellular growth and differentiation, the formation of extracellular matrix, and the immune function. TGF-βs belong to a larger family of structurally related proteins known as the TGF-β superfamily, which includes activins and bone morphogenetic proteins. TGF-β exerts the effects through binding to type I (TβR-I; 53 kDa) and type II (TβR-II; 75 kDa) serine/threonine kinase receptors. Overall structures of TβR-I and TβR-II are similar to each other. Preceding the kinase domain of TβR-I, there is a region termed the GS domain, which is conserved in type I receptors, but not in type II receptors. After ligand binding, TβR-I and TβR-II form a heteromeric receptor complex, which is most likely a heterotetramer composed of two molecules each of TβR-I and TβR-II. TβR-II transphosphorylates the GS domain of TβR-I, which then activates the TβR-I kinase and transduces signals. By yeast two-hybrid system, several proteins which interact with type I or type II receptors, and possibly transduce the signals for TGF-β, have been isolated. Mutations in the TβR-II gene have been identified in several carcinoma cells, which suggests that loss of the TβR-II protein is one of the mechanisms by which cancer cells acquire resistance to the growth inhibitory activity of TGF-β.

KEY WORDS: TGF-β, growth inhibition, immune suppression, serine/threonine kinase receptor, signal transduction.

THE TRANSFORMING GROWTH FACTOR (TGF)-β SUPERFAMILY

Proteins in the TGF-β superfamily are multifunctional cytokines that regulate the growth and differentiation of various types of cells [1, 2] (Fig. 1). Most members act as dimeric proteins. In each monomer they have seven invariant cysteine residues, one of which forms a disulphide bond between two monomeric peptides. The members in the TGF-β superfamily are produced as larger precursor proteins. The C-terminal mature domains with 110-140 amino acids form active dimers after cleavage from the N-terminal parts of the precursors.

TGF-β is a prototype of the proteins in the TGF-β superfamily [3, 4]. It inhibits the growth of most cell types, including hematopoietic cells, lymphocytes, epithelial cells, and endothelial cells. TGF-β is also known to induce the formation of extracellular matrix *in vitro* and *in vivo*. There are three mammalian isoforms of TGF-β, i.e. TGF-β1, -β2, and -β3. Targeted disruption of the TGF-β1 gene in mice caused the development of excessive inflammation in various organs, which led to death of the mice 2-3 weeks after birth [5, 6]. Thus, TGF-β1 plays an important role in the regulation of the immune function *in vivo*.

Activin was originally identified as proteins that stimulate the secretion of follicle stimulating hormone from pituitary cells [7]. Activin was later found to induce the formation of mesoderm in *Xenopus* embryos, and stimulate the differentiation of erythroid progenitor cells [8]. Activin is produced by bone marrow stromal cells, which suggests that it may function in a paracrine fashion for the differentiation of hematopoietic cells *in vivo*.

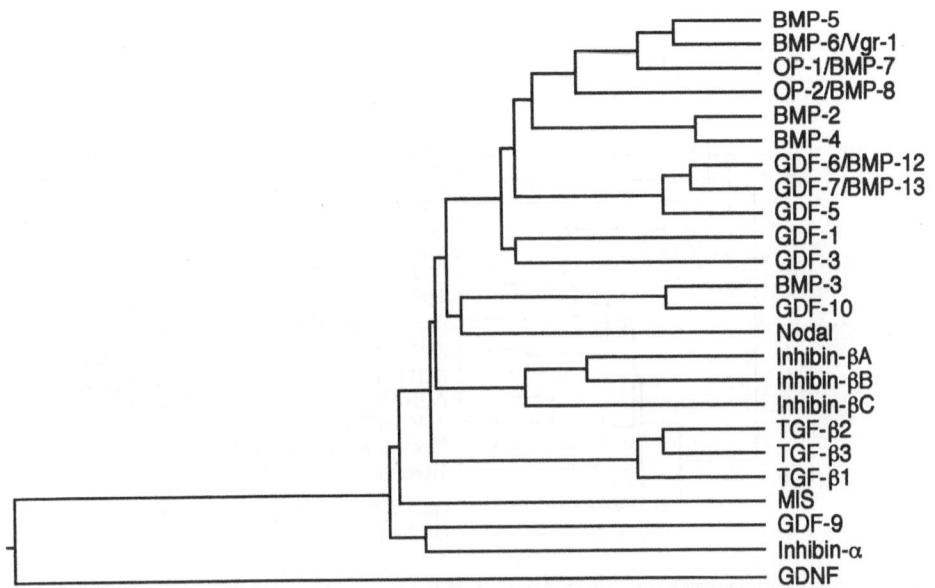

Fig. 1. Phylogenetic tree based on the amino acid sequences of the members in the TGF-β superfamily. Amino acid sequences were compared by the Clustal computer alignment program [53]. Only the *mammalian* members in the TGF-β superfamily are listed in this figure. Activins are dimers of inhibin-β chains, whereas inhibins are heterodimers of α and β chains. Bioactivity of the inhibin βC chain has not been determined. OP, osteogenic protein; GDF, growth/differentiation factor; MIS, Müllerian inhibiting substance, GDNF, glial cell line-derived neurotrophic factor.

Bone morphogenetic protein (BMP) is a family of proteins originally identified by their activity to induce bone formation *in vivo* [9-11]. They also act on various cell types, e.g. monocytes, neuronal cells and epithelial cells. Null mutation of the BMP-4 gene in mice revealed that BMP-4 may play an important role in early stages of hematopoiesis [12]. Since the formation of bone marrow takes place during the process of bone morphogenesis induced by BMPs, it is possible that certain other members in the BMP family may also act on hematopoietic progenitor cells.

TWO DIFFERENT TYPES OF SERINE/THREONINE KINASE RECEPTORS

Members in the TGF-β superfamily act through two different types of serine/threonine kinase receptors, type I and type II [13-16]. Both type I and type II receptors are composed of the N-terminal signal sequences, followed by short extracellular domains, single transmembrane domains, and intracellular domains containing serine/threonine kinase regions. Figure 2 shows a phylogenetic tree of serine/threonine kinase receptors. Type I and type II receptors form subfamilies in the serine/threonine kinase receptor family [17-19]. Thus far, eighteen serine/threonine kinase receptors have been identified in different species.

The type II receptors in mammals have molecular masses of more than 75 kDa, which is larger than the type I receptors at about 55 kDa. In the TGF-β receptor system, the TGF-β type II receptor (TβR-II) binds ligands in the absence of the TGF-β type I receptor (TβR-I), but it requires TβR-I for signal transduction (Fig. 3A). On the other hand, TβR-I does not bind ligands in the absence of TβR-II. Formation of heteromeric receptor complex between TβR-I and TβR-II is essential for signal transduction [18-21].

In the receptor system for *Drosophila* decapentaplegic (Dpp), a member in the BMP subgroup, a type I receptor (Thick veins) is larger than its type II receptor (Punt) [22]. Moreover, the hierarchy

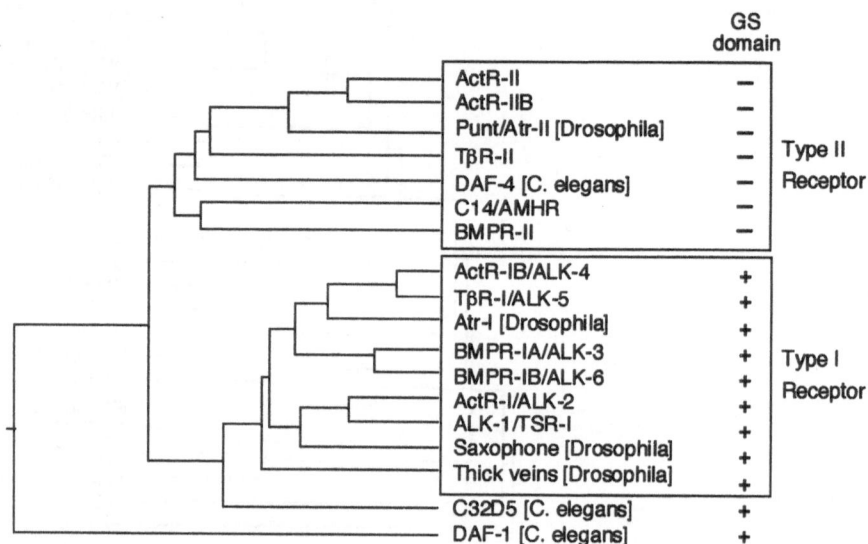

Fig. 2. <u>Relationship between the kinase domains of the serine/threonine kinase receptors.</u> Amino acid sequences were compared by the Clustal computer alignment program [53]. It is not yet determined whether DAF-1 and C32D5 act as type I receptors or not. ActR, activin receptor; AMHR, anti-Müllerian hormone receptor; ALK, activin receptor-like kinase; TSR, TGF-β superfamily receptor.

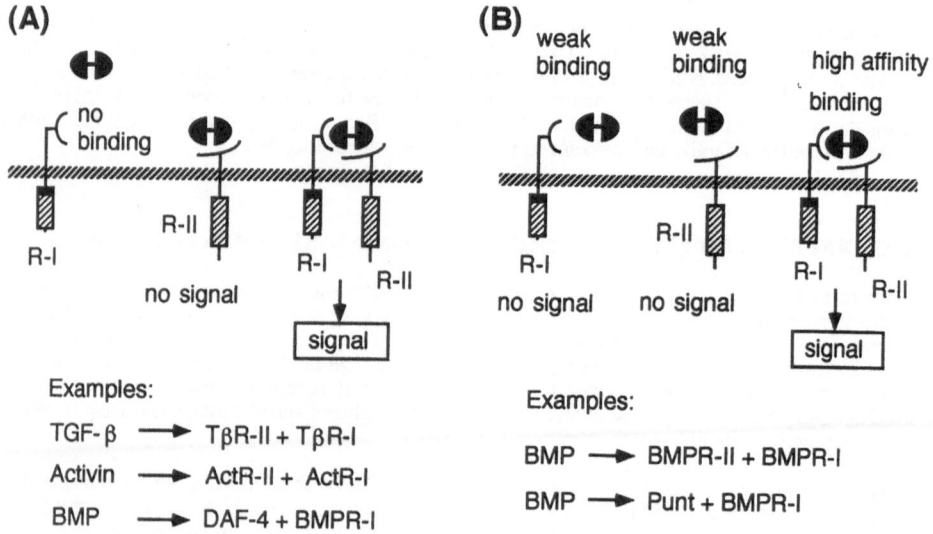

Fig. 3. <u>Binding of the proteins in the TGF-β superfamily to the type I and type II serine/threonine kinase receptors.</u> Only one molecule each of type I and type II receptors is shown in this scheme, but the heteromeric complex may be composed of hetero-oligomer, most likely a heterotetramer (see Fig. 5).

in the ligand binding observed in the TGF-β receptor system, is not observed in certain other systems. For example, osteogenic protein (OP)-1 weakly binds its type I (BMPR-IA and BMPR-IB) and type II (BMPR-II) receptors independently [23, 24], but the affinity is dramatically increased in the presence of both receptor types [25-27] (Fig. 3B). In the *Drosophila* Dpp receptor system, ligands bind the type I receptor (Thick veins) independently, whereas the type II receptor (Punt) requires the type I receptors for ligand binding [22]. Thus, neither the sizes of the receptors nor the hierarchy in ligand-binding can be applied for discrimination of the type I and type II receptors.

Preceding the kinase domains, all the type I, but not the type II receptors, have a highly conserved region, termed the GS domain, because of the presence of SGSGS motif (Fig. 4). The GS domain plays an important role in the signal transduction of serine/threonine kinase receptors. The presence or absence of the GS domain can, thus, be used to distinguish the class of serine/threonine kinase receptors.

MECHANISM OF THE TGF-β RECEPTOR ACTIVATION

TGF-β transduces signals by heteromeric complex of TβR-I and TβR-II. TβR-II is a constitutively active kinase. After the ligand binding to TβR-II, TβR-I binds to the TGF-β—TβR-II complex. The kinase of TβR-II transphosphorylates the GS domain in TβR-I, which then leads to the activation of the serine/threonine kinase of TβR-I and the intracellular signal transduction (Fig. 5) [28]. Thus, TβR-I acts as a downstream component of TβR-II, and TβR-I specifies signals in the serine/threonine kinase receptor system.

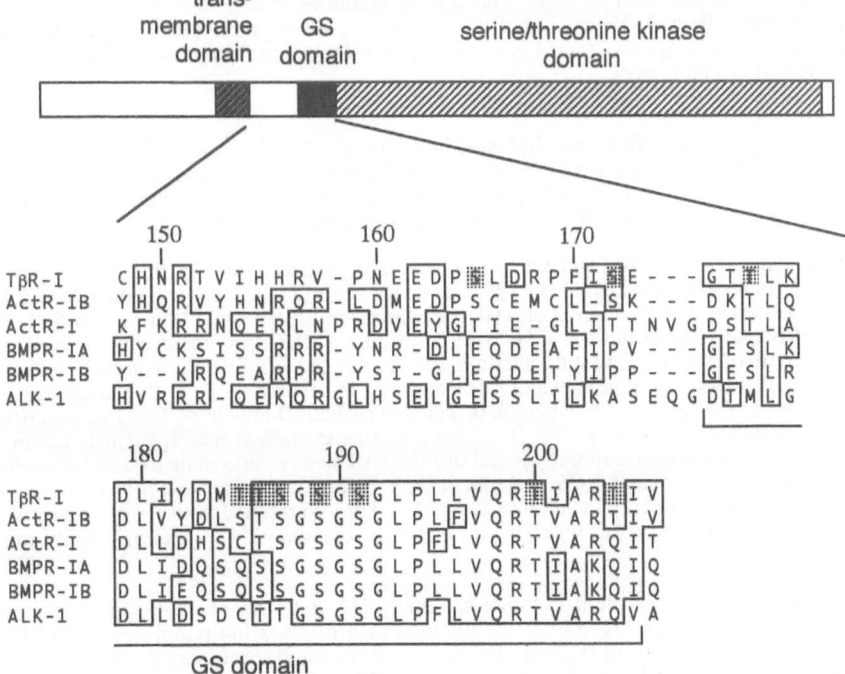

Fig. 4. Comparison of the amino acid sequences of the juxtamembrane domains of type I serine/threonine kinase receptors. Amino acid residues conserved in more than three of the type I receptors are boxed. Amino acid positions in TβR-I are indicated. The amino acid residues in TβR-I analyzed by mutation [34-36] are shaded.

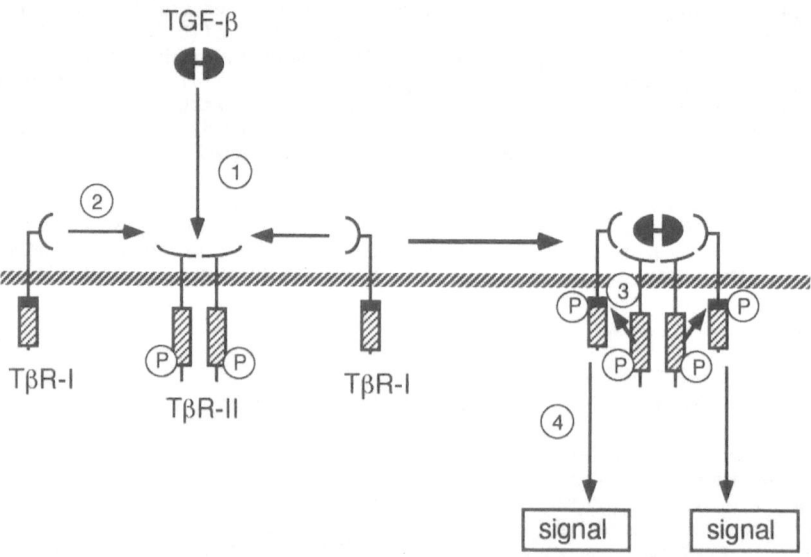

Fig. 5. <u>Mechanisms of the activation of serine/threonine kinase receptors.</u> 1) TGF-β binds to the type II receptor, which is a constitutively active kinase. 2) Then the type I receptor is recruited to the ligand—type II receptor complex. 3) The serine/threonine kinase of the type II receptor transphosphorylates the GS domain in the type I receptor, and 4) the type I receptor kinase is activated and transduces signals. In the ligand—receptor complex, probably two molecules each of type I and type II receptors exist.

TβR-II forms a homodimer (or homo-oligomer) in the presence and absence of ligands [29, 30]. After ligand binding, more than two molecules of TβR-I could be identified in the ligand—receptor complex [31]. Thus, TβR-I and TβR-II appear to form not a heterodimeric complex; instead, they may form a complex composed of two molecules each of TβR-I and TβR-II.

Intracellular domains of the type I and type II receptors have distinct roles. The intracellular domain of TβR-II can not be substituted by that of TβR-I, and vice versa [32, 33]. We and others have found that serine residues in the GS domain of TβR-I are imporant in the signal transduction [34, 35]. Mutations of two or more of the conserved serine residues in the GS domain caused the loss of signaling activity of TβR-I; however, mutations of the single serine residues did not affect its signaling activity. Moreover, Wieser *et al.* [35] have shown that mutation of Thr-204 to aspartic acid (T204D) results in the constitutive activation of TβR-I. The T204D mutant of TβR-I can transduce signals in the absence of TGF-β or TβR-II, which confirms the notion that TβR-I may act in the downstream of TβR-II. We have recently found that the juxtamembrane domain located between the transmembrane domain and the GS domain of TβR-I plays an important role in the signal transduction [36]. Interestingly, mutation of Ser-172 or Thr-176 resulted in the perturbation of the growth inhibitory signal, but not of the signal for matrix production. Thus, signaling activity can be separated at this portion.

In some cell types, including a pituitary tumor cell line, GH3, and certain hematopoietic cells, only ~60 kDa complexes could be seen by cross-linking experiments using radioiodinated TGF-β1. However, immunoprecipitation of the cross-linked complexes using specific antibodies to TβR-I or TβR-II revealed that these cells have TβR-I as well as TβR-II, and both receptor types could be co-immunoprecipitated by either antibodies [37, 38, and our unpublished data]. Thus, the apparent absence of TβR-II in these cells is due to poor cross-linking of ^{125}I-TGF-β to TβR-II, the reason for which remains to be elucidated. As far as we have investigated, all cells which respond to TGF-β have both TβR-I and TβR-II, and these two receptors are essential for signal transduction.

Activins bind two different types of type I receptors, ActR-I and ActR-IB. ActR-IB is most similar to TβR-I among the serine/threonine kinase receptor family, whereas ActR-I is less similar to them (Fig. 2). In the mink lung epithelial cells transfected with the receptor cDNAs, ActR-IB induced the growth inhibitory effect, whereas ActR-I did not [39]. Moreover, ActR-IB is a predominantly expressed type I receptor for activin in erythroid progenitor cells and pituitary cells [40], indicating that ActR-IB is responsible for cell differentiation and other metabolic effects in these cell types.

INTRACELLULAR COMPONENTS THAT INTERACT WITH SERINE/ THREONINE KINASE RECEPTORS

Intracellular components that transduce signals for serine/threonine kinase receptors are not fully determined yet. However, recent studies revealed that the yeast two-hybrid system is a powerful method to obtain proteins that interact with serine/threonine kinase receptors. Using the TβR-I intracellular domain as a bait, FKBP-12 [41, and our unpublished data] and farnesyltransferase-α (FT-α) [42] were shown to bind TβR-I.

FKBP-12 is a binding protein for immunosuppressants FK506 and rapamycin. FKBP-12 interacts with TβR-I as well as the other type I receptors. Binding was observed in the kinase-active TβR-I, but not in the kinase-defective mutant [41, and our unpublished data]. Moreover, the interaction between FKBP-12 and TβR-I could be prevented by excess amounts of FK506 [41]. However, phosphorylation of FKBP-12 by the type I receptors is not observed; thus, functional importance of FKBP-12 in the signal transduction pathway of serine/threonine kinase receptors remains to be elucidated.

FT-α is an enzyme subunit that is involved in farnesylation and geranylgeranylation of small G proteins, such as Ras, Rac, and Rho. Similar to FKBP-12, FT-α did not interact with the kinase-defective TβR-I [42]. The interaction was more prominent in the constitutively active TβR-I (T204D) than in the wild type TβR-I in the yeast system. Moreover, the TβR-I kinase induced the phosphorylation of FT-α. The functional role of the interaction between FT-α and the type I receptors remains to be determined, but the current observation strongly suggests the importance of FT-α in the signaling pathway of serine/threonine kinase receptors.

The intracellular domain of TβR-II was also used as a bait in yeast two-hybrid screening, and Chen *et al.* [43] have isolated a novel protein termed TRIP-1 (TGF-β-receptor interacting protein). TRIP-1 is structurally similar to WD-domain containing proteins, which are involved in protein-protein interaction. TRIP-1 binds to TβR-II, but not to ActR-II or type I receptors. Moreover, TRIP-1 is phosphorylated by TβR-II. Although the interaction and phosphorylation occur independently from the ligand-binding [43], the data suggest that TRIP-1 may play an important role in the signal transduction of TGF-β.

In addition, interaction between the intracellular domains of type I and type II receptors can be seen in the yeast two-hybrid system [44]. The interaction was observed only between type I and type II receptors, but not between type II receptors, or between type I receptors. The type I—type II receptor interaction observed in the two-hybrid system does not necessarily reflect the association that occurs physiologically in mammalian cells. For example, the ActR-I and TβR-II kinase domains interact with each other in the yeast system [44], but this is not seen in mammalian cells, except in the cells which are transfected with the receptor cDNAs and therefore overexpress the receptor molecules [19]. The interaction between type I and type II receptor intracellular domains can be used to obtain novel serine/threonine kinase receptors; a human BMP type II receptor (BMPR-II) was isolated by the yeast two-hybrid system using the TβR-I intracellular domain as a bait [26, 45].

TGF-β AND CANCER

Since TGF-β is a potent growth inhibitor for many different cell types, escape from the growth inhibition by TGF-β may lead to uncontrolled growth of cancer cells. Upregulation of the TGF-β receptors is sometimes observed during the progression of cancer [46]. However, recent data revealed that loss of TβR-II can be seen in various transformed cells, including T-cell malignancies,

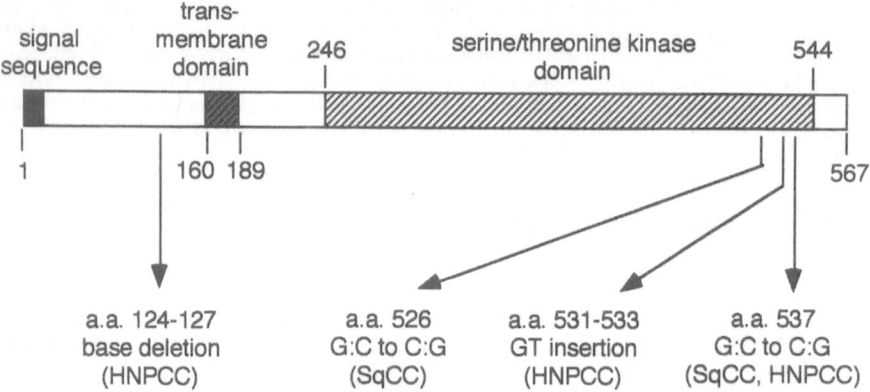

Fig. 6. Mutations in TβR-II. SqCC, squamous cell carcinoma.

gastric carcinoma, colon carcinoma, and squamous head and neck carcinoma [47-51, and our unpublished data].

In hereditary nonpolyposis colon cancer (HNPCC) with DNA repair defect, base deletion was seen in the 10 repeating adenines at nucleotides 709-718, which results in the truncation of TβR-II protein at amino acids 124-127 (Fig. 6) [49, 50]. Introduction of the wild type TβR-II gene into the TGF-β-resistant colon carcinoma cells resulted in the restoration, at least in part, of the responsiveness to TGF-β [52].

In addition, mutations in the serine/threonine kinase domain were seen in HNPCC and squamous head and neck carcinomas [49-51]. Mutation in Glu-526 to Gln resulted in the decreased TβR-II kinase activity, whereas that in Arg-537 to Pro (R537P) led to the increased kinase activity of TβR-II [51]. Despite the increased TβR-II kinase activity, the cells with the R537P mutant of TβR-II did not respond to TGF-β, but its mechanism remains to be determined. These data suggest that the TβR-II gene may be one of the major targets of mutation during the process of carcinogenesis.

PERSPECTIVES

Current studies led to the identification of various serine/threonine kinase receptors for the proteins in the TGF-β superfamily. Mechanisms of activation of serine/threonine kinase receptors have revealed the importance of transactivation of the type I receptors by the type II receptors. Future studies will be aimed at the further study on the identification of downstream components of the serine/threonine kinase receptors, and the elucidation of their intracellular signal transduction pathways. Moreover, understanding the TGF-β receptor and signal transduction pathway may allow us to design novel ways for the treatment of various disorders.

ACKNOWLEDGEMENTS: I would like to thank P. ten Dijke, T. Imamura, C.-H. Heldin (Ludwig Institute for Cancer Research, Uppsala, Sweden), M. Kawabata, H. Ichijo, M. Kato, H. Yamashita, and T. Okadome (the Cancer Institute, Tokyo) for collaboration. This work was in part supported by Grants-in-Aid from Ministry of Education, Science and Culture, Japan, and Haraguchi Memorial Cancer Research Fund.

REFERENCES

1. Miyazono K, ten Dijke P, Ichijo H, Heldin C-H (1994) Receptors for transforming growth factor-β. Adv Immunol 55: 181-220
2. Kingsley DM (1994) The TGF-β superfamily: new members, new receptors, and new genetic tests of function in different organisms. Genes Dev 8: 133-146
3. Roberts AB, Sporn MB (1990) The transforming growth factor-βs. In: Sporn MB, Roberts AB (eds) Peptide growth factors and their receptors, part I. Springer-Verlag, Berlin, pp 419-472
4. Sporn MB, Roberts AB (1992) Transforming growth factor-β: Recent progress and new challenges. J Cell Biol 119: 1017-1021
5. Shull MM, Ormsby I, Kier AB, Pawlowski S, Diebold RJ, Yin M, Allen R, Sidman C, Proetzel G, Calvin D, Annunziata N, Doetschman T (1992) Targeted disruption of the mouse transforming growth factor-β1 gene results in multifocal inflammatory disease. Nature 359: 693-699
6. Kulkarni AB, Huh C-G, Becker D, Geiser A, Lyght M, Flanders KC, Roberts AB, Sporn MB, Ward JM, Karlsson S (1993) Transforming growth factor β1 null mutation in mice causes excessive inflammatory response and early death. Proc Natl Acad Sci USA 90: 770-774
7. Mathews LS (1994) Activin receptors and cellular signaling by the receptor serine kinase family. Endocrine Rev 15: 310-325
8. Murata M, Eto Y, Shibai H, Sakai M, Muramatsu M (1988) Erythroid differentiation factor is encoded by the same mRNA as that of the inhibin βA chain. Proc Natl Acad Sci USA 85: 2434-2438
9. Wozney JM (1989) Bone morphogenetic proteins. Prog Growth Factor Res 1: 267-280
10. Reddi AH (1992) Regulation of cartilage and bone differentiation by bone morphogenetic proteins. Curr Opin Cell Biol 4: 850-855
11. Reddi AH (1994) Bone and cartilage differentiation. Curr Opin Genet Develop 4: 737-744
12. Winnier G, Blessing M, Labosky PA, Hogan BL (1995) Bone morphogenetic protein-4 is required for mesoderm formation and patterning in the mouse. Genes Dev 9: 2105-2116
13. Miyazono K, ten Dijke P, Yamashita H, Heldin C-H (1994) Signal transduction via serine/threonine kinase receptors. Seminars Cell Biol 5: 389-398
14. Massagué J, Attisano L, Wrana JL (1994) The TGF-β family and its composite receptors. Trends Cell Biol 4: 172-178
15. Derynck R (1994) TGF-β-receptor-mediated signaling. Trends Biochem Sci 19: 548-553
16. ten Dijke P, Miyaono K, Heldin C-H (1996) Signaling via hetero-oligomeric complexes of type I and type II serine/threonine kinase receptors. Curr Opin Cell Biol (in press)
17. ten Dijke P, Ichijo H, Franzén P, Schulz P, Saras J, Toyoshima H, Heldin C-H, Miyazono K (1993) Activin receptor-like kinases; A novel subclass of cell surface receptors with predicted serine/threonine kinase activity. Oncogene 8: 2879-2887
18. Franzén P, ten Dijke P, Ichijo H, Yamashita H, Schulz P, Heldin C-H, Miyazono K (1993) Cloning of a TGFβ type I receptor that forms a heteromeric complex with the TGFβ type II receptor. Cell 75: 781-792
19. ten Dijke P, Yamashita H, Ichijo H, Franzén P, Laiho M, Miyazono K, Heldin C-H (1994) Characterization of type I receptors for transforming growth factor-β and activin. Science 264: 101-104
20. Lin HY, Wang X-F, Ng-Eaton E, Weinberg RA, Lodish HF (1992) Expression cloning of the TGF-β type II receptor, a functional transmembrane serine/threonine kinase. Cell 68: 775-785
21. Wrana JL, Attisano L, Cárcamo J, Zentella A, Doody J, Laiho M, Wang X-F, Massagué J (1992) TGFβ signals through a heteromeric protein kinase receptor complex. Cell 71: 1003-1014
22. Letsou A, Arora K, Wrana JL, Simin K, Twombly V, Jamal J, Staehling-Hampton K, Hoffmann FM, Gelbart WM, Massagué J, O'Connor MB (1995) Drosophila Dpp signaling is mediated by the *punt* gene product: A dual ligand-binding type II receptor of the TGFβ receptor family. Cell 80: 899-908
23. ten Dijke P, Yamashita H, Sampath TK, Reddi AH, Estevez M, Riddle DL, Ichijo H, Heldin C-H, Miyazono K (1994) Identification of type I receptors for osteogenic protein-1 and bone morphogenetic protein-4. J Biol Chem 269: 16985-16988

24. Koenig BB, Cook JS, Wolsing DH, Ting J, Tiesman JP, Correa PE, Olson CA, Pecquet AL, Ventura F, Grant RA, Chen G-X, Wrana JL, Massagué J, Rosenbaum JS (1994) Characterization and cloning of a receptor for BMP-2 and BMP-4 from NIH 3T3 cells. Mol Cell Biol 14:5961-5974

25. Rosenzweig BL, Imamura T, Okadome T, Cox GN, Yamashita H, ten Dijke P, Heldin C-H, Miyazono K (1995) Cloning and characterization of a human type II receptor for bone morphogenetic proteins. Proc Natl Acad Sci USA 92: 7632-7636

26. Liu F, Ventura F, Doody J, Massagué J (1995) Human type II receptor for bone morphogenetic proteins (BMPs): extension of the two-kinase receptor model to the BMPs. Mol Cell Biol 15: 3479-3486

27. Nohno T, Ishikawa T, Saito T, Hosokawa K, Noji S, Hanse Wolsing D, Rosenbaum JS (1995) Identification of a human type II receptor for bone morphogenetic protein-4 that forms differential heteromeric complexes with bone morphogenetic protein type I receptor. J Biol Chem 270: 22522-22526

28. Wrana JL, Attisano L, Wieser R, Ventura F, Massagué J (1994) Mechanism of activation of the TGF-β receptor. Nature 370: 341-347 ,

29. Henis YI, Moustakas A, Lin HY, Lodish HF (1994) The types II and III transforming growth factor-β receptors form homo-oligomers. J Cell Biol 126: 139-154

30. Chen R-H, Derynck R (1994) Homomeric interactions between type II transforming growth factor-β receptors. J Biol Chem 269: 22868-22874

31. Yamashita H, ten Dijke P, Franzén P, Miyazono K, Heldin C-H (1994) Formation of hetero-oligomeric complexes of type I and type II receptors for transforming growth factor-β. J Biol Chem 269: 20172-20178

32. Okadome T, Yamashita H, Franzén P, Morén A, Heldin C-H, Miyazono K (1994) Distinct roles of the intracellular domains of transforming growth factor-β type I and type II receptors in signal transduction. J Biol Chem 269: 30753-30756

33. Vivien D, Attisano L, Wrana JL, Massagué J (1995) Signaling activity of homologous and heterologous transforming growth factor-β receptor kinase complexes. J Biol Chem 270: 7134-7141

34. Franzén P, Heldin C-H, Miyazono K (1995) The GS domain of the transforming growth factor-β type I receptor is important in signal transduction. Biochem Biophys Res Commun 207: 682-689

35. Wieser R, Wrana JL, Massagué J (1995) GS domain mutations that constitutively activate TβR-I, the downstream signaling component in the TGF-β receptor complex. EMBO J 14: 2199-2208

36. Saitoh M, Nishitoh H, Amagasa T, Miyazono K, Takagi M, Ichijo H (1996) Identification of important regions in the cytoplasmic juxtamembrane domain of type I receptor that separate signaling pathways of transforming growth factor-β. J Biol Chem (in press)

37. Yamashita H, Okadome T, Franzén P, ten Dijke P, Heldin C-H, Miyazono K (1995) A rat pituitary tumor cell line (GH3) expresses type I and type II receptors and other cell surface binding protein(s) for transforming growth factor-β. J Biol Chem 270: 770-774

38. Moustakas A, Takumi T, Lin HY, Lodish HF (1995) GH3 pituitary tumor cells contain heteromeric type I and type II receptor complexes for transforming growth factor β and activin-A. J Biol Chem 270: 765-769

39. Cárcamo J, Weis FMB, Ventura F, Wieser R, Wrana JL, Attisano L, Massagué J (1994) Type I receptors specify growth-inhibitory and transcriptional responses to transforming growth factor β and activin. Mol Cell Biol 14: 3810-3821

40. Yamashita H, ten Dijke P, Huylebroeck D, Sampath TK, Andries M, Smith JC, Heldin C-H, Miyazono K (1995) Osteogenic protein-1 binds to activin type II receptors and induces certain activin-like effects. J Cell Biol 130: 217-226

41. Wang T, Donahoe PK, Zervos AS (1994) Specific interaction of type I receptors of the TGF-β family with the immunophilin FKBP-12. Science 265: 674-676

42. Kawabata M, Imamura T, Miyazono K, Engel ME, Moses HL (1995) Interaction of the TGF-β type I receptor with farnesyl-protein transferase-α. J Biol Chem (in press)

43. Chen R-H, Miettinen PJ, Maruoka EM, Choy L, Derynck R (1995) A WD-domain protein that is associated with and phosphorylated by the type II TGF-β receptor. Nature 377: 548-552

44. Chen R-H, Moses HL, Maruoka EM, Derynck R, Kawabata M (1995) Phosphorylation-dependent interaction of the cytoplasmic domains of the type I and type II transforming growth factor-β receptors. J Biol Chem 270: 12235-12241

45. Kawabata M, Chytil A, Moses HL (1995) Cloning of a novel type II serine/threonine kinase receptor through interaction with the type I transforming growth factor-β receptor. J Biol Chem 270: 5625-5630

46. Yamada N, Kato M, Yamashita H, Nistér M, Miyazono K, Heldin C-H, Funa K (1995) Enhanced expression of transforming growth factor-β and its type I and type II receptors in human glioblastoma tissues. Int J Cancer 62: 386-392

47. Kadin ME, Cavaille-Coll MW, Gertz R, Massagué J, Cheifetz S, George D (1994) Loss of receptors for transforming growth factor β in human T-cell malignancies. Proc Natl Acad Sci USA 91: 6002-6006

48. Park K, Kim S-J, Bang Y-J, Park J-G, Kim NK, Roberts AB, Sporn MB (1994) Genetic changes in the transforming growth factor β (TGFβ) type II receptor gene in human gastric cancer cells: correlation with sensitivitiy to TGFβ. Proc Natl Acad Sci USA 91: 8772-8776

49. Markowitz S, Wang J, Myeroff L, Parsons R, Sun L, Lutterbaugh J, Fan RS, Zborowska E, Kinzler KW, Vogelstein B, Brattain M, Willson JKV (1995) Inactivation of the type II TGFβ receptor in colon cancer cells with microsatellite instability. Science 268: 1336-1338

50. Lu S-L, Akiyama Y, Nagasaki H, Saitoh K, Yuasa Y (1995) Mutations of the transforming growth factor-β type II receptor gene and genomic instability in hereditary nonpolyposis colorectal cancer. Biochem Biophys Res Commun 216: 452-457

51. Garrigue-Antar L, Munoz-Antonia T, Antonia SJ, Gesmonde J, Vellucci VF, Reiss M (1995) Missense mutations of the transforming growth factor β type II receptor in human head and neck squamous carcinoma cells. Cancer Res 55: 3982-3987

52. Wang J, Sun L, Myeroff L, Wang X, Gentry LE, Yang J, Liang J, Zborowska E, Markowitz S, Willson JKV, Brattain MG (1995) Demonstration that mutation of the type II transforming growth factor β receptor inactivates its tumor suppressor activity in replication error-positive colon carcinoma cells. J Biol Chem 270: 22044-22049

53. Higgins DG, Sharp PM (1989) Fast and sensitive multiple sequence alignments on a microcomputer. Comput Appl Biosci 5: 151-153

Anti-Apoptotic Role of Protein-Tyrosine Kinases During Granulocytic Differentiation of HL-60 Cells

Takuya Katagiri#, Kazunari K. Yokoyama†, Shinkichi Irie* and Koko Katagiri*#

#Department of Immunology, Center for Basic Research, The Kitasato Institute, 5-9-1 Shirokane, Minato-ku, Tokyo 108, Japan: †Tsukuba Life Science Center, The Institute of Physical and Chemical Research, 3-1-1 Koyadai, Tsukuba, Ibaraki 305, Japan; *Institute of Biomatrix, Nippi Inc., 1-1-1 Senju-Midori-chou, Adachi-ku, Tokyo 120, Japan

Summary

The human promyelocytic leukemia cell line HL-60 can be induced to differentiate towards neutrophils and subsequently die via apoptosis *in vitro*. In this paper, we investigated the roles of protein tyrosine kinases (PTKs) in retinoic acid (RA)-induced granulocytic differentiation of HL-60 cells. Accompanying the RA-induced differentiation, Lyn and Fgr PTKs were phosphorylated on their tyrosine residues and their activities were induced. The degree of both activities and tyrosine-phosphorylation of these PTKs was reduced to be minimal at day 5 when the HL-60 cells start to be dead by apoptosis. The inhibitors of PTKs, herbimycin A and genistine, were demonstrated to cause premature cell death of HL-60 cells in the presence of RA. The death was the consequence of an apoptotic process. The RA-treated HL-60 cells, when incubated with specific *c-lyn* or *c-fgr* antisense oligodeoxy-nucleotide, also underwent premature death. These data implicate that Lyn and Fgr PTKs prevent programmed cell death to promote granulocytic differentiation of HL-60 cells.

Key Words : apoptosis, retinoic acid, HL-60 cells, granulocytic differentiation, protein-tyrosine kinases (PTKs)

Introduction

The human promyelocytic leukemia cell line HL-60, upon stimulation with RA *in vitro*, undergoes differentiation towards neutrophils at day 3 to day 4 and dies via apoptosis at day 6 to day 8 (1). Neutrophil are the first cells to accumulate at the site of inflammation and plays a critical role in inducing various inflammatory events. As soon as neutrophils complete their roles at the inflammatory site, they die via apoptosis and are removed by macrophages to limit tissue injury since they release harmful molecules such as proteolytic enzymes. Therefore, molecular analysis for the events after stimulation of HL-60 cells with RA will provide a useful information on both the differentiation and the apoptosis of neutrophils. The protein tyrosine kinases (PTKs) play crucial roles in the intracellular signal transduction for growth and differentiation of the cells. Recently, we reported that PTKs play essential roles in TPA-induced monocytic differentiation of HL-60 cells (2,3,4), and that Ras and GAP complex function downstream of PTKs during the differentiation (5). In addition, our previous paper described the induction of *src* family PTKs, *lyn* and *fgr* mRNA during RA-induced granulocytic differentiation (2). We have therefore investigated the role of PTKs in the differentiation. In the current study, Lyn and Fgr PTKs were demonstrated to act, instead of Bcl-2, as anti-apoptotic agents to promote granulocytic differentiation of HL-60 cells.

Materials and Methods

Cells.   HL-60 cells were suspended with RPMI1640 medium containing 10% FCS. For differentiation experiments, growing cells were subcultured at a density of 2×10^5 cells/ml, and inducers were added to the medium at the following concentrations: $1\mu M$ for retinoic acid(RA)(Sigma Chemical Co., St. Louis, MO) and 10ng/ml for 12-O-tetradecanoyl phorbol-13-acetate (TPA) (Sigma). Herbimycin A (0.1 and 0.2μg/ml)(Gibco, Grand Island, NY) and genistein (10μg/ml) (Funakoshi Inc., Tokyo, Japan) were also added to the medium.

Immunoprecipitation. RA-treated cells (1×10^7) were collected by centrifugation and lysed at 0_o C for 60 min in 1 ml of lysis buffer (1% Triton X-100, 20mM Tris amino-methane, 150mM NaCl, 2mM EDTA, 2μg/ml aprotinin, 2μg/ml leupeptin, 1mM PMSF, 1mM Na3VO4, 10mM NaF; pH7.6). The supernatant was precleared by incubation with excess amount of protein G-Sepharose 4B (Pharmacia Fine Chemicals, Piscataway, NJ). The cleared lysate was incubated with specific antibodies and protein G-Sepharose 4B. The immunoprecipitates were washed with the lysis buffer extensively.

Immunoblotting. The 10μl of the cell lysate (10^6 cells) or the immunoprecipitated proteins were subjected to electrophoresis on 9% polyacrylamide/SDS gel. The transfer of the proteins to polyvinylidene difluoride membrane (PVDF, Pharmacia) and the blotting with specific antibody or ^{125}I-PY-20 was carried out. ECL (enhanced chemiluminescence) system (Amersham) or autoradiography was applied to detection.

Analysis of DNA fragmentation. DNA pellet obtained from HL-60 cells was resuspended in 200μl TE buffer, separated (5μg DNA per lane) by horizontal electrophoresis (2V/cm) in 1% agarose gel with running buffer containing 90mM Tris-HCl, 90mM boric acid, and 2mM EDTA pH8.0, stained with 0.5μg/ml ethidium bromide, and visualized under ultraviolet light.

Treatment of HL-60 cells with antisense phosphorothioate oligonucleotides (PONs). We synthesized antisense PONs complementary to position 142-162 of human *c-fgr* sequence (CCTGGAATGGGCTGTGTGTTC) and 292-312 of human *c-lyn* sequence (GGAAATATGGGATGTATAAAA). Sense PONs corresponding to each position were prepared as controls. Sense (S) or antisense (AS)*c-lyn* or S or AS *c-fgr* PONs was added to the culture medium for HL-60 cells at the concentration of 20μM. After 4 days of PONs treatment, the culture medium was replaced with fresh medium containing 20μM S or AS PONs, and 1μM of RA was added to the cultures.

Results

Tyrosine-phosphorylation of protein molecules during granulocytic differentiation.
By using immunoblotting with anti-phosphotyrosine antibody (PY-20), tyrosine-phosphorylation of protein molecules was investigated during RA-induced granulocytic differentiation of HL-60 cells (Fig. 1). Protein tyrosine phosphorylation was detected within 12 hours after the stimulation and reached a plateau at day 2 and declined thereafter to the minimum at day 5 (Fig. 1). As shown in Fig.1, the protein molecules of MW 53 to 56 kD were markedly tyrosine phosphorylated. To identify the tyrosine-phosphorylated proteins, we examined the tyrosine phosphorylation of Lyn (p53^{lyn} and p56^{lyn}) and Fgr (p55^{fgr}) because the kinetics of expressions of both PTKs were similar to those of tyrosine-phosphorylation of the 53 to 56 kD proteins (Fig.1). As shown in Fig.2 (left), Lyn and Fgr PTKs were highly tyrosine-phosphorylated in RA-treated cells, but not in TPA-treated cells. Absorption with anti-Lyn and anti-Fgr antibody plus protein G-Sepharose 4B demonstrated that the major tyrosine-phosphorylated proteins of MW 53 to 56 kD were Lyn and Fgr PTKs (Fig.2 right).

Effect of herbimycin A on granulocytic differentiation of HL-60 cells.
To know the role of tyrosine kinases in the RA-induced granulocytic differentiation of HL-60 cells, we investigated the effects of herbimycin A on the differentiation. By using a method of Giemza-Wright staining of the cells, we observed an apoptotic cell death of HL-60 cells treated with herbimycin A during RA-induced granulocytic differentiation. Apoptotic cell death of HL-60 cells treated with herbimycin A plus RA was confirmed by detecting the ladder pattern of DNA cleavage in these cells (Fig.3). In contrast, the DNA remained unfragmented in the preparation obtained from HL-60 cells treated with RA, herbimycin A, or TPA plus herbimycin A for 48 hrs.

Induction of apoptosis in lyn or fgr antisense PONs-treated HL-60 cells in the presence of RA.
As tyrosine kinases were demonstrated to be involved in the RA-induced apoptosis of HL-60 cells (Fig. 3), we focused on the two tyrosine kinases, Lyn and Fgr, and prepared antisense phosphorothioate oligonucleotides (PONs) specific for them. We confirmed the strong suppression of the expression of Lyn and Fgr PTKs in HL-60 cells by treatment of the cells with specific antisense PONs (data not shown). When the antisense PONs-treated HL-60 cells were stimulated with RA for 48 hr, more than 80% of the cells died with immature characteristics (Fig.4). However, sense PONs-treated HL-60 cells were demonstrated to have no indication of cell death. The cell death appeared to be characteristics of apoptosis under microscopic observation (data not shown).

Figure1. (upper) Protein-tyrosine
phosphorylation in HL-60 cells after
stimulation with retinoic acid.
The lysates from the HL-60 cells stimulated
with RA for 0, 1, 2 or 5 days were
immunoblotted with ^{125}I-labeled PY-20.
The autoradiograph was exposed for 24
hours at -80°C with an intensifier screen.
 (lower) Expressions of Lyn, Fgr and actin
in HL-60 cells after stimulation with RA.
The lysates from the HL-60 cells stimulated
with RA for 0, 1, 2 or 5 days were
immunoblotted with anti-Lyn, anti-Fgr and
anti-actin. The bands were detected by ECL
assay system.

Figure 2. Lyn and Fgr were major
phosphotyrosine-containing proteins in
RA-treated HL-60 cells. (left) The lysates
from the HL-60 cells treated with TPA or
RA for 48 hours were immunoprecipitated
with polyclonal anti-Lyn or anti-Fgr
antibodies and protein G-Sepharose 4B. The
immunoprecipitates were subjected to
electrophoresis, transferred to PVDF filter,
immunoblotted with ^{125}I-labeled PY-20
and autoradiographed. (right) The lysates
from RA-treated HL-60 cells were
immunoprecipitated with anti-Lyn plus
anti-Fgr (anti-Lyn+anti-Fgr) or rabbit IgG
(RIg). The supernatant was subjected to
SDS-PAGE, transferred to a PVDF filter,
and immunoblotted with ^{125}I-labeled PY-
20.

Fugure 3.   DNA fragmentation in the HL-
60 cells treated with RA plus herbimycin A.
The high molecular weight DNA extracted
from untreated HL-60 cells (None), from
HL-60 cells treated with 0.2µg/ml of
herbimycin A (H0.2), from HL-60 cells
induced to differentiate with 1µM of RA for
2 days (RA), from HL-60 cells induced to
differentiate with 10ng/ml of TPA (TPA)
for 2 days, from HL-60 cells treated with
TPA plus herbimycin A (TPA+H0.2) or
fragmented DNA from HL-60 cells treated
with RA plus herbimycin A (RA+H0.2) for
2 days were subjected to agarose gel
electrophoresis.

Figure 4.   Viability of HL-60 cells
cultured for 2 days in the absence (None) or
presence (RA) of RA after treatment with c-
lyn or c-fgr S or AS oligomer.   Cell
viability was assessed by the ability of the
cells to exclude trypan blue. The average
and SE of triplicate determination are
shown.

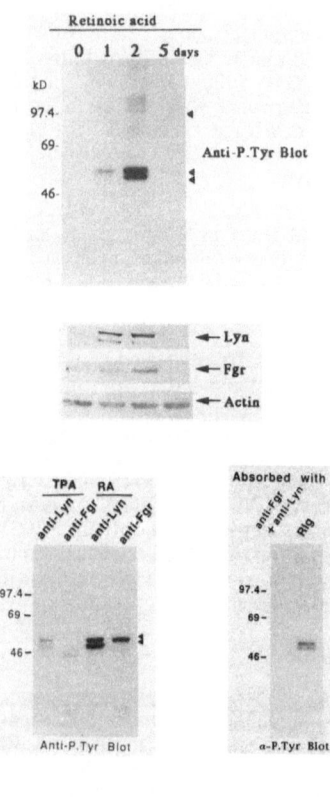

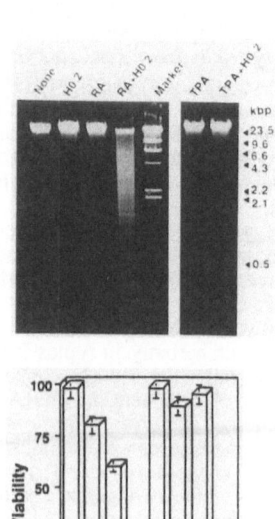

Discussion

The regulation system of apoptosis is highly organized and the balances between inducers and repressors determines the occurrence of apoptosis.   In the current study, two cytoplasmic tyrosine kinases, Lyn and Fgr were demonstrated to be members of the repressors for apoptosis of neutrophils.   Both Lyn and Fgr PTKs were shown to be induced and tyrosine-phosphorylated during differentiation of HL-60 cells towards neutrophils.   After completion of the differentiation, the expression of these PTKs was reduced to a minimum and the cells die via apoptosis.   Using antisense oligonucleotides specific for Lyn or Fgr PTK, it was demonstrated that inhibitiingexpression of either PTKs upon RA stimulation leads to premature cell death via apoptosis.   Consistent with the results, herbimycin A in combination with RA was exhibited to cause premature cell death of the HL-60 cells.   These data imply that Lyn and Fgr PTKs exert an anti-apoptotic effect to promote differentiation of HL-60 cells towards neutrophils.

In neutrophils, Lyn has been demonstrated to be activated and associated with PI3 kinase accompanying the stimulation with granulocyte macrophage-colony stimulating factor (GM-CSF). It was shown that granulocyte- colony stimulating factor (G-CSF) activated Lyn and Syk (p72^{syk}) both of which were then recruited into G-CSF receptor signaling complex in human peripheral neutrophils (6).   While, Fgr is associated with FcγIIR after stimulation with a chemotactic agonist on neutrophils and agonists of β2 integrin activation such as TNF, TPA and FMLP enhance the kinase activity of Fgr in human neutrophils (7). Our data on the anti-apoptotic role of Lyn and Fgr PTK in the granulocytic differentiation of HL-60 cells will add a new insight into the function of these PTKs in the neutrophils.

As RA induces growth arrest and terminal differentiation in some promyelocytic leukemia cell lines, RA has been utilized as a differentiation therapy for treatment of patients with acute promyelocytic leukemia (8).   In the current study, RA in combination with a small amount of herbimycin A was found to be a potent agent to induce apoptosis of the promyelocytic leukemia cell line HL-60. Although its validity and toxicity should be scrutinized using experimental animals, careful treatment with the combination of the agents will improve the remedial value exhibited by RA alone. For more specifically refined treatment, further studies on the molecular mechanisms of the anti-apoptotic function of tyrosine kinases are required.

REFERENCES

1. Martin, J., Bradley, J.G., and Cotter, T.G. (1990)
     Clin. Exp. Immunol.   **79**, 448-453.
2. Katagiri, K., Katagiri, T., Koyama, Y., Morikawa, M., Yamamoto, T., and Yoshida, T. (1991)
     J.Immonol.   **146**, 701-707.
3. Katagiri, K., Katagiri, T., Kajiyama, K., Uehara, Y., Yamamoto, T., and Yoshida, T. (1992)
     Cell. Immunol.   **140**, 282-294.
4. Katagiri, K., Katagiri, T., Kajiyama, K., Yamamoto, T., and Yoshida, T. (1993)
     J. Immunol.   **150**, 585-593.
5. Katagiri, K., Hattori, S., Nakamura, S., Yamamoto, T., Yoshida, T., and Katagiri, T. (1994)
     Blood   **84**, 1780-1789.
6. Corey, S. J., Burkhardt, A. L., Bolen, J. B., Geahlen, R. L., Tkatch, L. S., and Tweardy,
     D.,J. (1994)   Proc. Natl. Acad. Sci. USA   **91**, 4683-4687.
7. Berton, G., Fumagalli, L., Laudanna, C., and Sorio, C.   (1994)
     J. Cell Biol.   **126**, 1111-1121.
8. Castaigne,S., Chomienne,C., Daniel, M.T., Ballerini, P., Berger, R., Fenaux, P., and Degos,
     L. (1990)   Blood   **76**, 1704-1717

Fibronectin Rescues Bone Marrow Cells from Apoptosis with IgG

Kachio Tasaka, Hideshi Yoshikawa, and Toshiko Sakihama

Department of Parasitology & Immunology, Yamanashi Medical University, Shimokato, Tamaho, Nakakoma, Yamanashi, 409-38 Japan

SUMMARY

The FDC-P2/185-4 cell line (185-4) is an IL-3 dependent cell line derived from murine bone marrow. 185-4 cell began to die due to apoptosis 12 hours after depletion of IL-3. However, addition of fibronectin with normal IgG rescued the cells from apoptosis by an autocrine mechanism of IL-3. However neither fibronectin alone nor IgG alone induced IL-3. Addition of either RDG peptide or anti-integrin VLA-4 or anti FcγRIII mAb 2.4G2 blocked IL-3 induction, indicating that integrin VLA-5 and FcγRIII are both indispensable cell surface molecules for signal transduction. Other ECM, such as collagen and laminin had no such effect. Thus, fibronectin may play an important role in regulating hematopoietic cells in bone marrow by rescuing them from apoptosis in collaboration with IgG.

KEY WORDS: fibronectin, IL-3, FcR, integrin, bone marrow cell

INTRODUCTION

Fibronectin (FN) is a major extracellular matrix (ECM) and component, constituting the milieu of bone marrow. Here, we show that FN is not only a supportive material but also induces a signal to bone marrow cells via integrin(s) rescuing 185-4 cells from apoptosis by inducing cytokines with co-stimulation of FcγRIII.

MATERIALS AND METHODS

The FDC-P2 cell line was originally established by Dexter from DBA/2 mouse bone marrow as an IL-3 dependent cell line [1]. FDC-P2/185-4 cells were cloned from FDC-P2 cells in our laboratory as a responding cell line to the MRL/*lpr* mouse IgG [2]. Cell growth was measured by an MTT assay [3]. The anti-VLA-4 antibody, anti-integrin α5 mAb and Fab of anti-integrin α5 mAb were gifts from Dr. H. Yagita, Juntendo University. The anti FcγRII/III monoclonal antibody 2.4G2 was a gift from Dr. M. Inaba, Kansai Medical University.

RESULTS

Apoptosis of 185-4 cell occurred 12-24 hours after depletion of IL-3.

On depletion of IL-3 from the medium, the fragmentation of DNA, stained with PI, was detected 12 hours after by flow cytometry. Ladder formation of DNA was detected 24 hours after by

139

electrophoresis, showing apoptosis of 185-4 cells [4].

Anti-integrin α5 mAb rescued the cells from apoptosis but Fab did not.

After addition of anti-integrin α5 mAb to 185-4 cells in the absence of IL-3, the cells proliferated in a dose dependent manner, but the addition of the Fab of anti-integrin α5 mAb did not cause any cell proliferation, as shown in figure 1, indicating the necessity of FcR for cell growth.

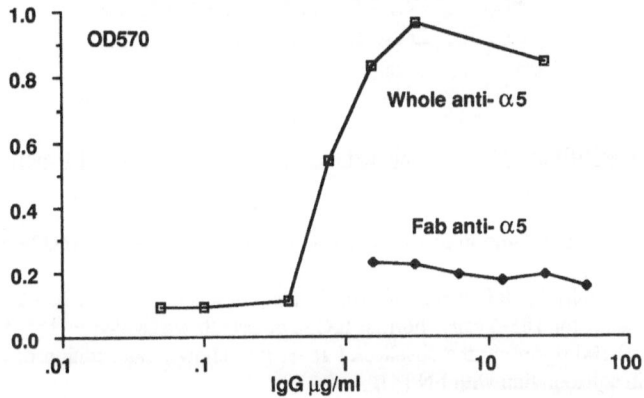

Fig.1 Whole anti-Integrin α5 mAb induced proliferation but Fab did not.

Anti IL-3 antisera inhibited the proliferation of 185-4 cells, induced by anti integrin α5 mAb.

Anti IL-3 rabbit antisera inhibited proliferation of 185-4 cells, induced by addition of anti integrin α5 mAb. Normal rabbit serum as a control had no such effect, suggesting that cell proliferation induced by anti integrin α5 mAb is due to an autocrine mechanism of IL-3 (Fig.2).

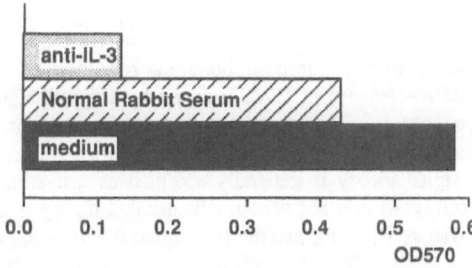

Fig.2 Anti IL-3 antiserum inhibited proliferation induced by anti-integrin α5 mAb.

Anti FcγR II/III mAb 2.4G2 inhibited the proliferation induced by anti integrin α5 mAb.

Anti FcγR II/III mAb 2.4G2 inhibited 185-4 cell proliferation induced by anti integrin α5 mAb. Normal rat IgG as a control had no such effect. This suggests that the signal via FcγRII/III of the 185-4 cell is indispensable for 185-4 cells to proliferate (Fig.3).

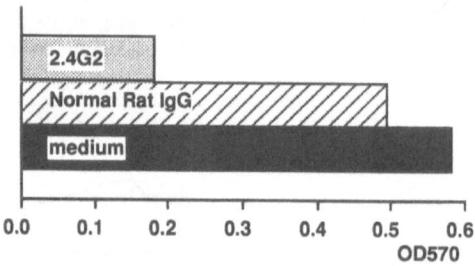

Fig.3   Anti FcγRII/III mAb 2.4G2 inhibited proliferation induced by anti-Integrin α5 mAb.

Fibronectin induced proliferation of 185-4 cells in the presence of normal IgG2a or IgG2b.

FcγR II/III has affinity for IgG2a and IgG2b. To analyze whether normal IgG2a or IgG2b provides enough stimulation for 185-4 cells, normal IgG2a or IgG2b was added to 185-4 cells with various doses of FN (0-100 µg/ml) in the absence of IL-3. It is shown that addition of either IgG induced proliferation in collaboration with FN [4].

Anti VLA-4 Ab or RGD inhibited 185-4 cell proliferation induced by   IgG2a or IgG2b in the presence of FN.

Anti VLA-4 mAb and RGD peptide are both inhibitors of FN for binding. Thus, to examine their effect on cell proliferation, anti VLA-4 mAb (10 µg/ml) or RGD in various concentrations(10-100 µg/ml) was added to 185-4 cells with IgG2a (1 µg/ml) or IgG2b (1 µg/ml) in the presence of FN. Both IgG2a and IgG2b, anti VLA-4 mAb or RGD (in a dose dependent manner) inhibited cell proliferation whereas control normal rat IgG or medium did not [4].

DISCUSSION

Herein, we present evidence that the murine bone marrow derived cell line FDC-P2/185-4 proliferates by an autocrine mechanism of IL-3, induced by the two signals of IgG and FN via FcγRIII and VLA-5 respectively. In our system VLA-4 is also involved in binding with FN as well as VLA-5. Another integrin family LFA-1 also had the same function (data not shown).   In T and B lymphocytes, the two signal theory is generally accepted as activating lymphocytes to induce cytokines, but   in other cell types it is not certain whether that theory is applicable or not. This is the first report to our knowledge showing that the two signal theory is applicable to other cell types such as myeloid precursor, 185-4 cells. Although mAb 2.4G2 cannot differentiate between FcγRII and FcγRIII, we have previously found that 185-4 cells have FcγRIII but not FcγRII by RT-PCR [4]. FcγRIII reportedly has a γ subunit which shares the TCR-CD3 complex and has a signal transduction function. Therefore, it is quite reasonable to assume that FcγRIII transduces a major signal like TCR and that the integrin molecule transduces a co-signal.   Integrin molecules are reportedly richer in immature hematopoietic cells than in mature cells [5]. Thus in bone marrow, where FN is abundant, integrin molecules on immature hematopoietic cells may play an important role together with IgG in the regulation of hematopoiesis, rescuing the cells from apoptosis.

REFERENCES

[1] Dexter TM, Garland J, Scott D, Scolnick E, Metcalf D (1980) Growth of factor-dependent hemopoietic precursor cell lines. J.Exp.Med.152:1036-1047

[2] Tasaka K, Sakihama T, Shirakura-Shibata Y, Matsuda S, Nakajima Y (1989) Proliferative activity of autoimmune MRL mouse serum IgG to interleukin 3 dependent line through autocrine mechanism.   Cell. Immunol. 121:317-327

[3] Mosmann TJ (1983) Rapid colorimetric assay for cellular growth and survival: Application to proliferation and cytotoxic assays.   J. Immunol. Methods. 65:55-63

[4] submitted for publication

[5] Papayannopoulou T, Brice M, Broudy VC, Zsebo KM (1991) Isolation of c-kit receptor-expressing cells from bone marrow, peripheral blood, and fetal liver : functional properties composite antigenic profile. Blood 78:1403-1412

Cytokine Gene Expression in Peripheral Blood Mononuclear Cells after Allogeneic Blood Stem Cell Transplantation

Junji Tanaka[1], Masahiro Imamura[1], Masaharu Kasai[2], Satoshi Hashino[1], Satoshi Noto[1], Sumiko Kobayashi[1], Keisuke Sakurada[1], Masahiro Asaka[1]

[1]Third Department of Internal Medicine, Hokkaido University School of Medicine, N15 W5, Kita-Ku, Sapporo 060, Japan. [2]Department of Internal Medicine, Sapporo Hokuyu Hospital, Higashi Sapporo 6-6, Shiroishi-Ku, Sapporo 003, Japan

SUMMARY

GVHD is one of the major complications of allogeneic bone marrow transplantation (allo BMT). Although it is mainly caused by donor T lymphocytes, cytokines play a central role in the regulation of immune responses, one manifestation of GVHD being the dysregulation of cytokines. Therefore, we have investigated inflammatory cytokine (IL-1β, IL-6, TNF-α), immunostimulatory cytokine (IL-2, IFN-γ) and immunosuppressive cytokines (IL-4, IL-10, IL-13) mRNA expression in peripheral blood mononuclear cells (PBMC) after allogeneic blood stem cell transplantation. This study shows that inflammatory cytokine mRNA expression in PBMC from severe GVHD ($\geq$grade III) patients increased compared with PBMC from allo BMT without severe GVHD and auto BMT patients. In contrast, immunosuppresive cytokine mRNA expression increased in patients without severe GVHD. On the other hand, immunostimulatory cytokine mRNA expression remained fairly consistent during GVHD. Therefore, it is suggested that the cytokine network system shifted to enhance inflammatory cytokines in severe GVHD patients, but to enhance the immunosuppresive cytokines in patients without severe GVHD.

KEY WORDS: bone marrow transplantation, cytokine, gene expression, graft-versus-host disease

INTRODUCTION

GVHD is one of the major complications of allogeneic bone marrow transplantation (allo BMT). Although it is mainly caused by donor T lymphocytes, cytokines play a central role in the regulation of immune responses, one manifestation of GVHD being the dysregulation of cytokines.[1-3] IL-2 and IFN-γ are critical in immunoresponse including alloresponse and also IL-1β, IL-6 and TNF-α are considered important in the development of clinical manifestation of GVHD. On the other hand, Th2 cytokines have suppressive effect on Th1 cells and inhibit immunoresponse. Therefore, we have investigated inflammatory cytokines such as interleukin (IL)-1β, IL-6 and TNF-α, immunostimulatory cytokines such as IL-2 and IFN-γ, and immunosuppressive cytokines such as IL-4, IL-10 and IL-13 mRNA expression in peripheral blood mononuclear cells (PBMC) after allo BMT by the method we have previously reported.[4-12]

PATIENTS AND METHODS

In this study, we analyzed twenty patients who received allo BMT from HLA matched donors. The conditioning regimens used were busulfan (4 mg/kg for 4 days) plus cyclophosphamide (60 mg/kg for 2 days) or cyclophosphamide (60 mg/kg for 2 days) and VP-16 (20 mg/ kg for 2 days) plus total body irradiation (12 Gy in 6 fractions). Allo BMT patients were administered cyclosporine A (3 mg/kg) and methotrexate (15 mg/m^2 for 1 day and 10 mg/kg for 3 days) as prophylaxis for GVHD. Mononuclear cells were obtained from heparinized fresh blood samples by centrifugation on a Ficoll-Hypaque gradient. Total RNA was then extracted from the cells using guanidine thiocyanate/phenol/chloroform. Each 5 μg of total RNA was reverse-transcribed with 600 U of murine Moloney leukemia virus reverse transcriptase (BRL, Grand Island, NY, USA) and 150 pmol of random hexamer. Each aliquot (1/20th) of the resulting cDNA was added to a reaction mixture containing 50 mM KCl, 10 mM Tris-HCl (pH 8.3), 1.5 mM MgCl$_2$, 0.01 % gelatin, 0.2 mM of deoxnucleotide triphosphates, 100 pmol of each primer and 2.5 U of Taq polymerase (Perkin Elmer Cetus, Norwalk, CT, USA).[4-9] Each mixture (100 μl) was overlaid with 50 μl of mineral oil and incubated in a thermal cycler for 1 min at 94 °C, 1 min at 60 °C and 2 min at 72 °C. After PCR amplification, 7 μl aliquots of the reaction mixture were removed and subjected to electrophoresis on 2 % agarose gel containing ethidium bromide. In this study, when cytokine mRNA expression could be detected after amplification of 20, 27 or 34 cycles for IL-1β, IL-2, IL-6, IFN-γ and TNF-α and 35, 40 or 45 cycles for IL-4, IL-10 and IL-13, they were defined as +++, ++, +, ± or -, according to increasing amounts of product detectable.

RESULTS

This study showed that IL-1β, IL-6 and TNF-α mRNA expression in PBMC from four severe GVHD patients (acute GVHD≥grade III and extensive chronic GVHD) were increased compared with in PBMC from nine patients without severe GVHD . In contrast, IL-4, IL-10 and IL-13 mRNA expression were not increased in five patients with severe GVHD compared with patients without severe GVHD. IL-2 was not detected in any patient in this assay. Also, IFN-γ expression was fairly consistent throughout the grades of GVHD (Table 1).

Table 1. Cytokine Gene Expression After Allo BMT

Clinical Status	IL-1β ≥+++	IL-6 ≥+	TNF-α ≥++	IL-2 -	IFN-γ ≥++	IL-4 ≥++	IL-10 + IL-13 ≥++
aGVHD ≤ II cGVHD(limited)	0/9 (0%)	0/9 (0)	1/9 (11)	9/9 (100)	3/9 (33)	5/14 (36)	11/12 (92)
aGVHD ≥ III cGVHD(extensive)	4/5 (80)	5/5 (100)	5/5 (100)	5/5 (100)	0/5 (0)	0/5 (0)	1/5 (20)

Abbreviations: aGVHD, acute graft-versus-host disease; cGVHD, chronic graft-versus-host disease; IFN, interferon; IL, interleukin; TNF, tumor necrosis factor.

DISCUSSION

Allo BMT is now frequently performed for the treatment of hematological malignancies and aplastic anemia. However, severe complications such as GVHD are frequent after allo BMT. Therefore, it is very important to diagnose and treat GVHD quickly and precisely.

GVHD may be induced when genetically disparate lymphocytes recognize the histocompatibility antigens of the host as foreign, become sensitized, and proliferate. They then attack the host skin, liver and gut, thereby producing the clinical syndrome of GVHD. Although this is mainly caused by donor T lymphocytes, cytokines play a central role in the regulation of immune responses, and one manifestation of GVHD is the dysregulation of cytokines. Cytokines produced by T lymphocytes, monocytes/macrophages, and fibroblasts play a central role in the immune response. It was considered that the dysregulated production of inflammatory cytokines was a primary mediator of clinical manifestation of acute GVHD.[1-3] The existence of type 1 T helper (Th1) and type 2 T helper (Th2) subsets of human CD4 T lymphocytes has been recently reported. It has also been reported that Th1 cells produce IL-2, IFN-γ and TNF-α while Th2 cells produce IL-4, IL-5, IL-6, IL-10 and IL-13.[13,14] Also, IL-4, IL-10 and IL-13 are usually considered to be important cytokines with inhibitory effects on Th1 cytokines and monokines. In addition, Th2 cells prevent LPS-induced lethality during murine graft-versus-host reaction. Th1 cytokines have an important role in the afferent phase of GVHD and Th1 response is critical for GVHD. However, Th1 response can be regulated by Th2 cytokines. In this study, we have demonstrated that IL-4, IL-10 and IL-13 gene expression in PBMC is suppressed in patients with severe GVHD but not in those without severe GVHD. In contrast, inflammatory cytokine gene expression increased in such severe GVHD patients. Therefore, it is thought that severe GVHD developed in allo BMT patients when the Th2 cytokines are suppressed and inflammatory cytokines are enhanced. Interestingly, IL-2 mRNA expression in PBMC was not detected by this assay despite being easily detected in the MLC system.[5-6] Therefore, IL-2 in PBMC itself may not be so upregulated in cyclosporine A administered allo BMT patients and IL-2 may be involved in afferent phase of GVHD as mainly autocrine manner and IL-2 receptor may be upregulated in severe GVHD patients[11]. Also, other cytokines such as IL-12[15] may represent a potent role in inducing severe GVHD without enhancing IL-2 mRNA expression in PBMC. In conclusion, the cytokine network system might shift to enhance inflammatory cytokines in severe GVHD patients, but shift to enhance immunosuppresive cytokines in patients without severe GVHD. Therefore, the cytokine network system has an important role in GVHD after allo BMT and influences the prognosis of BMT patients.

ACKNOWLEDGEMENTS

This work was supported in part by grants from the Idiopathic Disorders of Hematopoietic Organs Research Committee and Bone Marrow Transplantation Research Committee of the Ministry of Health and Welfare of Japan and a Grant-in-Aid for Scientific Research from the Ministry of Education, Science and Culture, Japan.

REFERENCES

1. Ferrara JLM, Deeg HJ. (1991) Graft versus host disease. N Engl J Med 324: 667-674.
2. Antin JH, Ferrara JLM. (1992) Cytokine dysregulation and acute graft-versus-host disease. Blood 80: 2964-2968.
3. Ferrara JLM. (1994) Paradigm shift for graft-versus-host disease. Bone Marrow Transplant. 14: 183.
4. Tanaka J, Imamura M, Kasai M, Masauzi N, Watanabe M, Matsuura A, Morii K, Kiyama Y, Naohara T, Higa T, Honke K, Gasa S, Sakurada K, Miyazaki T. (1993) Rapid analysis of tumor necrosis factor-alpha mRNA expression during veno-occlusive disease of the liver after allogeneic bone marrow transplantation. Transplantation 55: 430-432.
5. Tanaka J, Imamura M, Kasai M, Masauzi N, Matsuura A, Ohizumi H, Morii K, Kiyama Y, Naohara T, Higa T, Sakurada K, Miyazaki T. (1993) Cytokine gene expression in peripheral blood mononuclear cells during graft-versus-host disease after allogeneic bone marrow transplantation. Br J Haematol, 85: 558-565.
6. Tanaka J, Imamura M, Kasai M, Kobayashi S, Hashino S, Kobayashi H, Sakurada K, Miyazaki T. (1994) Cytokine gene expression in the mixed lymphocyte culture in allogeneic bone marrow transplantation as a predictive method for transplantation-related complications. Br J Haematol 87: 415-418.
7. Tanaka J, Imamura M, Kasai M, Zhu X, Kobayashi S, Imai K, Hashino S, Sakurada K, Miyazaki T. (1994) Cytokine gene expression by Concanavalin A-stimulated peripheral blood mononuclear cells after bone marrow transplantation: An indicator of immunological abnormality due to chronic graft-versus-host disease. Bone Marrow Transplant 14: 695-701.
8. Tanaka J, Imamura M, Zhu X, Kobayashi S, Imai K, Hashino S, Sakurada K, Kasai M, Higa T. (1994) Potential benefit of recombinant human granulocyte colony-stimulating factor-mobilized peripheral blood stem cells for allogeneic transplantation. Blood 84: 3595-3596.

9. Tanaka J, Imamura M, Kasai M, Sakurada K, Miyazaki T. (1995) Cytokine gene expression after allogeneic bone marrow transplantation. Leuk Lymphoma 16: 413-418.

10. Tanaka J, Imamura M, Kasai M, Sakurada K. (1995) Transplantation-related complications predicted by cytokine gene expression in the mixed lymphocyte culture in allogeneic bone marrow transplants. Leuk Lymphoma 19: 27-32.

11. Tanaka J, Imamura M, Kasai M, Zhu X, Kobayashi S, Hashino S, Higa T, Sakurada K, Asaka M. (1995) Cytokine receptor gene expression in peripheral blood mononuclear cells during graft-versus-host disease after allogeneic bone marrow transplantation. Leuk Lymphoma 19: 281-287.

12. Tanaka J, Imamura M, Kasai M, Zhu X, Kobayashi S, Hashino S, Higa T, Sakurada K, Asaka, M. Possible role of T cell surface molecule gene expression in the mixed lymphocyte culture for predicting trasnsplantation-related complications after allogeneic bone marrow transplantation. Eur J Haematol 55, 282-284, 1995.

13. Mosmann TR, Cherwinski H, Bond MW, Giedlin MA, Coffmann RL. (1986) Two types of murine helper T cell clone. 1.Definition according to profiles of lymphokine activities and secreted proteins. J Immunol 136: 2348-2357.

14. Salgame P, Abrams JS, Clayberger C, Goldstein H, Convit J, Modlin RL, Bloom BR. (1991) Differing lymphokine profiles of functional subsets of human CD4 and CD8 T cell clones. Science 254: 279-282.

15. Trinchieri G. (1994) Interleukin-12: A cytokine produced by antigen-presenting cells with immunoregulatory functions in the generation of T-helper cells type 1 and cytotoxic lymphocytes. Blood 84: 4008-4027.

In Vivo Effects of FLT-3 Ligand in Mice

Eishi Ashihara, Chihiro Shimazaki, Yoshikazu Sudo, Takehisa Kikuta, Hideyo Hirai, Toshoyuki Sumikuma, Noboru Yamagata, Hideo Goto, Tohru Inaba, Naohisa Fujita, and Masao Nakagawa[1]

[1]Second Department of Medicine, Kyoto Prefectural University of Medicine, 465 Kawaramachi-Hirokoji, Kamigyo-ku, Kyoto 602, Japan

SUMMARY

We investigated the effects of the administration of FLT-3 ligand (FL) on mobilization of hematopoietic stem and progenitor cells in mice. C57bl / 6J mice were injected subcutaneously with FL once a day for 5 days at doses of 20, 100, and 200 µg/kg. After the collection of peripheral blood, we determined the number of white blood cells (WBCs), and the formation of colony-forming cells (CFCs) in blood, bone marrow and spleen. The administration of FL at doses of 100 and 200 µg/kg increased the number of WBC up to 1.7- and 2.4-fold, respectively. Hematopoietic progenitor cells (HPCs) were mobilized into the blood dose-dependently. On Day 5, the number of HPCs was increased up to 2.2-, 2.8-, and 5.5-fold by the administration of FL at 20, 100, and 200 µg/kg, respectively. The number of HPCs in the bone marrow increased up to 1.9- to 3.8- fold. The number of HPCs in the spleen also increased up to 32-fold at a dose of 200 µg/kg FL. Mobilized peripheral blood mononuclear cells were transplanted into lethally irradiated mice and the number of CFU-S (Day 12) was scored. A dose-dependent mobilization of CFU-S (Day 12) into blood was observed. These observations suggest that FL can mobilize hematopoietic stem and progenitor cells into the blood of mice and those cells mobilized by FL may be applicable to peripheral blood stem cell transplantation.

KEY WORDS: FLT-3 Ligand (FL), mobilization, stem cell transplantation

INTRODUCTION

Hematopoietic stem cells and progenitor cells in the circulation increase in number after administration of several growth factors with or without cytotoxic agents [1]-[4]. The FLT-3 ligand (FL) is a ligand for FLT3/FLK2 tyrosine kinase receptor which is expressed in the hematopoietic stem cells and its cDNA is cloned by Lyman et al. [5] and Hannum et al.[6] independently. These investigators found that FL stimulates the proliferation of hematopoietic stem cells and primitive progenitors in combination with other growth factors in vitro [5]-[8]. But it has not been known whether in vivo administration of FL could mobilize hematopoietic stem and progenitor cells into blood. We investigated the effects of in vivo administration of FL on the mobilization of hematopoietic stem and progenitor cells in mice.

MATERIALS AND METHODS

Six to 8-week-old C57bl/6J mice were injected subcutaneously with Chinese hamster ovarian (CHO) cell-derived FL for 5 days. FL was kindly provided by Dr. Stewart D. Lyman (Immunex Corp., Seattle, WA, USA). The dosages of FL were 20, 100, and 200 µg/kg. Peripheral blood was collected and pooled on Days 0, 3, 5, 7, and 9, and we determined the number of WBCs with the differential counts. After peripheral blood had been collected, bone marrow and spleen cell suspensions were prepared and light density mononuclear cells were obtained by the gradient separation procedure. CFCs were estimated with a standard methylcellulose method using a recombinant mouse (rm) SCF, rmIL-3, rmGM-CSF, r human (h) G-CSF, and rhEpo (provided by Kirin Brewery, Tokyo, Japan). Peripheral blood mononuclear cells were transplanted into lethally irradiated mice and CFU-S (Day 12) were scored on each time point.

RESULTS

(1) Effects of FL on Circulating WBC: Administration of FL at a dose of 20 µg/kg did not increase WBCs, but at doses of 100 and 200 µg/kg FL increased WBCs up to 1.7- and 2.4-fold, respectively, as compared with control on Day 0 (Fig. 1). The increase in total WBC count by the administration of FL at a dose of 100 ʈg/kg was the result of an increase in lymphocytes, but the leukocytosis engendered by the administration of 200 µg/kg FL reflected an increase especially in neutrophils and monocytes.

(2) Effects of FL on Mobilization of Hematopoietic Progenitor Cells into the Circulation: The hematopoietic progenitor cells (HPCs) were mobilized into the blood in a dose-dependent fashion by FL (Fig. 2). On Day 5 after FL administration the number of HPCs in the blood increased up to 2.2-, 2.8-, and 5.5-fold at doses of 20, 100, and 200 µg/kg FL, respectively. Interestingly, animals given FL, 200 µg/kg, showed a 14.6-fold increase in the number of HPCs on Day 7 as compared with control on Day 0. Various CFCs (BFU-E, CFU-GM, and CFU-Mix) were mobilized into the blood dose-dependently by the administration of FL.

(3) Effects of FL on Progenitor Cell Number in Bone Marrow and Spleen: The number of HPCs in the bone marrow increased up to 1.9- to 3.8-fold, but not in a dose-dependent manner. The administration of FL led to an increase in the number of HPCs in the spleen on Day 5 up to 2.1- to 3.3-fold at doses of 20 and 100 µg/kg, respectively, and up to 32-fold at a dose of 200 µg/kg (data not shown).

(4) Effects of FL on CFU-S (Day 12) in Peripheral Blood: A dose-dependent mobilization of CFU-S (Day 12) into blood was observed. Administration of FL, at a dose of 20 µg/kg, did not mobilize CFU-S (Day 12) as compared with control, but at doses of 100 and 200 µg/kg, increased the number of CFU-S (Day 12) in peripheral blood up to 1.7- and 2.2-fold, respectively, on Day 5. On Day 7 after the administration of FL at a dose of 200 µg/kg, there was a striking increase in the number of CFU-S (Day 12) to 7.7-fold (Fig. 3).

DISCUSSION

The present studies demonstrated that in vivo administration of FL can enhance the leukocytosis and mobilize hematopoietic stem cells and progenitor cells into the blood in mice. Although in vivo administration of high doses of FL brought out a dramatic increase in the number of HPCs in the peripheral blood and the spleen, the number of HPCs in the bone marrow increased only slightly. Because the space for hematopoiesis in bone marrow is limited, the increase of HPCs in bone marrow might be small, with HPCs being distributed to the peripheral blood or spleen after the administration of FL. Otherwise, the total number of HPCs per mouse was increased as compared with the control (Day 0) after the administration of FL. Redistribution as well as in vivo expansion of HPCs in the mouse could be part of the mechanism of mobilization engendered by the administration of FL. It is noteworthy that the number of CFCs in the peripheral blood and the spleen, and the number of CFU-S (Day 12) in the peripheral blood was increased most on Day 7 when FL, at a dose of 200 µg/kg, was administered for 5 days. One explanation for this finding is that CHO cell-derived FL may have a long half-life in vivo (personal communication from Dr. Lyman). Another possibility is that the administration of FL may stimulate the production of other growth factors, leading indirectly to a proliferation of hematopoietic stem cells and progenitor cells. We concluded that FL could mobilize hematopoietic stem cells and progenitor cells into the blood in mice. SCF is reported to be more useful than G-CSF for mobilizing immature progenitor cells, but SCF induces the proliferation and maturation of mast cells[9]-[10], which leads to allergic reactions in humans. Otherwise, FL does not affect the growth of mast cells or their degranulation[11], so it is expected that in vivo administration of FL could induce far fewer allergic reactions than does SCF during the harvesting of the grafts for peripheral blood stem cell transplantation. Hematopoietic stem cells and progenitor cells mobilized by FL might be useful for peripheral blood stem cell transplantation. Further studies are warranted to determine whether FL could mobilize stem cells into the blood in humans and whether FL could have synergistic effects on mobilization with other growth factors such as G-CSF.

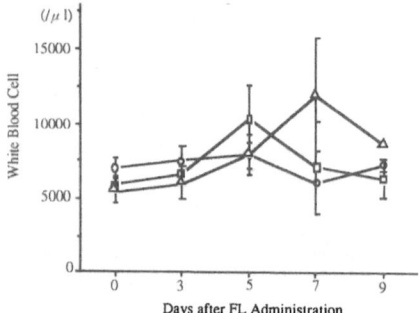

Fig. 1: Changes in the mean ± S.D. of total WBCs (A) during
administration of FL at 20 μ g/kg (○), 100 μ g/kg (□),
and 200 μ g/kg(△) for 5 days.

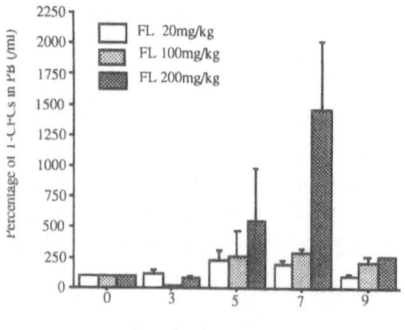

Fig. 2: Changes in the number of total CFCs in peripheral blood
during administration of FL at 20, 100, 200 mg/kg for 5 days.
Data are expressed as a percentage of total CFC numbers
on each time point for control mice on day 0 and show the
mean + S.D. .

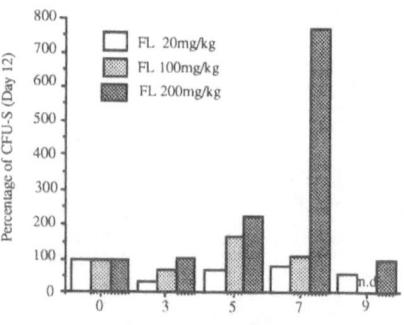

Fig. 3: Changes in the number of CFU-S (Day 12) during
administration of FL at 20, 100, and 200 mg/kg
for 5 days. Data are expressed as a percentage
of the value for control mice on day 0. n.d.: not
done

REFEENCES

[1]Molineux G, Pojda Z, Hampson IN, Lord BI, Dexter TM:Transplantation potential of peripheral blood stem cells induced by granulocyte colony-stimulating factor. Blood76:2153, 1990
[2]Neben S, Marcus K, Mauch P:Mobilization of hematopoietic stem cell and progenitor cell subpopulations from the marrow to the blood of mice following cyclophosphamide and/or granulocyte colony-stimulating factor. Blood 81:1960, 1993
[3]Ganser A, Lindermann A, Ottamann OG, Seipelt G HessU, Geissler G, Kanz L, Frisch J, Schulz G, Herrmann F, Mertelsmann R, Hoelzer D:Sequential in vivo treatment with two recombinant human hematopoietic growth factors (interleukin-3 and granulocyte-macrophage colony-stimulating factor) as a new therapeutic modality to stimulate hematopoiesis: Results of a Phase I study. Blood 79:2583, 1992
[4]Shimazaki C, Oku N, Ashihara E, Okawa K, Goto H, Inaba T, Ito K, Fujita N, Tsuji H,

Murakami S, Haruyama H, Nishio A, Nakagawa M:Collection of peripheral blood stem cells mobilized by high-dose Ara-C plus VP-16 or aclarubicin followed by recombinant human granulocyte-colony stimulating factor. Bone Marrow Transplant 10:341, 1992

[5]Lyman SD, James L, Bos TV, de Vries P, Brasel K, Gliniak B, Hollingsworth LT, Picha KS, McKenna HJ, Splett RR, Fletcher FA, Maraskovsky E, Farrah T, Foxworthe D, Williams DE, Beckmann P:Molecular cloning of a ligand for the flt3/flk-2 tyrosine kinase receptor:A proliferative factor for primitive hematopoietic cells. Cell 75:1157, 1993

[6]Hannum C, Culpepper J, Campbell D, McClanahan T, Zurawski S, Bazen JF, Kastelein R, Hudak S, Wagner J, Mattson J, Luh J, Duda G, Martina N, Peterson D, Menon S, Shanafelt A, Muench M, Kelner G, Namikawa R, Rennick D, Roncarolo M-G, Zlotnik A, Rosnet O, Dubreuil P, Birnbaum D, Lee F:Ligand for FLT3/FLK2 receptor tyrosine kinase regulates growth of haematopoietic stem cells and is encoded by variant RNAs. Nature 368:643, 1994

[7]Hudak S, Hunte B, Culpepper J, Menon S, Hannum C, Thompson-Snipe L, Rennick D:FLT3/FLK2 ligand promotes the growth of murine stem cells and the expansion of colony-forming cells and spleen colony-forming units. Blood 85:2747, 1995

[8]Lyman SD, James L, Johnson L, Brasel K, de Vries P, Escobar SS, Downey H, Splett R, Beckmann MP, McKenna HJ:Cloning of the human homologue of the murine flt3 ligand:A growth factor for early hematopoietic progenitor cells. Blood 83:2795, 1994

[9]Tsai M, Takeishi T, Thompson H, Langley KE, Zsebo KM, Metcalf DD, Geissler EN, Galli S:Induction of mast cell proliferation, maturation, and heparin synthesis by the rat c-kit ligand, stem cell factor. Proc Natl Acad Sci USA 88:6382, 1991

[10]Mitsui H, Furitsu T, Dvorak AM, Irani AA, Schwartz LB, Inagaki N, Takei M, Ishizaka K, Zsebo KM, Gillis S, Ishizaka T:Development of human mast cells from umbilical cord blood cells by recombinant   human and murine c-kit ligand. Proc Natl Acad Sci USA 90:735, 1993

[11]Lyman SD, Brasel K, Rousseau AM, Williams DE:The flt3 Ligand:A hematopoietic stem cell factor whose activities are distinct from steel factor, in Murphy MJ Jr (ed):Polyfunction of Hematopoietic Regiulators. The Metcalf Forum. Dayton, OH. AlphaMed Press, 1994, p 99

Gene Regulation
and Gene Therapy

Ribozyme-Mediated Reversal of Human Pancreatic Carcinoma Phenotype

Hiroshi Kijima, David Y. Bouffard and Kevin J. Scanlon

Section of Biochemical Pharmacology, Department of Medical Oncology, Montana Building, City of Hope National Medical Center, 1500 East Duarte Road, Duarte, California 91010, U.S.A.

SUMMARY

Point mutations in the *ras* gene have been found in approximately 90% of human pancreatic carcinomas. These alterations can be used as potential targets for specific ribozyme-mediated reversal of the malignant phenotype. We have evaluated the efficacy of a hammerhead ribozyme directed against codon 12 (GUU) of the activated K-*ras* gene in a Capan-1 human pancreatic carcinoma cell line using different delivery systems. Our results have demonstrated that the anti-K-*ras* ribozyme cloned into the pHß plasmid was able to efficiently suppress K-*ras* gene expression and to inhibit the proliferation of transfected Capan-1 cells. In contrast, the anti-K-*ras* ribozyme was less efficient against the Capan-1 cells when cloned into a pLNCX retroviral plasmid. In addition, our results showed that adenoviral-mediated expression of the ribozyme RNA was more effective than the two other plasmid vectors. Our studies have characterized different viral and non-viral delivery systems for the therapeutic application of an anti-K-*ras* ribozyme against a human pancreatic carcinoma cell line. In the near future, ribozymes could emerge as important therapeutic agents against human malignancies, and optimal delivery systems are necessary to achieve maximal gene therapy benefit.

KEY WORDS: catalytic RNA, *ras* oncogene, gene delivery systems, gene modulation, pancreatic neoplasm

INTRODUCTION

Recent advances in the understanding of the genetic mechanisms of carcinogenesis and the manipulation of gene expression have introduced new strategies for cancer therapeutics, *i.e.*, cancer gene therapy. Gene therapy of cancer is based on the specific correction of genetic abnormalities identified in human neoplasms. Strategies used to reverse cancer phenotypes have included the suppression of activated oncogenes or the restoration of normal suppressor genes. Currently, specific gene modulation using oligonucleotides has been characterized and defined as an important strategy for suppressing activated oncogenes [1-4].

Oligonucleotides capable of modulating specific gene expression include triplex DNA, antisense DNA/RNA and ribozymes (catalytic RNAs)[1]. Antisense-mediated gene modulation has been shown to be effective for gene therapy [5-7]. Ribozyme strategies have more advantages because of their site-specific cleavage activities and catalytic potentials [8]. In recent years, investigators have reported the efficacy of ribozymes against various oncogenes (*e.g.*, *ras*, c-*fos*, *BCR-ABL*), the drug resistance gene (*e.g.*, *mdr*1) and the human immunodeficiency virus-type 1 [3,4,9,10]. Our studies have previously demonstrated that anti-oncogene ribozymes effectively suppress the expression of targeted genes and cause reversal of the malignant phenotype in human cancer cell

153

lines [11-18]. Because of their *in vitro* effectiveness, anti-oncogene ribozymes have been proposed to have potential clinical utilities as anticancer agents. However, one of the most important issues pertaining to the clinical application of ribozymes is an effective gene delivery system [18]. Certain gene transfer systems such as retroviral vectors have been shown to be effective for targeting hematopoietic cells, while only a few studies have demonstrated efficient *in vivo* delivery systems against human solid tumors [18-20].

In this study, we have investigated the *in vitro* efficacy of a hammerhead ribozyme against the activated K-*ras* oncogene in a human pancreatic carcinoma cell line containing the K-*ras* mutation. For future clinical trials of gene modulation using ribozymes, we have evaluated a highly-efficient adenoviral-mediated delivery system of the anti-K-*ras* ribozyme. This delivery system shows promise for the therapeutic application of the anti-K-*ras* ribozyme as a clinical agent against human pancreatic carcinoma.

MATERIALS AND METHODS

Cells

The human pancreatic carcinoma cell line, containing a homozygous K-*ras* mutation (GTT), was obtained from ATCC: Capan-1 (#ATCC HTB79; adenocarcinoma). The cell line and its transformants were maintained in RPMI medium containing 10% fetal bovine serum and supplemented with 100 IU/ml penicillin and 100 μg/ml streptomycin. The cells were grown in monolayers and passed by trypsinization weekly. The cells were found to be free of mycoplasma contamination when tested with a Mycoplasma Rapid Detection System (GEN-PROBE, San Diego, CA) every three months. Thymidine uptake studies were used to determine the rate of [^{3}H]-labeled thymidine incorporation into trichloroacetic acid-precipitable material; the tumor cells (5 x 10^3 cells/35 mm dish) were grown for 48 hours, then incubated for two hours with [^{3}H] thymidine (10^6 cpm/dish), washed, precipitated with acid and counted. Colony formation in soft agar was performed as follows: the tumor cells were plated in triplicate at 5 x 10^3 cells/35 mm dish onto 0.3% agarose and supplemented with 1%, 10% or 20% fetal bovine serum. Colonies were counted two weeks after seeding.

Synthetic nucleotides

Oligodeoxynucleotides were synthesized and used for the construction of the ribozyme-expressing plasmids and for the reverse transcription-polymerase chain reaction (RT-PCR) assay, as well as for the detection of gene expression by hybridization as previously described [13]. Oligonucleotides for cloning the anti-K-*ras* ribozyme into the pHß plasmid and pACCMVpLpA adenoviral shuttle vector (with flanking *Sal*I and *Hind*III sites) were K*ras*Rz-1,

5'-TCG ACT ACG CCC TGA TGA GTC CGT GAG GAC GAA ACA GCT A-3'
and K*ras*Rz-2,

5'-AGC TTA GCT GTT TCG TCC TCA CGG ACT CAT CAG GGC GTA G-3'
Oligonucleotides for cloning the anti-K-*ras* ribozyme into the pLNCX retroviral plasmid (with flanking *Hind*III and *Cla*I sites) were K*ras*Rz-3,

5'-AGC TTT ACG CCC TGA TGA GTC CGT GAG GAC GAA ACA GCT AT-3' ;
and K*ras*Rz-4,

5'-CGA TAG CTG TTT CGT CCT CAC GGA CTC ATC AGG GCG TAA-3'.
Primers to detect ribozyme expression were

pHß-PCR-1, 5'-AGC ACA GAG CCT CGC CTT T-3' and
pHß-PCR-2, 5'- GTC TGG ATC CCT CGA AGC-3';

pLNCX-PCR-1, 5'-GAG ACG CCA TCC ACG CTG TT-3' and
pLNCX-PCR-2, 5'-CAG GTG GGG TCT TTC ATT CC-3';
pACCMV-PCR-1, 5'-GCG TGT ACG GTG GGA GGT CT-3' and
pACCMV-PCR-2, 5'-GTT TCG TCC TCA CGG ACT CAT-3';
the probe was Rz-probe, 5'- CTC ACG GAC TCA TCA GG-3'.
Primers to detect c-K-*ras* oncogene expression were
Kras-1, 5'-GAC TGA ATA TAA ACT TGT GG-3' and
Kras-2, 5'-CTA TTG TTG GAT CAT ATT CG-3';
the probe was Kras-S, 5'-TCT GAA TTA GCT GTA TCG TC-3'.
Primers to detect PGK gene expression were
PGK-3, 5'-AGT CGG TAG TCC TTA TGA GC-3' and
PGK-4, 5'-CAG CAG GAT GAC AGA CCC AG-3';
the probe was PGK-S, 5'-GAA CTC AAA TCT CTG CTG GG-3'.

Double-stranded DNA cycle sequencing

The genomic DNA of the Capan-1 cells was isolated using TRIzol Reagent (Gibco BRL, MD). DNA sequencing using dsDNA Cycle Sequencing System (Gibco BRL) was performed to detect the mutation of c-K-*ras* oncogene in codon 12.

Plasmid construction (Figs. 1 and 2)

The pHß Apr-1 neo (pHß) plasmid was obtained from Dr. L. Kedes (USC, Los Angeles, CA)[21,22]. The anti-K-*ras* ribozyme was cloned into the plasmid pHß using two synthetic single-stranded oligodeoxynucleotides (KrasRz-1, KrasRz-2) with flanking *Sal*I and *Hind*III restriction sites. Primers for screening cell lines to detect the presence of pHß/anti-K-*ras* ribozyme were pHß-PCR-1 and pHß-PCR-2 as mentioned above. The pLNCX retroviral plasmid was obtained from Dr. D. Miller (Fred Hutchinson Cancer Research Center, Seattle, WA)[23,24]. The anti-K-*ras* ribozyme was cloned into the pLNCX plasmid using two synthetic single-stranded oligodeoxynucleotides (KrasRz-3, KrasRz-4) with flanking *Hind*III and *Cla*I restriction sites. Primers for screening cell lines to detect the presence of pLNCX/anti-K-*ras* ribozyme were pLNCX-PCR-1 and pLNCX-PCR-2. The pACCMVpLpA adenoviral shuttle vector was provided by Dr. R. Gerard (University of Texas Southwestern, Houston, TX)[25]. The anti-K-*ras* ribozyme was cloned into the pACCMVpLpA adenoviral vector using two synthetic single-stranded oligodeoxynucleotides (KrasRz-1, KrasRz-2) with flanking *Sal*I and *Hind*III restriction sites. Primers for screening cell lines to detect the presence of the pACCMVpLpA/anti-K-*ras* ribozyme were pACCMV-PCR-1 and pACCMV-PCR-2 as mentioned above.

Transfection studies

Subconfluent Capan-1 cells were transfected with the pHß or pLNCX plasmid by electroporation according to a protocol provided by IBI (New Haven, CT). The transfected cells were selected for integration of plasmid in growth media containing 500 μg/ml of G418 sulfate for 4 weeks. Selected G418-resistant colonies were grown and screened for expression of the ribozyme by RT-PCR assay.

Generation of recombinant adenovirus

The low passage 293 E1A transcomplementing cell line was obtained from Dr. F. Graham (McMaster University, Hamilton, Ontario, Canada) and maintained in DMEM media containing 10% fetal bovine serum and supplemented with 100 IU/ml penicillin and 100 μg/ml streptomycin [18,26]. To generate the recombinant anti-K-*ras* ribozyme-containing adenovirus, the shuttle

156

plasmid pACCMVpLpA and the adenoviral packaging plasmid pJM17 (provided Dr. F. Graham, McMaster University) were co-transfected into the 293 cell line using a commercial cationic liposome vector (Lipofectin Reagent, Gibco BRL). Transfected cells were maintained until onset of cellular cytopathic effects. The newly generated recombinant adenovirus was plaque-purified three times by a standard method [25,26].

RT-PCR assay

Poly(A) mRNAs were isolated using FastTrack mRNA Isolation Kit (Invitrogen, San Diego, CA). RT-PCR was performed according to a commercially available protocol (Perkin Elmer, Norwalk, CT), and was used to detect the ribozyme, c-K-*ras*, and phosphoglycerate kinase (PGK) gene expression [13]. The specific PCR products were size-fractionated by horizontal agarose gel electrophoresis, and transferred under vacuum to a nylon membrane (Hybond-N+, Amersham, IL). Hybridization was carried out with the aforementioned probes radiolabeled by 5' end-labeling method.

RESULTS

pHß plasmid

Double-stranded DNA cycle sequencing of Capan-1 genomic DNA demonstrated a GTT homozygous mutation at codon 12 of the K-*ras* gene which encodes for a valine (unpublished data). The GTT mutation offers a cleavable site for an anti-K-*ras* hammerhead ribozyme (Fig.1). The anti-K-*ras* ribozyme was cloned into the pHß plasmid (pHß/K*ras* Rz) and transfected into Capan-1 human pancreatic carcinoma cells by electroporation (Fig.2).

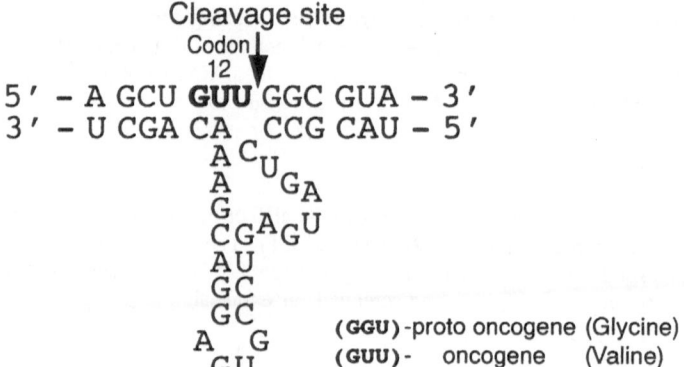

Fig. 1 <u>Schema of the anti-K-*ras* ribozyme and its substrate</u>. The hammerhead ribozyme against K-*ras* codon 12 targets the GUU mutant mRNA sequence of K-*ras* codon 12, encoding valine. The GGU wild-type sequence encoding glycine is not cleaved by the ribozyme.

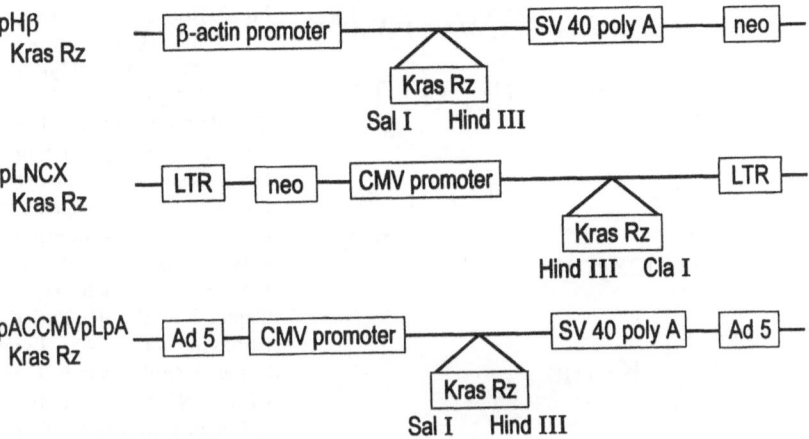

Fig. 2 <u>Schema of the plasmid constructions encoding the anti-K-*ras* ribozyme</u>. The pHß-Apr1 plasmid is driven by the human ß-actin promoter; the pLNCX retroviral vector has the CMV promoter; and the pACCMVpLpA adenoviral shuttle vector is driven by the CMV promoter.

Expression of the ribozyme was demonstrated in isolated G418-resistant clones by RT-PCR. A significant decrease of K-*ras* mRNA was shown in the Capan-1 cells transfected with pHß/K*ras* Rz (Fig.3). The semi-quantitative RT-PCR assay demonstrated that the K-*ras* mRNA was decreased in the transformants 4- to 8-fold more than in the Capan-1 parental cells. Western blotting of the K-*ras* p21 protein data suggested a corresponding decrease with the inhibition of K-*ras* mRNA (data not shown). Alteration of growth characteristics was observed by the generation time measurement, [3H] thymidine incorporation assay and soft agar colony formation assay (Table 1). In the transformants with pHß/K*ras* Rz, the generation time was longer by 1.6 to 2.2 times compared to the parental cells, ranging from 91 to 122 hours. The Capan-1 transformants/pHß K-*ras* ribozyme showed 43 to 54% decrease in [3H]thymidine incorporation. The colony formation assay showed that the transformants were substantially decreased in number as compared to the control cells (54 to 59% decrease).

pLNCX retroviral plasmid

The anti-K-*ras* ribozyme was cloned into the pLNCX retroviral plasmid (pLNCX/K*ras* Rz) and transfected into the Capan-1 cells by electroporation (Fig.2). Expression of the ribozyme was displayed in G418-resistant clones by RT-PCR. K-*ras* gene expression was slightly decreased in the Capan-1 cells transfected with pLNCX/K*ras* Rz, though each transformant exhibited abundant expression of the anti-K-*ras* ribozyme (Fig.3). In the transformants with pLNCX/K*ras* Rz, the generation time was slightly longer by 1.1 to 1.3 times compared to the parental cells, ranging from 62 to 70 hours (Table 1). The Capan-1 transformants/pLNCX K-*ras* ribozyme showed 35 to 44% decrease in [3H] thymidine incorporation. Colony numbers of Capan-1 transformants in soft agar were decreased as compared to the control cells (33 to 52% decrease).

Gene expression (RNA-PCR)
Capan-1 (codon 12, GTT)

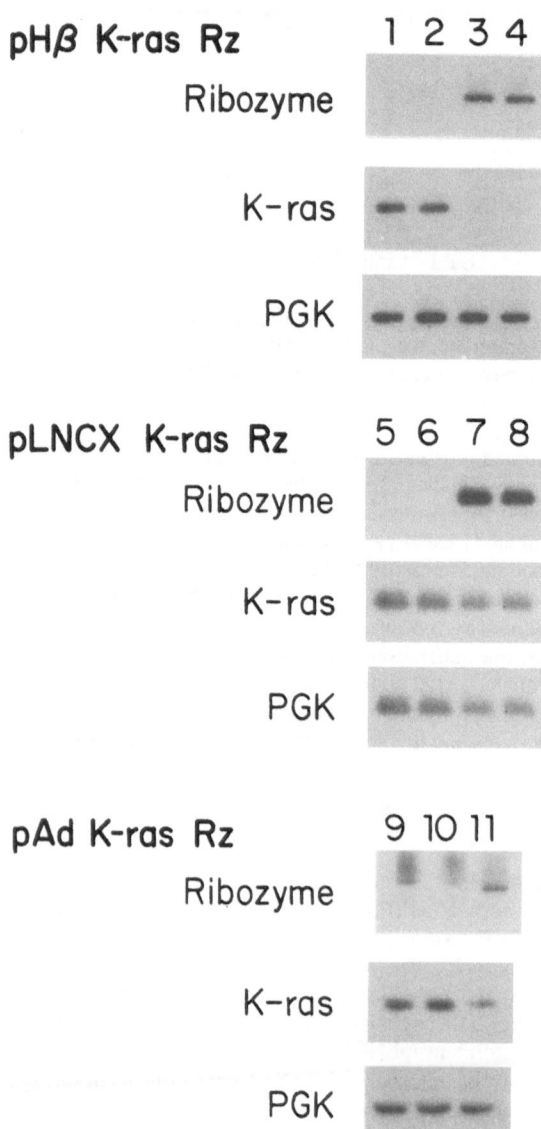

pHβ K-ras Rz

Ribozyme

K-ras

PGK

pLNCX K-ras Rz

Ribozyme

K-ras

PGK

pAd K-ras Rz

Ribozyme

K-ras

PGK

Fig. 3 <u>Relevant gene expression in the Capan-1 pancreatic carcinoma cell line by RT-PCR.</u>

Template RNA of each lane was 6.3 ng; the PCR product of each lane was shown after 30 cycles of RT-PCR. Lane 1, Capan-1 cells; Lane 2, Capan-1 with pHß vector only;Lane3,Capan-with pHß/anti-K-*ras* ribozyme clone #1; Lane 4, Capan-1 with pHß/anti-K-*ras* ribozyme clone #2; Lane 5, Capan-1 cells; Lane 6, Capan-1 with pLNCX vector only; Lane 7, Capan-1 with pLNCX/anti-K-*ras* ribozyme clone #3; Lane 8, Capan-1 with pLNCX/anti-K-*ras* ribozyme clone #4; Lane 9, Capan-1 cells; Lane 10, Capan-1 infected with recombinant Ad dl312 (E1A- control); Lane 11, Capan-1 infected with Recombinant Ad/anti-K-*ras* ribozyme. Each ribozyme transformant was shown to exhibit abundant expression of the ribozyme (Lanes 3, 4, 7, 8 and 11). In the Capan-1 cells with pHß/anti-K-*ras* ribozyme, the ribozyme diminished the K-*ras* gene expression of Capan-1 cells which have a cleavable mutant sequence for the ribozyme; meanwhile, in the pLNCX/anti-K-*ras* ribozyme transformants, the ribozyme did not significantly downregulate the K-*ras* gene expression. In the Capan-1 cells infected with Ad/anti-K-*ras* ribozyme, the ribozyme downregulated the K-*ras* gene expression of Capan-1 cells. Each cell line (Lanes 1 to 11) was shown to exhibit similar Expression of the phosphoglycerate kinase (PGK) gene.

Table 1. Growth characteristics of pancreatic carcinoma cells

Cell Line	GT[1] (Hrs)	(^{3}H)Thd[2] (%)	SAC[3] 1%	10%	20%
pHβ transformants					
Capan-1	56	100	0	82	101
Capan-1/pHβ only	60	85	0	78	90
Capan-1/pHβ K*ras* Rz #1	122	46	0	26	41
Capan-1/pHβ K*ras* Rz #2	91	57	0	29	46
pLNCX transformants					
Capan-1	55	100	0	82	101
Capan-1/pLNCX only	59	86	0	76	88
Capan-1/pLNCX K*ras* Rz #3	62	65	0	46	68
Capan-1/pLNCX K*ras* Rz #4	70	56	0	27	48
recombinant Ad transformants					
Capan-1	59	100	8	91	121
Capan-1/Ad dl312 (E1-)	60	99	6	78	111
Capan-1/Ad K*ras* Rz	255	53	0	2	21

[1] GT (Hrs), generation time (hours).

[2](^{3}H)Thd (%), the rate of ^{3}H-labeled thymidine incorporation assay.

[3]SAC, soft agar colony formation assay with 1% to 20% fetal bovine serum.

[1-3] Experiments were performed at least twice in duplicate. Standard deviation was less than 10%.

Recombinant adenoviral vector

A recombinant adenovirus was constructed to encode the anti-K-*ras* ribozyme (Fig.2). This methodology for recombinant adenovirus construction is based on *in vivo* homologous recombination between the adenoviral shuttle vector pACCMVpLpA and the adenoviral packaging plasmid pJM17 (18). The adenoviral shuttle vector containing the anti-K-*ras* ribozyme, pACCMVpLpA/K*ras* Rz, was constructed and used to derive the corresponding adenoviral vector. The adenoviral vector is predicted to contain the anti-K-*ras* ribozyme expression cassette inserted in place of the deleted adenoviral E1 sequence. The PCR assay of viral DNA demonstrated the presence of the anti-K-*ras* ribozyme in the recombinant adenovirus (data not shown).

The adenoviral-mediated suppression of cancer cell growth was evaluated in the absence of any selection pressure, in contrast to the previous studies with the pHß and the pLNCX plasmid. The Capan-1 cells were cultured in 60-mm dishes and infected with the recombinant adenovirus encoding the anti-K-*ras* ribozyme (Ad-K*ras* Rz) at 200 plaque-forming units (PFU)/cell. The Capan-1 cells infected with Ad-K*ras* Rz exhibited expression of the anti-K-*ras* ribozyme and decreased K-*ras* gene expression (Fig.3). In the Capan-1 cells infected with Ad-K*ras* Rz, the generation time (255 hours) was significantly longer by 4.3 times compared to the parental cells (59 hours) (Table 1). The Capan-1 transformants/Ad-K*ras* Rz showed 47% decrease in [^{3}H] thymidine incorporation. Colonies of Capan-1 transformants in soft agar were substantially decreased in number as compared to the control cells (82% decrease).

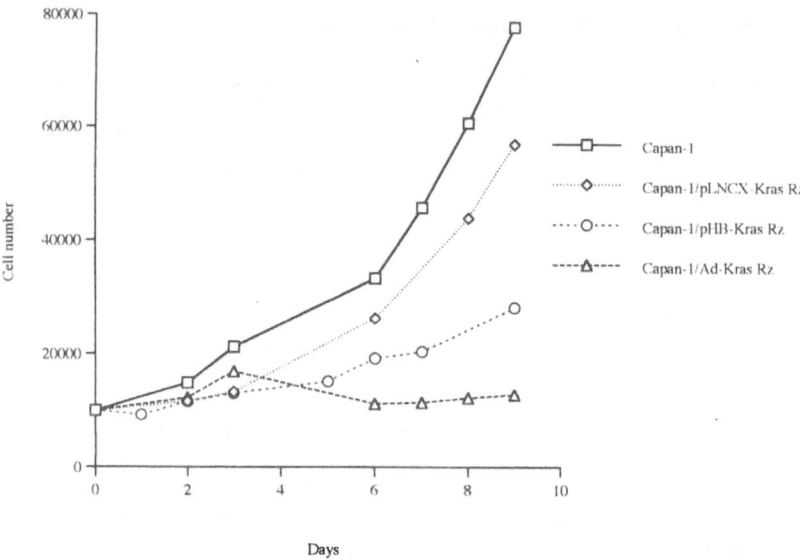

Fig. 4. <u>Growth curve of the Capan-1 pancreatic carcinoma cell lines</u>. The growth suppression effect by Ad/anti-K-*ras* ribozyme was greater than the pHß/anti-K-*ras* ribozyme and retroviral pLNCX/anti-K-*ras* ribozyme.

DISCUSSION

Human cancers have been shown to possess alterations in oncogene function which may be caused by point mutations, amplification or overexpression [27,28]. A point mutation in the *ras* oncogene family activates its p21 gene product, and affects cell growth resulting in malignant transformation [29]. Mutations within the *ras* gene have been frequently observed in human cancers, including approximately 90% of pancreatic adenocarcinomas, 40-50% of colon adenocarcinomas and 30% of lung adenocarcinomas [30-32]. Therefore, the mutant *ras* gene could become a specific target for cancer gene modulation, resulting in reversal of the malignant phenotype. Ribozymes have previously been shown to be selective in discriminating mutated oncogenes from proto-oncogenes and efficacious in reversing the transformed phenotype [13-17].

In the present study, we have shown the efficacy of a hammerhead ribozyme against mutant K-*ras* gene, using different vector systems, in the Capan-1 human pancreas carcinoma cell line. Recently, two groups have demonstrated the efficiency of antisense DNA/RNA directed against K-*ras* to inhibit the human pancreatic tumor growth in cultured cell systems [33] and an *in vivo* mice model [34]. Compared to antisense-mediated strategies, the advantages of hammerhead ribozymes are their catalytic activity, site-specific cleavage and the ability to discriminate a single base mutation [3,4,8-10,35]. We have previously demonstrated that an anti-H-*ras* ribozyme has efficiently inhibited the mutant H-*ras* gene expression but not the H-*ras* proto-oncogene expression [16,17] in several human carcinoma cell lines as well as transformed NIH3T3 cells [13-18]. Ribozyme kinetic studies have shown that adding bases to the flanking sequence can increase site specificity, and decrease the dissociation step between the ribozyme and its substrate [10,36,37]. Based on our kinetic studies, we have optimized the anti-K-*ras* ribozyme with a 12-base optimal length flanking sequences to maximize the turnover rate of the ribozyme and enhance its efficacy. As mentioned previously, the Capan-1 cell line has a GTT homozygous mutation of the K-*ras* gene (codon 12) which is a target for the ribozyme. Our results show that the anti-K-*ras* ribozyme has suppressed the expression of the mutant K-*ras* mRNA in the Capan-1 cells and also reversed their malignant phenotype.

To have optimal ribozyme expression and activity in cultured cell lines and for *in vivo* studies, it is necessary to design effective delivery systems [19]. Fundamentally, the methods used for gene delivery are physical transfection and viral transduction [20]. To express the anti-K-*ras* ribozyme in cultured Capan-1 cells, we have cloned it into the pHß plasmid driven by the human ß-actin promoter [21,22]. The pHß has been shown to strongly express the anti-K-*ras* ribozyme (Fig.3). In the selected Capan-1 clones transfected with the pHß/K*ras* Rz, the generation time was significantly longer by 1.6 to 2.2 times. For *in vitro* ribozyme studies, the pHß plasmid is thought to be an appropriate vector.

For the clinical application of ribozyme-mediated gene therapy to become feasible, we must exploit effective *in vivo* vector systems. Recent advances in gene delivery systems have not been extensive, but researchers have examined the *in vivo* use of retroviral vectors and reported their usefulness in transfecting hematopoietic cells [19,20,38-40]. We have cloned the anti-K-*ras* ribozyme into the pLNCX retroviral plasmid and transfected it into the Capan-1 cells by electroporation [23,24]. Ribozyme-expressing clones were selected after G418 screening and RT-PCR assay. However, these transformants did not show significant downregulation of K-*ras* mRNA, and their generation time was not significantly longer than the parental cell lines (only 1.1 to 1.3 times). We speculate that although this retroviral plasmid works well for hematopoietic cells, it fails to be effective in the pancreatic carcinoma cells. Roth and colleagues have reported that another retroviral vector LNSX driven by a ß-actin promoter was relatively effective in human lung cancer cells [6,7]. Recently, Yoshida *et al.* have also observed the inhibition of pancreatic tumor dissemination using a liposome-mediated gene transfer of antisense K-*ras* construct cloned into a LNSX retroviral plasmid driven by a SV40 promoter [34]. In further studies, therefore, we intend to replace the CMV promoter of our retroviral plasmid pLNCX/K*ras* Rz by another, such as the ß-actin promoter or SV40 promoter, and re-evaluate its utility compared to antisense oligonucleotides.

Adenoviral vectors, as well as retroviral vectors, have recently been used in clinical trials for gene therapy [19,20,25,26]. The recombinant adenoviruses are characterized by (i) epichromosomal gene expression in the targeted cells; (ii) infection of both dividing and non-dividing target cells; and (iii) production of high viral titers. One disadvantage of adenoviral vectors is their transient expression (two to six weeks) compared to retroviral vectors. Our *in vitro* studies demonstrated that the recombinant adenovirus Ad-K*ras* Rz almost completely suppressed cell growth of the Capan-1 cells. The growth suppression effect by the Ad-K*ras* Rz was significantly better than the pHß/K*ras* Rz and the retroviral pLNCX/K*ras* Rz (Fig.4). The pACCMVpLpA adenoviral plasmid is derived from human adenovirus serotype 5 and driven by the CMV promoter/enhancer element [25], while the pLNCX retroviral vector is driven by the retroviral long terminal repeat and CMV promoter [23]. We supposed that the different vector constructions and the different gene delivery systems (electroporation vs. infection) caused the different efficacy between the pLNCX/K*ras* Rz and Ad-K*ras* Rz. However, there was no selection pressure for the adenovirus studies in comparison to the plasmid studies. In addition, the significant growth suppression by the Ad-K*ras* Rz was achieved using less adenovirus (*i.e.*,200 PFU/cells) in comparison with our previous study of adenoviral-mediated delivery of the anti-*ras* ribozyme in the EJ bladder carcinoma cells which used 500 PFU/cell [18]. We speculate that the recombinant adenovirus is an effective vector for delivering the ribozyme to human cancers. In addition, the Ad-K*ras* Rz does not have the ability to replicate in the infected cells because it was constructed to encode the anti-K-*ras* ribozyme in place of the deleted E1 sequence. The Ad-K*ras* Rz could have highly-efficient delivery and minimal pathogenic effects in other organs. Based on this data, we conclude that the recombinant adenovirus Ad-K*ras* Rz may be an appropriate viral vector system for ribozyme-mediated gene therapy of human pancreatic carcinoma.

ACKNOWLEDGEMENTS

We thank Ms. Carol Polchow for preparing the manuscript. This research was supported by a grant from the state of California Tobacco-Related Disease Research Program (4RT-0297) and a Terry Fox Research Fellow Award (from the National Cancer Institute of Canada-Award #6597) supported with funds provided by the Terry Fox Run for Dr. David Bouffard. Dr. Hiroshi Kijima's present address is:Tokai University School of Medicine, Department of Pathology, Bohseidai, Isehara, Kanagawa, 259-11, Japan.

REFERENCES

1. Scanlon KJ, Ohta Y, Ishida H, Kijima H, Ohkawa T, Kaminski A, Tsai J, Horng G, Kashani-Sabet M (1995) Oligonucleotide-mediated modulation of mammalian gene expression. FASEB J 6:1288-1296
2. Helene, C (1994) Control of oncogene expression by antisense nucleic acids. Eur J Cancer 30A:1721-1726
3. Kashani-Sabet M, Scanlon KJ (1995) Application of ribozymes to cancer gene therapy. Cancer Gene Ther 2:213-221.
4. Christoffersen RE, Marr JJ (1995) Ribozymes as human therapeutic agents. J Med Chem 38:2023-2037
5. Mercola D, Cohen JS (1995) Antisense approaches to cancer gene therapy. Cancer Gene Ther 2: 47-59
6. Georges RN, Mukhopadhyay T, Zhang Y, Yen N, Roth JA (1993) Prevention of orthotopic human lung cancer growth by intratracheal instillation of a retroviral antisense K-*ras* construct. Cancer Res 53:1743-1746
7. Zhang Y, Mukhopadhyay T, Donehower LA, Georges RN, Roth JA (1993) Retroviral vector-mediated transduction of K-*ras* antisense RNA into human lung cancer inhibits expression of the malignant phenotype. Human Gene Ther 4:451-460
8. Symons RH (1994) Ribozymes. Curr Opin Structural Biol 4:322-330
9. Castanotto D, Rossi JJ, Sarver N (1994) Antisense catalytic RNAs as therapeutic agents. Adv Pharmacol 25:289-317
10. Kijima H, Ishida H, Ohkawa T, Kashani-Sabet M, Scanlon KJ (1995) Therapeutic applications of ribozymes. Pharmacol Ther 68:247-267
11. Scanlon KJ, Jiao L, Funato T, Wang W, Tone T, Rossi JJ, Kashani-Sabet M (1991) Ribozyme-mediated cleavage of c-*fos* mRNA reduces gene expression of DNA synthesis enzymes and metallothionein. Proc Natl Acad Sci USA 88:10591-10595
12. Scanlon KJ, Ishida H, Kashani-Sabet M (1994) Ribozyme-mediated reversal of the multidrug-resistant phenotype. Proc Natl Acad Sci USA 91:11123-11127
13. Kashani-Sabet M, Funato T, Tone T, Jiao L, Wang W, Yoshida E, Kashfian BI, Shitara T, Wu AM, Moreno JG, Traweek ST, Ahlering TE, Scanlon KJ (1992) Reversal of the malignant phenotype by an anti-*ras* ribozyme. Antisense Res Dev 2:3-15
14. Kashani-Sabet M, Funato T, Florenes VA, Fodstad O, Scanlon KJ (1994) Suppression of the neoplastic phenotype *in vivo* by an anti-*ras* ribozyme. Cancer Res 54:900-902
15. Tone T, Kashani-Sabet M, Funato T, Shitara T, Yoshida E, Kashfian BI, Horng M, Fodstad O, Scanlon KJ (1993). Suppression of EJ cells tumorigenicity. In Vivo 7:471-476
16. Ohta Y, Tone T, Shitara T, Funato T, Jiao L, Kashfian BI, Yoshida E, Horng H, Tsai P,

Lauterbach K, Kashani-Sabet M, Florenes VA, Fodstad O, Scanlon KJ (1994) H-*ras* ribozyme-mediated alteration of the human melanoma phenotype. Ann N Y Acad Sci 716:242-253

17. Funato T, Shitara T, Tone T, Jiao L, Kashani-Sabet M, Scanlon KJ (1994) Suppression of H-*ras*-mediated transformation in NIH3T3 cells by a *ras* ribozyme. Biochem Pharmacol 48:1471-1475

18. Feng M, Cabrera G, Deshane J, Scanlon KJ, Curiel DT (1995) Neoplastic reversion accomplished by high efficiency adenoviral-mediated delivery of an anti-*ras* ribozyme. Cancer Res 55:2024-   2028

19. Jolly D (1994) Viral vector systems for gene therapy. Cancer Gene Ther 1:51-64

20. Hodgson CP (1995) The vector void in gene therapy. Biotechnology 13:222-225

21. Gunning P, Leavitt J, Muscat G, Ng S-Y, Kedes L (1987) A human ß-actin expression vector system directs high-level accumulation of antisense transcripts. Proc Natl Acad Sci USA 84:4831-4835

22. Ng S-Y, Gunning P, Eddy R, Ponte P, Leavitt J, Show T, Kedes L (1985) Evolution of the functional human ß-actin gene and its multi-pseudo gene family: Conservation of noncoding regions and chromosomal dispersion of pseudogenes. Mol Cell Biol 5:2720-2732

23. Miller AD, Rosman GJ (1989) Improved retroviral vectors for gene transfer and expression. Biotechniques 7:980-990

24. Miller DG, Adam MA, Miller AD (1990) Gene transfer by retrovirus occurs in cell that are actively replicating at the time of infection. Mol Cell Biol 10:4239-4242

25. Becker TC, Noel RJ, Coats WS, Gomez-Foix AM, Alam T, Gerard RD, Newgard CB (1994) Use of recombinant adenovirus for metabolic engineering of mammalian cells. Methods Cell Biol 43:161-189

26. Graham FL, Prevec L (1991) Manipulation of adenovirus vectors. Methods Mol Biol 7:109-128

27. Egan SE, Weinberg RA (1993) The pathway to signal achievement. Nature 365:781-783

28. Slamon DJ, deKernion JB, Verma IM, Cline MJ (1984) Expression of cellular oncogenes in human malignancies. Science 224:256-262

29. Barbacid M (1987) *ras* genes. Annu Rev Biochem 56:779-827

30. Bos JL (1989) *ras* oncogenes in human cancer: A review. Cancer Res 49:4682-4689

31. Almoguera C, Shibata D, Forrester K, Martin J, Arnheim N, Perucho M (1988) Most human carcinomas of the exocrine pancreas contain mutant c-K-*ras* genes. Cell 53:549-554

32. Tada M, Yokosuka O, Omata M, Ohto M, Isono K (1990) Analysis of *ras* gene mutations in biliary and pancreatic tumors by polymerase chain reaction and direct sequencing. Cancer 66:930-935

33. Carter G, Gilbert C, Lemoine NR (1995) Effects of antisense oligonucleotides targeting K-*ras* expression in pancreatic cancer cell lines. Int J Oncol 6:1105-1112

34. Aoki K, Toshida T, Sugimura T, Terada M (1995) Liposome-mediated *in vivo* gene transfer of antisense K-*ras* construct inhibits pancreatic tumor dissemination in the murine peritoneal cavity. Cancer Res 55:3810-3816

35. Koizumi M, Hayase Y, Iwai S, Kamiya H, Inoue H, Ohtsuka E (1989) Design of RNA enzymes distinguishing a single base mutation in RNA. Nucleic Acids Res 17:7059-7071

36. Hershlag D (1991) Implications of ribozyme kinetics for targeting the cleavage of specific RNA molecules *in vivo*: more isn't always better. Proc Natl Acad Sci USA 88: 6921-6925

37. Bertrand E, Pictet R, Grange T (1994) Can hammerhead ribozymes be efficient tools to inactivate gene function? Nucleic Acids Res 22:293-300

38. Anderson WF (1992) Human gene therapy. Science 256:808-813

39. Sarver N, Cantin EM, Chang PS, Zaia JA, Ladne PA, Stephens DA, Rossi JJ (1990) Ribozymes as potential anti-HIV-1 therapeutic agents. Science 247:1222-1225

40. Yu M, Ojwang J, Yamada O, Hample A, Rapapport J, Looney D, Wong-Staal F (1993) A hairpin ribozyme inhibits expression of diverse strains of human immunodeficiency virus type-1. Proc   Natl Acad Sci USA 87:6340-6344

A GENE THERAPY FOR PANCREATIC CANCER

Teruhiko Yoshida, Kazunori Aoki, Takashi Sugimura and Masaaki Terada

National Cancer Center Research Institute, 5-1-1 Tsukiji, Chuo-ku, Tokyo 104, Japan

SUMMARY

Pancreatic cancer is often resistant to conventional treatment, and the development of a new therapeutic strategy has been eagerly awaited. Characteristically, K-*ras* point mutation is observed at a high incidence in human pancreatic cancer. To determine if it is feasible to suppress the growth of pancreatic cancer by counteracting mutated K-*ras*, we constructed a plasmid vector expressing antisense K-*ras* RNA and transfected into human pancreatic cancer cells by lipofection. The *in vitro* growth was significantly suppressed for the antisense K-*ras*-transfected pancreatic cancer cells, but not for the sense K-*ras*-transfected cells. Immunoblot analysis showed a reduction of up to 20 % of K-*ras* specific p21 protein the antisense K-*ras*-transfected cells. There was no evidence of the induction of a massive apoptosis or the presence of a bystander effect. In an *in vivo* treatment model for peritoneal dissemination, the AsPC-1 pancreatic cancer cells were transplanted to the peritoneal cavity of nude mice at day 1. At day 4, the antisense K-*ras*-vector /lipopolyamine (DOGS) complex was injected intra-peritoneally 3 times every 12hrs. At day 28, 9 of the 10 sense K-*ras*-injected mice developed peritoneal dissemination and/or solid tumor formation on the pancreas or liver; in contrast, only 2 of the 12 mice treated with the antisense K-*ras* vector showed any evidence of intraperitoneal tumors. Although PCR screening indicated that the injected DNA was distributed to various organs except the brain, treatment-related toxicity was observed neither macroscopically nor microscopically. This study showed that the liposome-mediated *in vivo* gene transfer of antisense K-*ras* construct may be a useful therapeutic strategy for a subset of pancreatic cancer.

KEY WORDS: pancreatic cancer, antisense K-*ras*, lipopolyamine, gene therapy

INTRODUCTION

Pancreatic cancer remains as one of the most refractory cancers today and has a prognosis of less than 10% 3-year survival rate[1, 2]. The factors contributing to this poor prognosis include: 1) the difficulty of early diagnosis due to its anatomical location and lack of specific early symptoms [3]; 2) the tendency of the tumor to spread rapidly to the surrounding vital organs [4]; 3) the frequent occurrence of metastasis even from a small primary tumor less than 2 cm in diameter [3, 4]; and 4) non-surgical interventions, such as conventional chemo-, radio-, endocrine or immune therapy, are rarely successful [2, 5, 6]. Pancreatic cancer ranks fifth as a cause of cancer-related mortality in Japan and the United States. In Japan, the death rate for pancreatic cancer has risen sharply from 2.5 per 100,000 population in 1960 to 9.6 in 1991. Development of a new therapeutic strategy for pancreatic cancer is one of the most urgent issues in medicine today.

Characteristically, about 70-90% of human pancreatic cancers have been reported to harbor K-*ras* point mutation, more than 95% of which are located in codon 12 with the remainder at codon 13 [7-10]. The K-*ras* mutation could occur in the very early phase of pancreatic ductal carcinogenesis, because the mutation has also been found in mucous cell hyperplasia [11, 12]. It is conceivable that K-ras point mutation is related to the initiation of carcinogenesis, but not to the malignant progression of the pancreatic cancer. Moreover, it has been demonstrated in many cancers that a full-blown malignant transformation is completed upon the accumulation of multiple genetic changes during the multistep carcinogenesis. Pancreatic cancer is not an exception, and the reported genetic abnormalities include: abnormalities of *p53* and *p16* genes [13, 14], loss of expression of the *DCC* gene, somatic mutation of the *APC* gene [15], over-expression of acidic and basic fibroblast growth factors and microsatellite instability. In this study, we examined if the suppression of the function of the mutated K-*ras* gene alone effectively inhibits *in vitro* and *in vivo* growth of the pancreatic cancer cells [16]. We have also addressed the effective *in vivo* gene transfer based on the lipofection method.

MATERIALS AND METHODS

Cells and plasmids

The human pancreatic cancer cell line, AsPC-1, was maintained in an RPMI-1640 medium with 10% fetal bovine serum. AsPC-1 has a G to A transition at the second position of the K-ras codon 12 (GGT: glycine to GAT: aspartic acid).

The backbone retroviral vector plasmid LNSX was a kind gift from Dr. A. Dusty Miller (Seattle, Washington) [17] (Fig. 1).

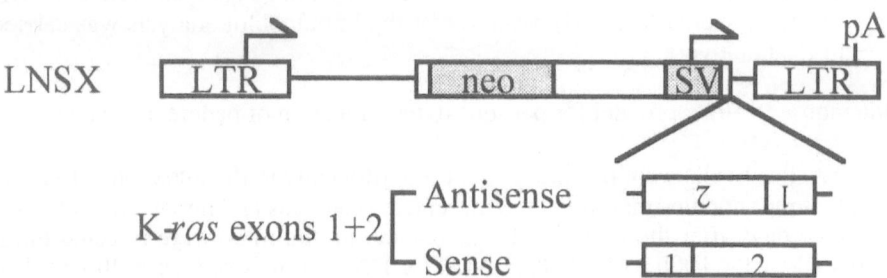

Fig. 1   LNSX-based expression plasmid for the K-*ras* cDNA fragment in antisense (AS-K-*ras*-LNSX) or sense (S-K-*ras*-LNSX) orientation.

A K-*ras* cDNA fragment spanning from nucleotide # 171 in the first exon to nucleotide # 517 in the third exon was cloned by reverse transcriptase-PCR from normal human placental mRNA. The *Cla*I and *Avr*II sites were attached to 5' and 3' ends of the cDNA, respectively. The 347-bp K-*ras* cDNA fragment was subcloned to the downstream of the internal SV40 early promoter on the LNSX vector in antisense (AS-K-ras-LNSX) or sense (S-K-*ras*-LNSX) orientation (Fig. 1). The K-ras expression unit was sequenced in full by the dideoxynucleotide chain termination method.

DNA transfection

The AS-K-*ras*-LNSX or S-K-*ras*-LNSX plasmid was transduced into the AsPC-1 human pancreatic cancer cell line by liposome-mediated transfection using a cationic liposome containing 2,3-dioleyloxy-N-[2(sperminecarboxamido)ethyl]-N, N-dimethyl-1-propanaminium trifluoroacetate and dioleoyl phosphatidylethanolamine (lipofectAMINE; GIBCO). Forty-eight hours after transfection, G418 selection was started, and several G418-resistant colonies were isolated. The remaining colonies were pooled and grown as a mixture. AsPC-1-AS (4.4), AsPC-1-AS (4.3) and AsPC-1-AS (4.9) are the single cell clones of AsPC-1 transduced with AS-K-*ras*-LNSX.

RNA blot and immunoblot analysis for K-*ras* expression

RNA blot analysis was performed on 2μg of poly(A)+ RNA. The sense and antisense strand-specific RNA probes were prepared by in vitro transcription of the 372-bp K-*ras* cDNA fragment spanning the first and second exon sequences as the template, which had been subcloned into a Bluescript vector. Hybridization was performed in 50% formamide, 5x Denhardt's solution, 0.1% SDS, 5x SSPE and 100mg/ml of salmon testis DNA at 42°C for 16 hr. The filters were then washed in 0.1x SSC and 0.1% SDS at 65°C. K-*ras* p21 immunoblot analysis was performed on cell lysates prepared in RIPA buffer (10mM Tris-HCl, pH7.4, 1% deoxycholate, 1% Nonidet-40, 150mM NaCl, 0.1% SDS, 0.2mM phenylmethylsulfonyl fluoride, 1μg/ml aprotinin, 1μg/ml leupeptin). 80μg of protein was immunoblotted by a K-*ras* specific p21 monoclonal antibody (Oncogene Science) and developed by enhanced chemiluminescence system (ECL). Serial dilution of the sample on the same blot and quantification of the band intensity by image analysis based on NIH Image software (ver. 1.52, NIH) assured that the immunoblot analysis was carried out semi-quantitatively.

Nude mouse treatment model for peritoneal dissemination of pancreatic cancer

6×10^5 AsPC-1 cells were transplanted intra-peritoneally to the nude mice, forming multiple tumor nodules mainly on the mesentery, pancreas and hepatic hilus by day 28. Three days after the tumor cell transplantation, the mice were injected intra-peritoneally with 100μg of AS-K-*ras*-LNSX DNA complexed with 400nmol of DOGS lipopolyamine [18] at 12hr intervals 3 times. Twenty-eight days after the AsPC-1 transplantation, the mice were sacrificed and examined for tumor development in the peritoneal cavity. Distribution of the vector DNA was examined by Southern blot and PCR analyses of the DNA extracted from the brain, lung, heart, liver, pancreas, spleen, kidney, testis, stomach, small intestine, colon, skeletal muscle and bone marrow at day 24 of DNA/lipopolyamine injection. One microgram of DNA was amplified by the primers specific to the LNSX vector sequence. For Southern blot analysis, the genomic DNA was digested by *KpnI*, which should yield the internal 3378-bp fragment from the K-*ras*-LNSX plasmid, irrespective of its presence as the episomal or integrated form.

RESULTS

Antisense K-*ras*-induced reduction of K-*ras* p21 protein expression

AsPC-1 cells were transfected either with antisense K-*ras* vector AS-K-*ras*-LNSX or sense K-*ras*-LNSX to generate AsPC-1-AS and AsPC-1-S cells, respectively. Several clones of AsPC-1-AS cells were isolated by G418 selection. First, Southern blot analysis confirmed the integration of the intact vector sequence in most of the clones. RNA blot hybridization with the strand-specific sense or antisense K-*ras* RNA probe detected a stable expression of the 3.5-kb antisense or sense K-*ras* RNA, which is considered to be the read-through transcript from the 5' LTR (not shown). Immunoblot analysis using the K-*ras* specific p21 monoclonal antibody showed a reduction of up to 20% of the K-*ras* p21 protein in the cloned AsPC-1-AS cells compared with the parental AsPC-1 cells. Furthermore, in the pooled AsPC-1-AS cells, the K-*ras* p21 protein was also decreased. Parental AsPC-1 cells and AsPC-1-S cells had identical expression of K-*ras* p21 (data not shown).

In vitro growth suppression of the antisense K-*ras*-transfected pancreatic cancer cells

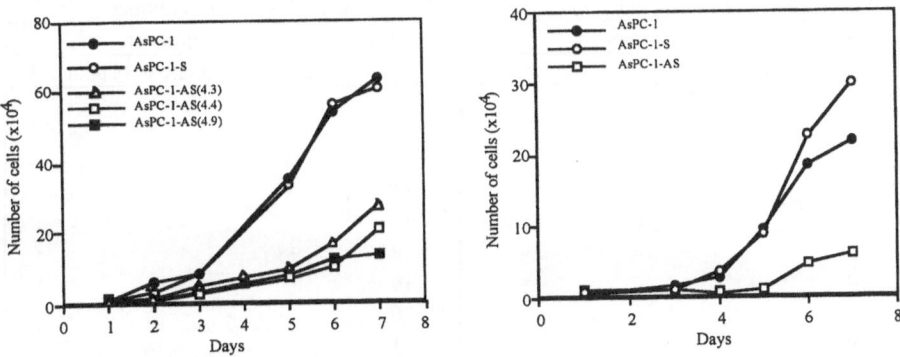

Fig. 2   *In vitro* growth curve of AsPC-1-AS and AsPC-1-S, antisense and sense K-*ras*-transfected AsPC-1 cells, respectively. 1×10^4 cells were seeded in duplicate in 6-well plates, and viable cells were counted at the indicated period of culture time by trypan blue dye exclusion assay. Left panel showed three antisense-expressing clones, 4.3, 4.4 and 4.9. Right panel compares pools of multiple G418-resistant colonies.

The antisense K-*ras* transfected AsPC-1 cells grew more slowly than the sense K-*ras* transfected control, which showed essentially the same growth rate as the parental AsPC-1 cells (Fig. 2). The antisense-induced growth inhibition was apparent even for the pooled population of the transfected cells, which may bmore closely mimic the in vivo treatment situation (Fig. 2, right panel).

The antisense K-*ras*-transfected AsPC-1 cells did not show significant apoptosis when stained with bisBENZIMIDE fluorochrome. Nor was the bystander effect identified by *in vitro* co-culture of the AsPC-1-AS and AsPC-1 cells; 0.5×10^4 cloned AsPC-1-AS were co-cultured with an equal number of the parental AsPC-1 cells in 6-well plates. The growth curve of the mixture was between those of the AsPC-1-AS and parental AsPC-1 cells (data not shown).

Inhibition of peritoneal dissemination by lipofection-mediated in vivo transfer of AS-K-*ras*-LNSX

The above data suggested the feasibility of suppressing pancreatic cancer cell growth by inhibiting single genetic abnormality, K-*ras* mutation. Of the 22 nude mice transplanted with the AsPC-1 cells in the peritoneal cavity, 10 were injected with the sense S-K-*ras*-LNSX, and 12 with antisense AS-K-*ras*-LNSX vectors three days after tumor inoculation. As shown in Table 1, direct intra-peritoneal injection of AS-K-*ras*-LNSX plasmid/ DOGS lipopolyamine complex suppressed tumor formation significantly as compared to the injection of the S-K-*ras*-LNSX vector (p <0.005). Histological examination of the small intestine, colon and pancreas of mice treated with AS-K-*ras*-LNSX revealed no evidence of AsPC-1-derived tumor formation.

Table 1. Tumor development in the peritoneal cavity of the mice treated with K- *ras* vectors

Antisense K-*ras* injected mice				Sense K-*ras* injected mice			
Mouse No.	Tumors on			Mouse No.	Tumors on		
	mesentery	pancreas	hepatic hilus		mesentery	pancreas	hepatic hilus
1	-	-	-	13	++	++	+
2	-	-	-	14	++	+++	+
3	-	-	-	15	+	+	-
4	-	-	-	16	+	-	+
5	-	-	-	17	-	-	-
6	-	-	-	18	++	-	-
7	++[a]	-	-	19	-	++	+
8	-	-	-	20	+	-	-
9	-	-	-	21	+	-	-
10	-	-	-	22	++	+	-
11	-	+	-				
12	-	-	-				
#mice with tumor/ total	2/12			#mice with tumor/ total	9/10		

[a]Tumors were grades as: +, <3mm in size and <3 in number; ++, 3-10mm in size or 3-10 in number; +++, >10mm in size or >10 in number.

Distribution of injected DNA and organ toxicity

PCR analysis showed that the injected DNA was present in multiple organs except for the brain at day 24 after injection. However, Southern blot analysis failed to detect the internal $KpnI$ fragment of the vector, suggesting that the vector is present at about 1/100-1/1000 copies in the normal tissues. No treatment-related toxicity was observed in any treated mice macroscopically nor microscopically on hematoxylin- and eosin-stained histological sections.

DISCUSSION

In sum, the gene transfer of the plasmid expressing antisense K-*ras* RNA suppressed K-*ras* p21 protein production and suppressed the pancreatic cancer cell growth *in vitro* and *in vivo*. Furthermore, it was suggested that the direct intraperitoneal injection of DNA: lipopolyamine complex is an efficient way of introducing genes *in vivo*. Although the small amount of the injected vector was widely distributed among normal tissues at day 24 after DNA injection, no apparent organ damage was identified, suggesting that this strategy is feasible and useful in certain settings of clinical treatment of pancreatic cancer, such as adjuvant therapy to surgical resection.

Comparison of the p21 level and the growth rate for each clone of antisense-transfected AsPC-1 suggested that the reduction of the K-*ras* p21 protein is proportional to the growth inhibition attained. By contrast, no evidence of increased apoptosis in AsPC-1-AS was identified by bisBENZIMIDE fluorochrome staining. Thus, the mechanism of the population growth suppression may not be the direct killing effect of the antisense K-*ras* RNA but the slowing down of the cell growth induced by the reduction of the mutated p21 protein, presumably the critical biochemical feature by which the pancreatic cancer cells continue to grow. We also investigated whether the antisense-expressing cells could inhibit the growth of the surrounding non-transduced populations, i.e., bystander effect. The co-culture of the AsPC-1-AS and the parental AsPC-1 cells did not show the growth inhibitory effect of the transduced cells on the non-transduced cells. This observed lack of any significant bystander effect should necessitate a very high efficiency of the gene transfer to the *in vivo* target cancer cells in order to achieve any therapeutic impact based on this strategy.

In this context, it was rather unexpected that we observed a significant suppression of the peritoneal and pancreatic tumor formation following the direct intraperitoneal injection of the AS-K-*ras*-LNSX: lipopolyamine complex. Gene transfer by liposome *in vivo* has certain limitations such as a low transduction efficiency and transient nature of the expression [19]. Presumably, the large amount of injected DNA to tumor cells might have enabled the efficient in vivo gene transfer in this particular experimental design. Liposome-mediated *in vivo* gene transfer deserves further extensive study because it has a number of advantages over the viral vectors; there is no possibility of the generation of replication competent virus; the liposome vector will be much more stable in the protein and cell-rich malignant ascites and in the blood stream; there is no acute toxicity or immune reaction such as those experienced for adenovirus vectors; virus-based gene transfer would be less prone to problems than multiple injections; vector production is less costly and less cumbersome.

In the nude mouse study using different cancer cells, it has been observed that the first adhesion of cancer cells to peritoneal mesothelium takes place between day 5 and day 7 day following intraperitoneal inoculation of the cancer cells The cancer cells then start proliferating and infiltrating the muscle layer on days 9 to 11 [20, 21]. It is conceivable that the primary target of the AS-K-*ras*-LNSX/lipopolyamine injected at day 3 or 4 is the initial adherence step of the AsPC-1 cells to the peritoneal mesothelium and pancreas. The peritoneal dissemination and local regional recurrence are the most frequent modes of recurrence after surgical resection of pancreatic cancer [22, 23]. Thus, the prevention and treatment of peritoneal dissemination are one of the most important issues in the treatment of pancreatic cancer. This study suggested that the intraperitoneal injection of the antisense K-*ras* expression construct complexed with liposome is effective in an early stage of carcinomatous peritonitis as an adjuvant therapy to the surgical restriction of the pancreatic cancer.

RNA blot analysis by the strand specific RNA probes showed that the size of the major antisense or sense K-*ras* RNA was 3.5 Kb, which was considered to be a read-through message from the promoter in 5' LTR of the LNSX vector. It thus remains to be shown which antisense sequence-containing transcript is essential for the suppression of the p21 protein, and whether the long overhang of the read-through antisense message has any functional significance. Re-designing and construction of the expression plasmid would be necessary to enhanc of the inhibitory effect on the growth of pancreatic cancer cells.

It has been reported that the K-*ras* gene mutation pattern in pancreatic cancer shows a geographical difference. In Japan, the most frequently detected mutation is a GGT to GAT transition at codon 12 [8, 10]. In the Netherlands, by contrast, mutations of this codon to TGT, GTT and GAT have been shown to occur essentially at an equal incidence [24]. In addition to the AsPC-1 cells, which have a GGT to GAT transition, we have also confirmed that another pancreatic cancer cell line, MIAPaCa-2, which has a GGT to TGT mutation, responded in vitro to our antisense-K-*ras* treatment [16]. It is expected that our strategy, the expression of the wild type K-*ras* cDNA fragment in the antisense orientation, would be useful in suppressing the proliferation of pancreatic cancer cells irrespective of the type of their K-*ras* mutation. This point marks an advantage to the other approach to target a specific mutated K-*ras* mRNA such as the ribozyme method, which can cleave only 3' to XUX-G sequences [25].

To address the inadvertent vector delivery to normal tissues, we performed Southern blot and PCR analysis for the evidence of the vector DNA in major organs of the treated mice. The PCR analysis, but not Southern blot analysis, showed that the injected DNA was delivered to various organs except the brain at least at day 24 after DNA injection. The different time point has not been examined.

Liposomes injected into the peritoneal cavity enter the lymphatics and then the blood circulation [19, 26, 27] to be distributed to the extra-peritoneal organs. The blood brain barrier may have blocked the liposome entry to the brain. Even though we did not find any evidence to suggest any macroscopic or microscopic toxicity in the treated mice, further examinations are required to define in which type of cells the injected DNA is present in tissues, how long DNA stays in the testis and ovary, and whether DNA is integrated into the genome of the spermatozoa and oocytes.

ACKNOWLEDGMENTS

This work was supported in part by a Grant-in-Aid for the 2nd Term Comprehensive 10-Year Strategy for Cancer Control from the Ministry of Health and Welfare, by Grants-in-Aid for Cancer Research from the Ministry of Health and Welfare and from the Ministry of Education, Science and Culture. We thank Dr. A. Dusty Miller for providing the LNSX vector. We are also grateful to Drs. Makoto Tsukamoto and Takahiro Ochiya for discussions and technical advice.

REFERENCES

1. Yamaguchi K, Enjoji M (1989) Carcinoma of the pancreas: a clinicopathologic study of 96 cases with immunohistochemical observations. Jpn. J. Clin. Oncol. 19:14-22
2. Warshaw AL, Fernandez-del Castillo C (1992) Pancreatic carcinoma. [Review]. N. Engl. J. Med. 326:455-65
3. Cohn I Jr. (1990) Overview of pancreatic cancer, 1989. [Review]. International Journal of Pancreatology 7:1-11
4. Ozaki H (1992) Improvement of pancreatic cancer treatment from the Japanese experience in the 1980s. [Review]. International Journal of Pancreatology 12:5-9
5. Arbuck SG (1990) Overview of chemotherapy for pancreatic cancer. [Review]. International Journal of Pancreatology 7:209-22
6. Dobelbower RR, Bronn DG (1990) Radiotherapy in the treatment of pancreatic cancer. [Review]. Baillieres Clinical Gastroenterology 4:969-83
7. Almoguera C, Shibata D, Forrester K, Martin J, Arnheim N, Perucho M (1988) Most human carcinomas of the exocrine pancreas contain mutant c-K-ras genes. Cell 53:549-54
8. Mariyama M, Kishi K, Nakamura K, Obata H, Nishimura S (1989) Frequency and types of point mutation at the 12th codon of the c-Ki-ras gene found in pancreatic cancers from Japanese patients. Jpn. J. Cancer Res. 80:622-6
9. Grunewald K, Lyons J, Frohlich A, et al. (1989) High frequency of Ki-ras codon 12 mutations in pancreatic adenocarcinomas. Int. J. Cancer 43:1037-41
10. Nagata Y, Abe M, Motoshima K, Nakayama E, Shiku H (1990) Frequent glycine-to-aspartic acid mutations at codon 12 of c-Ki-ras gene in human pancreatic cancer in Japanese. Jpn. J. Cancer Res. 81:135-40

11. Yanagisawa A, Ohtake K, Ohashi K, et al. (1993) Frequent c-Ki-ras oncogene activation in mucous cell hyperplasias of pancreas suffering from chronic inflammation. Cancer Res. 53:953-6

12. DiGiuseppe JA, Hruban RH, Offerhaus GJ, et al. (1994) Detection of K-ras mutations in mucinous pancreatic duct hyperplasia from a patient with a family history of pancreatic carcinoma. American Journal of Pathology 144:889-95

13. Scarpa A, Capelli P, Mukai K, et al. (1993) Pancreatic adenocarcinomas frequently show p53 gene mutations. American Journal of Pathology 142:1534-43

14. Liu Q, Yan YX, McClure M, Nakagawa H, Fujimura F, Rustgi AK (1995) MTS-1 (CDKN2) tumor suppressor gene deletions are a frequent event in esophagus squamous cancer and pancreatic adenocarcinoma cell lines. Oncogene 10:619-22

15. Horii A, Nakatsuru S, Miyoshi Y, et al. (1992) Frequent somatic mutations of the APC gene in human pancreatic cancer. Cancer Res. 52:6696-8

16. Aoki K, Yoshida T, Sugimura T, Terada M (1995) Liposome-mediated in vivo gene transfer of antisense K-ras construct inhibits pancreatic tumor dissemination in the murine peritoneal cavity. Cancer Res 55:3810-6

17. Miller AD, Rosman GJ (1989) Improved retroviral vectors for gene transfer and expression. Biotechniques 7:980-2

18. Behr JP, Demeneix B, Loeffler JP, Perez-Mutul J (1989) Efficient gene transfer into mammalian primary endocrine cells with lipopolyamine-coated DNA. Proc. Natl. Acad. Sci. USA 86:6982-6

19. Hug P, Sleight RG (1991) Liposomes for the transformation of eukaryotic cells. [Review]. Biochim. Biophys. Acta 1097:1-17

20. Birbeck MSC, Wheatley DN (1965) An electron microscopic study of the invasion of ascites tumor cells into the abdominal wall. Cancer Res. 25:490-497

21. Buck RC (1973) Walker 256 tumor implantation in normal and injured peritoneum studied by electron microscopy, scanning electron microscopy, and autoradiography. Cancer Res. 33:3181-8

22. Kayahara M, Nagakawa T, Ueno K, Ohta T, Takeda T, Miyazaki I (1993) An evaluation of radical resection for pancreatic cancer based on the mode of recurrence as determined by autopsy and diagnostic imaging. Cancer 72:2118-23

23. Westerdahl J, Andren-Sandberg A, Ihse I (1993) Recurrence of exocrine pancreatic cancer--local or hepatic? Hepato Gastroenterology 40:384-7

24. Smit VT, Boot AJ, Smits AM, Fleuren GJ, Cornelisse CJ, Bos JL (1988) KRAS codon 12 mutations occur very frequently in pancreatic adenocarcinomas. Nucl. Acids Res. 16:7773-82

25. Haseloff J, Gerlach WL (1988) Simple RNA enzymes with new and highly specific endoribonuclease activities. Nature 334:585-91

26. Ellens H, Morselt H, Scherphof G (1981) In vivo fate of large unilamellar sphingomyelin-cholesterol liposomes after intraperitoneal and intravenous injection into rats. Biochim. Biophys. Acta 674:10-8

27. Parker RJ, Sieber SM, Weinstein JN (1981) Effect of liposome encapsulation of a fluorescent dye on its uptake by the lymphatics of the rat. Pharmacology 23:128-36

Adoptive Immunotherapy with Cytokine Gene-modified Cytotoxic T Lymphocytes

Junko Abe[1], Hiroaki Wakimoto[1,2], Yoko Yoshida[1], Satoshi Okabe[1,3], Rikiya Tsunoda[4], Masaru Aoyagi[2], Kimiyoshi Hirakawa[2], and Hirofumi Hamada[1]

[1]Department of Molecular Biotherapy Research, Cancer Chemotherapy Center, Cancer Institute, 1-37-1 Kami-Ikebukuro, Toshima-ku, Tokyo 170; [2]Department of Neurosurgery and [3]First Department of Surgery, Tokyo Medical and Dental University, Bunkyo-ku, Tokyo 113; [4]Department of Anatomy, Fukushima Medical College, Fukushima-shi, Fukushima 960-12, Japan.

SUMMARY

Adoptive immunogene therapy of cancer is not widely studied, although it has been proposed as a promising strategy for cancer gene therapy. One of the major obstacles to this approach is the difficulty in introducing cytokine genes efficiently into T lymphocytes. We developed adoptive immunotherapy models with murine tumor-specific cytotoxic T lymphocytes (CTL). By using adenoviral vectors, we achieved up to 100% gene transduction of murine T lymphocytes. Treatment of mice with the CTL genetically modified to produce IL-2 resulted in reduction of tumor metastasis and longer survival from intracerebral tumor death. Through a comparative study on the antitumor effects of CTL genetically modified with a variety of cytokine genes, transduction with interferon-g gene showed a prominent increase in therapeutic efficacy of CTL in both metastatic and subcutaneous tumor models. Further additive effect was obtained by the adoptive cellular therapy in combination with vaccination of cytokine gene-modified tumor cells. Our findings provide a hopeful strategy of adoptive immunotherapy for human cancers.

Key Words: Adoptive Immunotherapy, Cytotoxic T lymphocyte, Adenoviral Vector, Interleukin-2, Interferon-g

INTRODUCTION

Along with vaccination using tumor cells as antigens, adoptive cellular therapy is a major strategy of cancer immunotherapy [1-3]. In the adoptive immunotherapy, autologous (or syngeneic) immunocompetent cells are expanded in vitro, and transferred to the tumor-bearing host [1,2]. During the period of ex vivo cell culture, antitumor immune response is selectively augmented, leading to circumvention of immunosuppressive conditions which are often present in tumor-bearing host (reviewed in ref. 4). A marking study demonstrated, however, that adoptively transferred tumor-infiltrating lymphocytes (TIL) were rapidly cleared from the circulation and inefficiently localized to tumor sites, exerting insufficient therapeutic efficacy [5]. In the face of the unsuccessful results of clinical studies, it is essential to develop novel modalities to improve therapeutic efficacies of the adoptive therapy [6,7].

Genetic transduction of the effector cells with cytokine genes has been proposed as a promising approach to improve antitumor activity, although investigations involving genetic modification of effector T cells have been hampered by the technical difficulties

174

[6]. It has remained unknown which cytokines are beneficial for cancer therapy when they are expressed in cytotoxic T lymphocytes (CTL). Using newly developed recombinant adenoviral vectors, we have achieved highly efficient gene transfer into tumor-specific CTL, and demonstrated that the production of IL-2 in the TIL enhanced the efficacy of adoptive therapy [7]. Further, we attempted to determine what cytokines were beneficial for adoptive cellular therapy when expressed in CTL. Through testing the effects of a variety of cytokines, we found that treatment of mice with the CTL producing interferon-g resulted in the most efficient suppression of tumor growth. The antitumor effect of the adoptive therapy with interferon-g -producing CTL were further augmented by the combined therapy with vaccination of irradiated, gene-modified tumor cells.

MATERIALS AND METHODS

Tumor cell lines and animals. B16F10, a metastatic subline of murine melanoma B16 originally developed by I. Fidler [8], was maintained in Dulbecco's modified Eagle's medium supplemented with 10% fetal calf serum and 2 mM glutamine. Colon-26 adenocarcinoma line was cultured in the same conditions. Female C57BL/6, (C57BL/6 x DBA/2)F1 (BDF1), and BALB/c mice, purchased from Charles River Japan, Atsugi, were used at the age of 6 to 8 weeks.

Preparation of TIL. Preparation of TIL was done as described [9-11] with some modifications. Freshly digested B16 melanoma tumor was suspended at 5×10^7 cells/ml in the complete culture medium (CM) at 4 ° C. CM consisted of RPMI 1640 with 10% heat-inactivated fetal bovine serum, 2mM L-glutamine, 5×10^{-5}M 2-mercaptoethanol, 100 U/ml penicillin, 100 mg/ml streptomycin, 0.5 mg/ml amphotericin B, 10mM 3-(N-morpholino)propanesulfonic acid, and 70 IU/ml recombinant human IL-2 provided by Shionogi Pharmaceuticals Co., Osaka. Cells were mixed with an equal volume of anti-CD8-conjugated immunomagnetic beads at 1×10^8/ml and incubated for 2 h at 4° C. Beads with attached cells were pelleted, washed three times with cold CM, suspended at 1×10^7 beads/ml in CM, plated in 24-well tissue culture plates and incubated at 37 ° C in 5% CO_2. By day 1, the beads, which had separated from the cells, were pelleted and discarded. All cultures were stimulated on day 1 with 2 x 10^5 irradiated (10,000 rads) tumor cells and 1×10^6 irradiated (3,000 rads) normal mouse splenocytes per well. The in vitro stimulation was repeated every 7 to 14 days. Cultures were split when confluent and were replated at 2×10^5 cells/ml in fresh CM. Cultures received fresh CM every 2 to 3 days.

Irradiation of Cells. Tumor cells and splenocytes were irradiated with a HITACHI MBR-1505R X-ray generator.

Flow Cytometry. Flow cytometry of cells was performed with a FACScan (Becton-Dickinson). The anti-mouse CD3 monoclonal antibody MAB1442 was purchased from Chemical International Inc. Hybridoma cell lines which produce anti-mouse CD8 (53-6.72, ATCC TIB105), anti-mouse CD4 (GK1.5, ATCC TIB207), anti-mouse NK (PK136, ATCC HB191) were purchased from American Type Culture Collection (ATCC). Ascites fluids containing monoclonal antibodies were prepared as described [12]. The R-phycoerythrin (R-PE)-labelled anti-H-2K^b (AF6-88.5) and FITC-labelled anti-H-2D^b (KH95) monoclonal antibodies were purchased from Pharmingen (San Diego, CA).

IL-2 Bioassay.   IL-2 bioassay was done as described [13].   Briefly, CTL were plated in 96-well tissue culture plates at 1×10^4 cells per well in a final volume of 0.2 ml growth medium supplemented with various concentrations of IL-2.   After incubation for 20 h, cells were pulsed with $1 \mu Ci$ [^{3}H]-thymidine per well and incorporation of the isotope was measured 4 h later.

Cytotoxicity Assay.   Cytotoxicity against B16 melanoma cells was assessed using b-D-galactosidase enzyme assay.   First, B16 cells were marked with a reporter lacZ gene by retroviral infection.   Approximately 90% of the cells expressed b-D-galactosidase. 3×10^5 of B16 cells were cocultured with various numbers of the TIL for 18 h in 24-well plates.   Then the detached tumor cells were discarded and β-D-galactosidase activity of the B16 cells which remained adhesive on the plates was assayed by the method described [14].   The percentage of detached cells was calculated as:

% detached cells = (1- experimental data / data of the well without effector cells) x 100.

^{51}Cr Release Assay.   CTL-mediated cytotoxicity against YAC-1 lymphoma cells (ATCC, TIB160) and P815 mastocytoma cells (ATCC, TIB64) was measured by the standard 4 h-^{51}Cr release assay as described [15].   The anti-mouse CD3 monoclonal antibody from the hybridoma 145-2C11 (ATCC, CRL1975) was used at a final concentration of 1/4000 dilution of ascites.

Retrovirus-mediated Gene Transduction.   To introduce a marker gene into cultured cells, we used ΨCRIP/MFGlacZ [16,17], which produces the replication-defective retrovirus containing lacZ gene.   Retrovirus-mediated gene transduction was carried out as previously described [16].   To estimate the percentage of cells expressing the newly introduced gene, we assayed duplicate cell culture plates for the presence of β-D-galactosidase by using 5-bromo-4-chloro-3-indolyl β-D-galactopyranoside (X-gal) as substrate.   Cleavage of this substrate by β-D-galactosidase yields a blue precipitate, which results in diffuse staining of transduced cells.

Adenovirus-mediated Gene Transduction.   The recombinant adenoviruses were constructed by homologous recombination between the expression cosmid cassette and the parental virus genome.   The method of generating recombinant adenovirus was a modification of the method of Saito et al. [18] and the detailed procedure will be published elsewhere (Miyake, S. et al., unpublished).   Briefly, an expression cosmid cassette was constructed by inserting the expression unit [19], comprised of the cytomegalovirus enhancer plus chicken β-actin promoter, a cDNA coding sequence, and the rabbit β-globin poly(A) signal sequence, into the SwaI site of pAdex1w which is a 42 kb cosmid containing 31 kb adenovirus type 5 genome lacking E1A, E1B, and E3 genes.   The expression cosmid cassette and adenovirus DNA-terminal protein complex were cotransfected into 293 cells (ATCC, CRL1573) by calcium phosphate precipitation method.   Incorporation of the expression cassette into the isolated recombinant virus was confirmed by digestion with appropriate restriction enzymes.   The recombinant viruses were subsequently propagated with 293 cells and the viral solution was stored at -80 ° C.   The titers of viral stocks were determined by plaque assay on 293 cells. For in vitro infection of adenoviruses, the medium was discarded from the cells seeded in 12-well culture plates, and 150 ml of viral stock was added to each well.   After incubation for 1 h at 37 ° C, growth medium was added and cells were cultured for 2 to 3 days.

Intracerebral Tumor Model.   BDF1 mice were transplanted into the right parietal lobe of the brain with 1×10^3 B16 cells mixed with 3×10^4 cells of the CD8+TIL with or without gene transduction. The antitumor effect was assessed by the survival of the mice.

Treatment model against lung metastasis. For adoptive therapy, TIL were infected with recombinant adenovirus as described [7] at a multiplicity of infection (m.o.i.) of 500 and used 24 h after the infection. Two days after the challenge with intravenous injection of tumor cells, genetically modified TIL at various E/T ratios were injected intravenously.′ For vaccination with tumor cells, irradiated (10,000 rads) genetically modified tumor cells (5 x 10^5) were prepared as described [20] and injected subcutaneously in the left flank of mice 2 days after the challenge. Sixteen days after the B16 challenge or 18 days after the Colon-26 challenge, mice were sacrificed and metastatic tumor nodules in the lung were counted under microscopic observation. Animal experiments were repeated at least twice. Statistical analysis was performed by the Mann-Whittney's U test.

Treatment against subcutaneous tumor. Mice were challenged subcutaneously in the right flank with 2 x 10^5 B16F10 cells. Two days after the challenge, mice were treated with intravenous injection of TIL with or without genetic transduction. Tumor growth was monitored by measuring the longest diameter and the perpendicular diameter of the mass, and scored by using the formula $(0.4)(a \times b^2)$ where a is the longer diameter and b is the shorter diameter [21]. Mice were sacrificed when challenge tumors exceeded 2 cm (longer diameter) or severe ulceration or bleeding developed as described previously [16]. Animal experiments were repeated at least twice.

Quantitative measurement of murine interferon-γ. This was done by using an in vitro enzyme-linked immunosorbent assay kit obtained from Endogen, Cambridge MA.

RESULTS

I. GENETIC TRANSDUCTION OF MURINE CD8+CTL. CD8+TIL were isolated from subcutaneous B16 melanoma tumor by using immunomagnetic beads. The cells were cultured with periodical in vitro stimulations with irradiated B16 tumor cells and mouse spleen cells. Flow cytometry revealed that the TIL consisted of Thy1-, CD3- and CD8-positive, CD4- and NK-negative T lymphocytes (Fig. 1).

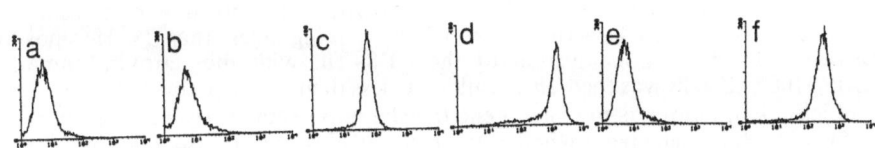

Fig.1 Characterization of the TIL. A, Flow cytometry of the TIL. Cells were stained with *a*, control serum; *b*, anti-NK; *c*, anti-CD3; *d*, anti-Thy1.2; *e*, anti-CD4; and *f*, anti-CD8 monoclonal antibodies. The ordinate and abscissa represent cell number and fluorescence intensity, respectively.

The CD8-positive TIL were IL-2-dependent, as determined by [^{3}H]-thymidine uptake assay (Fig. 2a). Half maximal growth stimulation was obtained at 4 IU/ml of IL-2. By microscopic observation, the B16 tumor monolayer was substantially damaged by the TIL after 1 day and completely disappeared after 2 days of cocultivation. Cytotoxicity assay using b-galactosidase enzyme test confirmed this microscopic observation (Fig. 2b). Murine YAC-1 lymphoma cells, which are susceptible to natural killer activity, were not damaged by the CD8+TIL (Fig. 2c). P815 mastocytoma cells, which are often used as target cells of CTL, were killed by the CD8+TIL only when they were cocultured in the presence of anti-CD3 antibody (Fig. 2c). Taken together, these results indicate that the CD8+TIL were CTL with specific cytotoxicity against B16 melanoma cells.

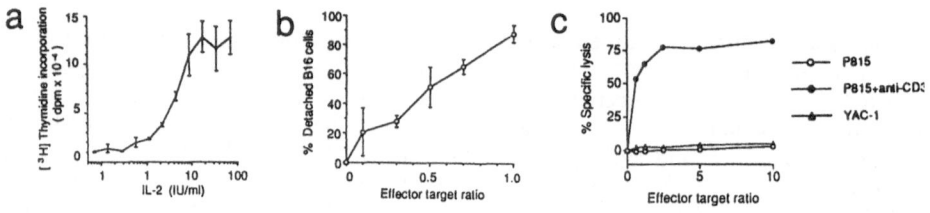

Fig.2 Growth and cytotoxicity of the TIL. *a*, IL-2-dependent growth of the CD8+TIL. *b*, The CD8+TIL-mediated cytotoxicity against B16 cells. *c*, Cytotoxicity assay against P815 and YAC-1 cells. Data represent the mean and the standard deviation of triplicate determinations.

To develop an animal model for adoptive immunogene therapy, we attempted to genetically modify the CD8+TIL. Retrovirus-mediated gene transduction is widely used in human gene therapy protocols [6]. Using a reporter recombinant retrovirus MFGlacZ (Fig. 3a), we attained highly efficient gene transfer into murine fibroblasts (Fig. 3b), as well as B16 melanoma cells (data not shown). In contrast, gene transduction efficiency of the murine CD8+TIL was very low, resulting in less than 1% lacZ-positive CD8+TIL (Fig. 3c). Cocultivation of the CD8+TIL with the retrovirus producer ψCRIP/MFGlacZ cells was tried, also resulting in less than 1% gene transduction. Thus, the efficiency of retrovirus-mediated gene transfer into murine CTL was very poor. It remains to be fully elucidated whether the cause of this poor transduction lies in the difficulty in the virus entry or the expression of the coded gene following the viral entry. We next tried an adenoviral vector derived from human adenovirus type 5 (Fig. 3d). With a reporter adenovirus Adex1CALacZ, lacZ gene expression was observed in nearly 100% of the CD8+TIL (Fig. 3f). We also attained efficient gene transduction of murine CD4+TIL and primary-cultured lymphocytes from lymph nodes, indicating that the feasibility of gene transduction by the recombinant adenovirus is not limited to the CD8+TIL (data not shown).

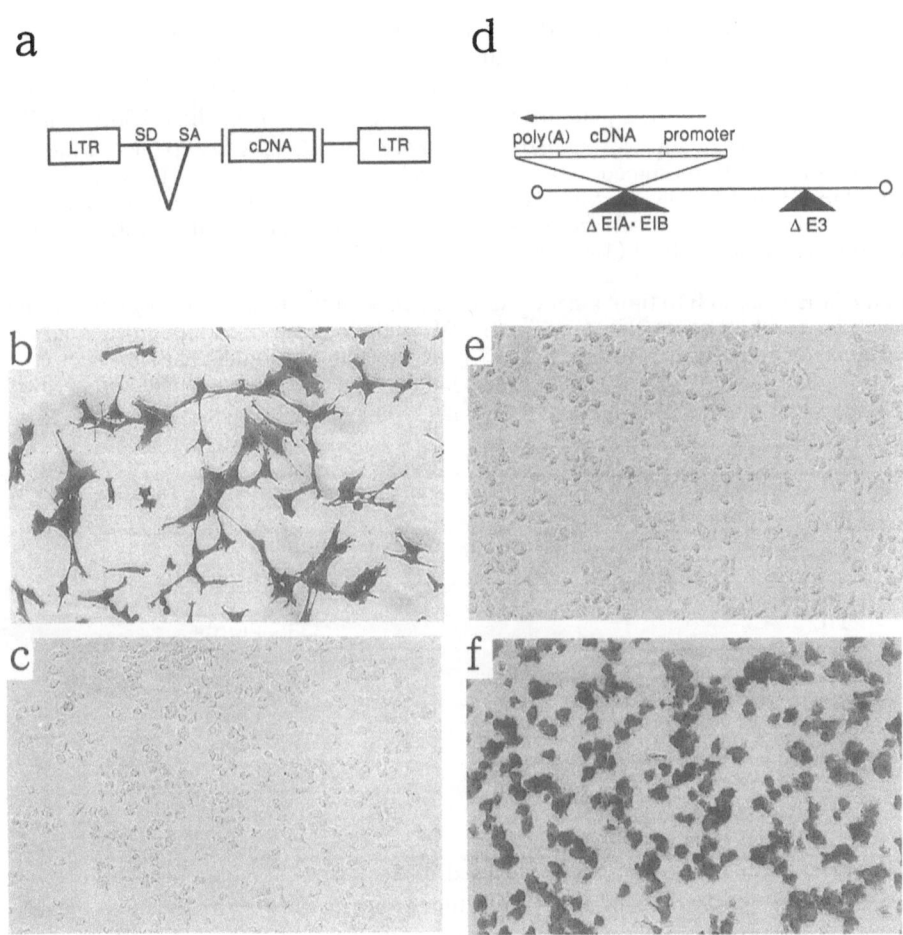

Fig.3   Recombinant virus-mediated gene transduction.   *a*, Structure of the recombinant retroviral vector.   The retroviral MFG vector was originally developed by R.C. Mulligan [16].   A 3.1 kb DNA fragment encoding the *E. coli* β-D-galactosidase (lacZ) was inserted into MFG to generate MFGlacZ.   *b*, X-gal staining of NIH3T3 fibroblasts infected with MFGlacZ.   *c*, X-gal staining of the CD8+TIL infected with MFGlacZ.   *d*, Structure of the Adex1 vector.   In place of E1A and E1B, an expression unit composed of a promoter, a cDNA, and a poly(A) signal was introduced to generate the Adex1 expression vector.   *e*, X-gal staining of the CD8+TIL infected with Adex1w, which lacks the lacZ expression cassette.   *f*, X-gal staining of the TIL infected with Adex1CAlacZ.

II. ADOPTIVE IMMUNOTHERAPY WITH CD8+CTL PRODUCING IL-2.

Since IL-2 and IL-7 are known as potent stimulators for CTL, recombinant adenoviruses encoding murine IL-2 and IL-7 were generated for in vivo studies. By infection of these viruses, we obtained gene-modified TIL that secrete more than 3,000 IU/ml/10^6 cells/24h of IL-2 and 2 ng/ml/10^6 cells/24h of IL-7, respectively, while the nontransduced TIL produced undetectable level of these cytokines. Treatment of mice with the TIL genetically modified to produce IL-2 resulted in further reduction in the number of metastatic tumor nodules than the nontransduced TIL, while IL-7 gene transduction had no effect (Table 1).

In the intracerebral B16 tumor model, mice treated with the IL-2-producing TIL survived much longer than control mice, while the TIL without gene transduction showed only marginal therapeutic effect (Fig.4). IL-7 gene transduction, again, had no effect in this model (data not shown). These results indicate that in vivo viability or cytotoxic activity of the TIL was augmented by IL-2 gene transduction.

Table 1 Antitumor effect of cytokine gene-transduced TIL in the B16F10 lung metastasis model

Effector	Effector/target ratio	Mean number of lung metastatic nodules (SE)	
control	0	465	(24)
TIL (4×10^5)	1	333	(76)[a]
TIL/IL2 (4×10^5)	1	219	(79)[b]
TIL/IL7 (4×10^5)	1	306	(128)
TIL (4×10^6)	10	30	(8)[c]
TIL/IL2 (4×10^6)	10	17	(9)[d]
TIL/IL7 (4×10^6)	10	41	(18)

Non-paired Student's t-test (SAS) was used to determine the significance of the data: [a]$p<0.01$ compared with the group without treatment; [b]$p<0.02$ compared with the group treated with TIL (4×10^5); [c]$p<0.01$ compared with the group without treatment or treated with TIL (4×10^5); [d]$p<0.01$ compared with the group treated with TIL (4×10^6). Seven mice were used for each group. Representative data from one of the two independent experiments are shown.

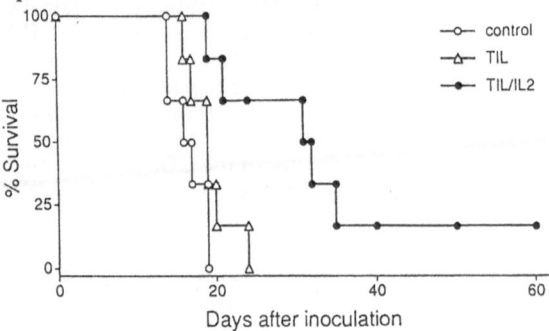

Fig.4 Effect of the IL-2 gene-transduced TIL in the intracerebral B16 tumor model. Representative data from one of the two independent experiments are shown.

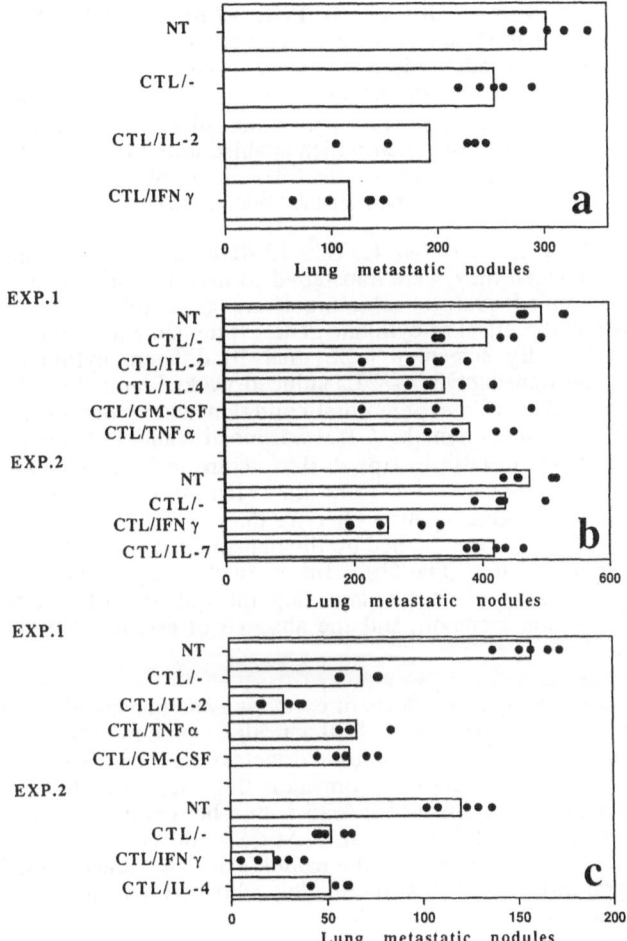

Fig.5 Effect of cytokine gene transduction of CTL in lung metastatic models.
a, Treatment against B16 lung metastasis with TIL/B16 transduced with IL-2 or interferon-γ. Mice were intravenously injected with 3×10^5 B16 cells, followed 2 days later by intravenous injection of 4.5×10^6 of TIL/B16 (E/T 15) without gene transduction (CTL/-), with IL-2 gene transduction (CTL/IL-2), or with interferon-γ gene transduction (CTL/IFNγ). Control mice were injected with the same volume of saline (nontreated, NT). The points represent the number of metastatic nodules of individual mouse, and the bar shows the mean of five determinations. **b**, Treatment against B16 lung metastasis with TIL/B16 transduced with cytokine genes. Mice were intravenously injected with 4×10^5 B16 cells, followed 2 days later by intravenous injection of 4×10^6 of TIL/B16 (E/T 10) without gene transduction (CTL/-), with genetic transduction of IL-4, GM-CSF, TNF-α, interferon-γ, and IL-7. **c**, Treatment against Colon-26 lung metastasis with TIL/C26 transduced with cytokine genes. Mice were intravenously injected with 2×10^4 Colon-26 cells, followed 2 days later by intravenous injection of 2×10^5 of TIL/C26 (E/T 10) without gene transduction (CTL/-), with genetic transduction of IL-2, TNF-α, GM-CSF, interferon-γ and IL-4.

III. COMPARATIVE STUDIES ON THE EFFECTS OF CYTOKINES[5]. For comparative studies on the effects of cytokines expressed in CD8+CTL, we generated a panel of recombinant adenoviruses derived from human adenovirus type 5 with expression cassettes [18,19] containing a variety of cytokines essentially as described previously [7]. In general, high titer viral stock solutions with more than 10^9 plaque-forming unit (pfu)/ml were obtained, which enabled us to perform highly efficient (nearly 100%) genetic transductions of murine CTL as confirmed by X-gal staining of the lymphocytes transduced with a reporter lacZ adenovirus.

Treatment with gene-modified CTL. TIL/B16 demonstrated only an insufficient antitumor effect when they were transferred to mice bearing B16 metastatic tumors in the lung [7]. An adequate effector/target ratio (E/T) of 10 was chosen in order to sensitively detect the effect of cytokine gene expression which enhanced the antitumor activity of CTL. By screening more than 10 different cytokines, we found that interferon-γ gene transduction of CTL induced marked reduction of metastatic nodule formation (Fig. 5a). In an experimental condition where the effect of nontransduced CTL was 10 - 20% reduction, the CTL transduced with interferon-γ exerted 60 - 75% reduction of lung metastases ($p < 0.01$ compared with nontransduced CTL). Experiments were repeated for more than five times and the interferon-γ gene transduction was reproducibly more effective than the IL-2 gene transduction ($p < 0.05$). No significant effects were obtained by the transduction with other cytokines; i.e., IL-4, GM-CSF, TNF-α, and IL-7 (Fig. 5b). The ineffectiveness of these cytokines could be attributed to a variety of causes, including the quantity of secreted cytokines, the duration of cytokine secretion, and the absence of essential factors such as IL-2 or interferon-γ.

Adoptive immunotherapeutic effects of cytokine gene transductions on lung metastasis of Colon-26 were also examined. In this model, again, transduction of TIL/C26 with interferon-γ or IL-2 gene induced a marked increase in their antitumor effect, leading to efficient suppression of metastasis formation (Fig. 5c). No therapeutic effects were obtained by the transductions of TIL/C26 with other cytokine genes, including TNF-α, GM-CSF, IL-4 (Fig. 5c), IL-1a, IL-6, IL-7, M-CSF, and G-CSF (data not shown). The fact that similar effects were seen in the models using two tumors of different origin (i.e., B16 and Colon-26) suggests that the findings obtained here are generally applicable to a variety of cancers.

Next we examined the therapeutic effect of cytokine gene transduction of CTL on their activities against established subcutaneous B16 tumor. As shown in Fig. 6, TIL/B16 without genetic transduction (E/T 30) revealed only a limited inhibitory effect against established solid tumors. The IL-2 gene transduction gave a significant increase in antitumor activity of CTL ($p < 0.05$ compared with nontransduced CTL on day 16). The most prominent antitumor effect was obtained by the CTL transduced with interferon-γ gene. Almost complete suppression of tumor growth was observed during the first two weeks after the administration of interferon-γ -producing CTL ($p < 0.01$ compared with the groups treated with IL-2 gene-modified CTL or nontransduced CTL on day 16) (Fig. 6).

---

[5]Abe, J., Wakimoto, H., Tunoda, R., Okabe, S., Yoshida, Y., Aoyagi, M., Hirakawa, K., and Hamada, H. In vivo antitumor effect of cytotoxic T lymphocytes engineered to produce interferon-γ by adenovirus-mediated genetic transduction. Biochem. Biophys. Res, Comm. in press

The level of interferon-γ secretion in vitro from interferon-γ gene-modified CTL was as high as 110 ng/ml per 10^5 cells per 48 h. Serum concentrations of interferon-γ from mice treated with CTL with or without the cytokine gene transduction were monitored.The interferon-γ concentration was the highest during the initial 2 to 3 days after the injection of CTL transduced with interferon-γ; ~8 - 10 ng/ml was observed by intravenous injection of 6 x 10^6 of the interferon-γ-producing CTL (Fig.7).

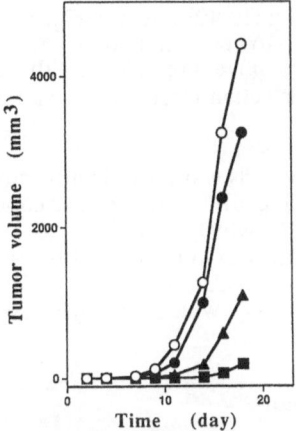

Fig.6   Therapeutic effect of CTL transduced with cytokine genes on the B16 subcutaneous tumor.   2 x 10^5 B16 cells were transplanted subcutaneously into mice. On day 2, mice were confirmed of the presence of visible subcutaneous tumors was confirmed, and the mice, randomized into groups each consisting of five, and treated with 6 x 10^6 TIL/B16 (E/T 30) with or without genetic transduction.   The data represent the mean tumor volume of each group treated with control saline (O), with nontransduced TIL/B16 (●), with TIL/B16 transduced with either IL-2 (▲) or interferon-γ(■) gene.

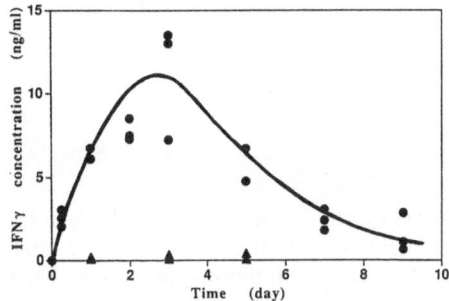

Fig.7   Serum concentration of interferon-γ in mice injected with CTL.   Mice were injected intravenously with 6 x 10^6 TIL/B16 (E/T 30) with or without interferon-γ gene transduction.   Each point demonstrates the serum concentration of interferon-γ of an individual mouse administered with nontransduced TIL/B16 (   ), or TIL/B16 transduced with interferon-γ gene (●).   Experiments were repeated twice and similar results were obtained.

In contrast, the mean serum concentration of interferon-γ from control mice injected with 6×10^6 of nontransduced CTL was 230 ± 230 pg/ml, which was comparable to the level with that of normal mice (130 ± 130 pg/ml), indicating that the rise in serum concentration of interferon-g was due to the effect of the genetic modification of CTL.

In vitro effect of interferon-g on B16 cells.   Flow cytometry analysis showed that the B16 melanoma line used in this study was MHC class I negative ($< 1\%$ positive; Fig. 8A, a).   However, the MHC class I induction was detectable at as early as 4 h after the addition of 10 ng/ml interferon-g (18.8% positive; Fig. 8A, b).   Both H-2K^b and H-2D^b were strongly induced in the B16 cells cultured in vitro for 24 h in the presence of 10 ng/ml of interferon-γ (99.9% positive; Fig. 8A, c).   The induction of the MHC class I molecules is one of the possible action mechanisms of interferon-γ leading to the in vivo therapeutic efficacy.

The in vitro growth of the B16 cells was only slightly suppressed in the presence of 10 ng/ml interferon-γ as shown in Fig. 8B.   The systemic concentration of interferon-g was, at the most, ~10 ng/ml (Fig. 7), which is unlikely to be high enough for the direct inhibition of the in vivo growth of B16 tumor.   However, it remains possible that the interferon-g -producing CTL accumulates in the tumor lesions, resulting in much higher local concentrations of interferon-γ   which directlyly suppresses the growth of the B16 tumor.

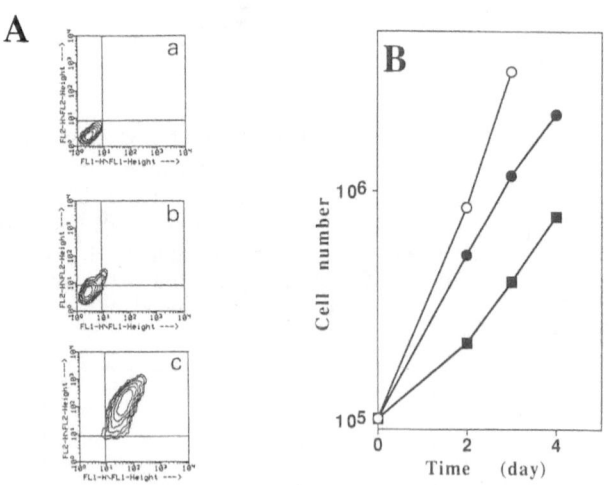

Fig.8   In vitro effects of interferon-γ on B16 cells.   **A**, Induction of MHC class I by interferon-γ.   The data demonstrate the flow cytometric analysis of B16 cells cultured in the presence of 10 ng/ml murine interferon-γ for 0 h, **a**; 4 h, **b**; and **c**; 24 h, .   Ordinate, fluorescence intensity stained with R-phycoerythrin (R-PE)-labelled anti-H-2K^b; abscissa, fluorescence intensity stained with FITC-labelled anti-H-2D^b.   **B**, Growth suppression by recombinant interferon-γ.   B16 cells were cultured in the medium without interferon-γ (○), with 10 ng/ml interferon-γ added on day 0 (●), or with 10 ng/ml interferon-γ added on day 0 followed by exchanges of the medium containing 10 ng/ml interferon-γ on day 1, 2, and 3 (■).   The data show the mean cell numbers of triplicate determinations.

Adoptive transfer of CTL in combination with gene-modified tumor vaccination.
In the previous studies on cytokine gene-modified tumor vaccination , a remarkable
antitumor response was induced by tumor cells transduced with GM-CSF gene
[16,20,31,32]. In this study, we examined the effect of interferon-γ gene-transduced
CTL in combination with GM-CSF-producing B16 tumor vaccine in the lung metastatic
model. Only a slight suppression (~15%) of metastasis was observed when mice were
treated with nontransduced CTL (Fig. 9). Vaccination with the GM-CSF-producing
tumor vaccine demonstrated a significant therapeutic effect; ~50% reduction of lung
metastatic nodules was achieved. The combined use of the GM-CSF-producing tumor
vaccine with the CTL significantly enhanced the antitumor activity. The interferon-g
gene-transduced CTL in combination with GM-CSF gene-modified tumor vaccine
resulted in the most efficient suppression of metastatic nodule formation (~85%
reduction in the number of metastatic nodules; $p < 0.01$ compared with the group treated
singly with the interferon-γ-transduced CTL; $p < 0.01$ compared with the group treated
singly with the GM-CSF-producing tumor vaccine) (Fig. 9).

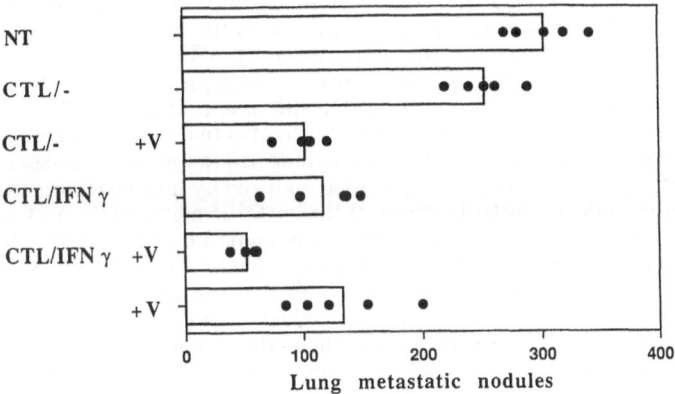

Fig.9 Therapeutic effect of adoptive therapy in combination with GM-CSF -
producing tumor vaccine in the B16 lung metastasis. Mice were first intravenously
injected with 3×10^5 B16 cells. Two days after the challenge they were intravenously
injected with 4.5×10^6 of TIL/B16 (E/T 15) without gene transduction (CTL/-), or with
interferon-γ gene transduction (CTL/ IFNγ). Control mice were injected with the same
volume of saline (nontreated, NT). For vaccination with tumor cells, irradiated (10,000
rads) GM-CSF -producing tumor cells (5×10^5) were inoculated subcutaneously in the
left flank of mice 2 days after the challenge, either alone (V) or in combination with
adoptive cellular therapies (CTL/-+V or CTL/IFNγ +V).

DISCUSSION

The transduction of tumor-specific CTL with interferon-γ gene demonstrated a
prominent augmentation of antitumor immunity in the adoptive cellular therapy in B16

melanoma as well as Colon-26 adenocarcinoma models (Fig. 5). Although the IL-2 gene transduction also showed increases in antitumor activity of CTL (Table 1, Fig. 4-6; ref. 7), the antitumor effect by the CTL augmented by the interferon-γ gene transduction was superior to that by the IL-2 gene transduction in the B16 treatment models against lung metastasis (Fig. 5a) or established subcutaneous tumors (Fig. 6). Nearly complete suppression of subcutaneous tumor growth was observed during the first two weeks after the adoptive therapy with interferon-γ gene-modified CTL.

Interferon-γ is a pleiotropic cytokine with a number of actions on many cell types (for reviews, see ref. 22,23). Recombinant interferon-γ has been reported to demonstrate some antitumor activity when administered systemically to tumor-bearing hosts [22,23]. Previous reports showed an increase in tumor suppression in vitro [24] and in vivo [25] by a glioma-specific murine CTL line transfected with interferon-γ gene. Several mechanisms are attributable to the efficacy of interferon-γ gene transduction of CTL in our adoptive therapy model: 1) interferon-γ could activate the adoptively transferred CTL in an autocrine or a paracrine manner; 2) interferon-γ could regulate specific effector mechanisms by direct actions on host helper T cells, NK cells or cytotoxic T cells; 3) amplified expression of MHC class I molecules on the tumor cells (Fig. 8A) could enhance the host antitumor response as well as the tumor susceptibility to CTL; 4) interferon-γ could upregulate the expression of MHC class II or costimulator molecules (e.g., B7-1)[26] in the host antigen-presenting cells (APC; i.e., monocytes/macrophages, dendritic cells) and/or the nonprofessional APC (i.e., epithelial, endothelial, and connective tissue cells), leading to effective tumor-antigen presentation to T lymphocytes; 5) interferon-γ could induce the expression of specific tumor-associated antigens on tumor cells which are recognized by host immunocompetent cells. In addition to the effects similar to those of the systemic administration of recombinant cytokines, more advantageous therapeutic effects could be anticipated in the adoptive transfer of the gene-modified CTL as a cytokine delivery system. Tumor-specific CTL transduced with cytokine gene(s) could possibly localize in the tumor lesions and/or regional lymph organs, leading to a high-dose local cytokine delivery to tumor cells as well as host immunocompetent cells. Since the systemic concentration of the cytokine could remain relatively low in the face of a very high local concentration, the adverse effects encountered in the high-dose systemic administration [27-30] could be controlled to minimal levels without losing the therapeutic efficacies.

A potent therapeutic effect was obtained by the combination of the interferon-g -producing CTL and the GM-CSF gene-transduced tumor vaccine (Fig. 9). Administration of the irradiated gene-modified tumor cells could work as a specific immunomodulator, keeping the CTL in an activated state with specificity against tumor antigens. GM-CSF is supposed to stimulate the professional APC of the host [16,20,31,32], leading to a tumor-specific activation of CD4+ helper T cells, which could eventually stimulate the tumoricidal activities of the CD8+CTL of both the adoptive and host origin.

Our findings could have important implications to the clinical application of specific immunotherapy for cancers. In order to achieve long-term suppression of tumor growth or ultimately cure of the disease, it would be desirable to perform the adoptive therapy accompanied with a tumor-specific immunization (i.e., gene-modified tumor cell vaccination [6,33], or tumor antigen-based vaccination) [6 34]. The specific immunization would support the survival and maintain the specific antitumor activity of the adoptively transferred T lymphocytes. In the meantime, the immunization could activate the host immune-responsive cells, which lead to the specific tumoricidal response and long-term memory against the tumor antigen. Vaccinations with irradiated tumor cells intensified by cytokine gene transduction (i.e., GM-CSF [16,20],

GM-CSF plus IL-4 [31]) are the candidates for the specific immunizations.

Since the mechanisms for tumor rejection could involve a highly regulated host immune system, therapeutic advantages may not necessarily be attained by simply increasing the dosage of a single therapeutic modality (i.e., adoptively transferred CTL, or gene-modified tumor cell vaccines). Indeed, it has been reported that the optimal levels of cytokine production are essential for the tumor vaccines to elicit adequate host responses [32,35,36]. It remains as an important future project to determine the optimal dosage and schedule of the adoptive immunotherapy. From technical points of view, further investigations are required concerning the methods of large-scale culture and genetic transduction of human CTL, as well as the preparation of tumor-based vaccines.

Acknowledgements
We thank Dr. K. Hanada for helpful discussions; Dr. I. Saito for providing pAdex1, and Adex1CAlacZ; Dr. J. Miyazaki for pCAGGS.

REFERENCES

1. Topalian, S.L. and Rosenberg, S.A. Adoptive cellular therapy: basic principles. pp178-196, in DeVita, V.T.Jr., Hellman, S., and Rosenberg, S.A. eds. Biologic Therapy of Cancer, Lippincott, Philadelphia, 1991.
2. Rubin, J.T., and Lotze, M.T. Adoptive cellular immunotherapy of cancer. pp379-410, in Mitchell, M.S. ed. Biological Approaches to Cancer Treatment: Biomodulation, McGraw-Hill, New York, 1993.
3. Greenberg, P.D. Adoptive T cell therapy of tumors: mechanisms operative in the recognition and elimination of the tumor cells. Adv. Immunol. 49: 281-355, 1991.
4. Schreiber, H. Tumor immunology. pp1143-1178, in Paul, W.E. ed. Fundamental Immunology, 3rd. ed., Raven Press, New York, 1993.
5. Rosenberg, S.A., Aebersold, P., Cornetta, K., Kasid, A., Morgan, R.A., Moen, R., Karson, E.M., Lotze, M.T., Yang, J.C., Topalian, S.L., Merino, M.J., Culver, K., Miller, A.D., Blaese, R.M., and Anderson, W.F. Gene transfer into humans: Immunotherapy of patients with advanced melanoma, using tumor-infiltrating lymphocytes modified by retroviral gene transduction. N. Engl. J. Med. 323: 570-578, 1990.
6. Dranoff, G. and Mulligan, R.C. Gene transfer as cancer therapy. Adv. Immunol. 58: 417-454, 1995.
7. Nakamura, Y., Wakimoto, H., Abe, J., Kanegae, Y., Saito, I., Aoyagi, M., Hirakawa, K., and Hamada, H. Adoptive immunotherapy with murine tumor-specific T lymphocytes engineered to secrete interleukin-2. Cancer Res. 54: 5757-5760, 1994.
8. Fidler, I.J. Biological behavior of malignant melanoma cells correlated to their survival in vivo. Cancer Res. 35: 218-224, 1975.
9. Alexander, R.B. and Rosenberg, S.A. Long term survival of adoptively transferred tumor-infiltrating lymphocytes in mice. J. Immunol. 145, 1615-1620, 1990.
10. Matis, L.A., Bookman, M., and Rosenberg, S.A. Cloning with antigens and interleukin 2 of murine T lymphocytes having distinct functions. Methods Enzymol. 150, 342-351, 1987.
11. Livingstone, A., and Fathman, C.G. Murine T cell clones. Methods Enzymol. 150, 325-333, 1987.
12. Goding, J.W. Monoclonal Antibodies: Principles and Practice. Academic Press, London, 1983.
13. Mishell, B.B. and Shiigi, S.M. Selected Methods in Cellular Immunology, W.H. Freeman & Co., San Francisco, 1980.

14. Sambrook, J., Fritsch, E.F., and Maniatis, T. Molecular Cloning. Cold Spring Harbor Laboratory Press, 1983.

15. Nakayama, E., Shiku, H., Takahashi, T., Oettgen, H.F., and Old, L.J. Definition of a unique cell surface antigen of mouse leukemia RL 1 by cell-mediated cytotoxicity. Proc. Natl. Acad. Sci. USA 76, 3486-3490, 1979.

16. Dranoff, G., Jaffee, E., Lazenby, A., Golumbek, P., Levitsky, H., Brose, K., Jackson, V., Hamada, H., Pardoll, D., and Mulligan R.C. Vaccination with irradiated tumor cells engineered to secrete murine granulocyte-macrophage colony-stimulating factor stimulates potent, specific, and long-lasting anti-tumor immunity. Proc. Natl. Acad. Sci. USA 90: 3539-3543, 1993.

17. Danos, O. and Mulligan, R.C. Safe and efficient generation of recombinant retroviruses with amphotropic and ecotropic host ranges. Proc. Natl. Acad. Sci. USA 85, 6460-6464, 1988.

18. Saito, I., Oya, Y., Yamamoto, K., Yuasa, T. and Shimojo, H. Construction of nondefective adenovirus type 5 bearing a 2.8-kilobase hepatitis B virus DNA near the right end of its genome. J. Virol. 54, 711-719, 1985.

19. Niwa, H., Yamamura, K. and Miyazaki, J. Efficient selection for high-expression transfectants with a novel eukaryotic vector. Gene 108, 193-200, 1991.

20. Abe, J., Wakimoto, H, Aoyagi, M., Hirakawa, K., and Hamada, H. Cytokine gene-modified tumor vaccination intensified by a streptococcal preparation OK-432. Cancer Immunol. Immunother. 41: 82-86, 1995.

21. Attia, M.A.M., and Weiss, D.W. Immunology of spontaneous mammary carcinomas in mice V. Acquired tumor resistance and enhancement in strain A mice infected with mammarytumor virus. Cancer Res. 26: 1787-1800, 1966.

22. Kurzrock, R., Talpaz, M., and Gutterman, J.U. Interferons–a, b, g: basic principles and preclinical studies. pp247-274, in DeVita, V.T.Jr., Hellman, S., and Rosenberg, S.A. eds. Biologic Therapy of Cancer, Lippincott, Philadelphia, 1991.

23. Borden, E.C., Witt, P.L., Paulnock, D.M., and Grossberg, S. Antitumor effects of interferons: mechanisms and therapeutic activity. pp440-476, in Mitchell, M.S. ed. Biological Approaches to Cancer Treatment: Biomodulation, McGraw-Hill, New York, 1993.

24. Nishihara, K., Miyatake, S., Sakata, T., Yamashita, J., Kikuchi, H., Kawade, Y., Zu, Y., Namba, Y., Hanaoka, M., and Watanabe, Y. Augmentation of tumor targeting in a line of glioma-specific mouse cytotoxic T-lymphocytes by retroviral expression of mouse g-interferon complementary DNA. Cancer Res. 48: 4730-4735, 1988.

25. Miyatake, S., Nishihara, K., Kikuchi, H., Yamashita, J., Namba, Y., Hanaoka, M., and Watanabe, Y. Efficient tumor suppression by glioma-specific murine cytotoxic T lymphocytes transfected with interferon-g gene. J. Natl. Cancer Inst. 82: 217-220, 1990.

26. Freedman, A.S., Freeman, G.J., Rhynhart, K. and Nadler, L.M. Selective induction of B7/BB-1 on interferon-g stimulated monocytes: a potential mechanism for amplification of T cell activation. Cell. Immunol. 137: 429-437, 1991.

27. Terrell, T.G. and Green, J.D. Comparative pathology of recombinant murine interferon-g in mice and recombinant human interferon-g in cynomolgus monkeys. Int. Rev. Exp. Pathol. 34B: 73-101, 1993.

28. Steinmann, G.G., Rosenkaimer, F., and Leitz G. Clinical experiences with interferon-a and interferon-g Int. Rev. Exp. Pathol. 34B: 193-207, 1993.

29. Harada, Y., and Yahara, I. Pathogenesis of toxicity with human-derived interleukin-2 in experimental animals. Int. Rev. Exp. Pathol. 34A: 37-55, 1993.

30. Anderson, T.D., Hayes, T.J., Powers, G.D., Gately, M.K., Tudor, R., and Rushton, A. Comparative toxicity and pathology associated with administration of recombinant IL-2 to animals. Int. Rev. Exp. Pathol. 34A: 57-77, 1993.

31. Wakimoto, H., Abe, J., Nakamura, Y., Kanegae, Y., Saito, I., Aoyagi, M., Hirakawa, K., and Hamada, H. Enhanced antitumor effects by vaccines and IL-2-secreting cytotoxic T lymphocytes. p164 in Gene Therapy, Cold Spring Harbor

Laboratory Press, New York, 1994.
32. Abe, J., Wakimoto, H., Yoshida, Y., Aoyagi, M., Hirakawa, K., and Hamada, H. Antitumor effect induced by GM-CSF gene-modified tumor vaccination: Comparison of adenovirus- and retrovirus-mediated genetic transduction. J. Cancer Res. Clin. Oncol. 121: 587-592, 1995.
33. Pardoll, D.M. Paracrine cytokine adjuvants in cancer immunology. Annu. Rev. Immunol. 13: 399-415, 1995.
34. Boon, T., De Plaen, E., Lurquin, C., Van Den Eynde, B., Van Der Bruggen, P., Traversari, C., Amar-Costesec, A., and Van Pel, A. Identification of tumor rejection antigens recognized by T lymphocytes. pp23-37, in McMichael, A.J. and Bodmer, W.F. eds., Cancer Surveys: A New Look at Tumour Immunology, Vol. 13, Cold Spring Harbor Laboratory Press, New York, 1992.
35. Schmidt, W., Schweighoffer, T., Herbst, E., Maass, G., Berger, M., Schilcher, F., Schaffner, G., and Birnstiel, M. Cancer vaccines: The interleukin 2 dosage effect. Proc. Natl. Acad. Sci. USA 92: 4711-4714, 1995.
36. Fakhrai, H., Shawler, D.L., Gjerset, R., Naviaux, R.K., Koziol, J., Royston, I., and Sobol, R.E. Cytokine gene therapy with interleukin-2-transduced fibroblasts: Effects of IL-2 dose on anti-tumor immunity. Hum. Gene Ther. 6: 591-601, 1995.

Gene Transfer to Hematopoietic Progenitor and Stem Cells: Progress and Problems

CE Dunbar, M Fox, J O'Shaughnessy, S Doren, RVB Emmons, T Soma, JM Yu, C Carter, S Sellers, K Hines, K Cowan, NS Young, AW Nienhuis

Hematology Branch, National Heart, Lung, and Blood Institute, National Institutes of Heath, Bethesda, MD USA

Introduction

The hematopoietic stem cell has been an obvious target for gene therapy technologies because of its ability to permanently reconstitute all the lineages of the hematopoietic and immune systems after transplantation. Many different congenital and acquired diseases could theoretically be treated by introducing a new gene into stem cells.[1-4] Retroviral vectors are currently the only gene transfer system with the appropriate characteristics of chromosomal integration and stable helper-free producer cell lines that can be used clinically in protocols targetted at hematopoietic stem cells. In rodent models, investigators have demonstrated efficient and reproducible gene transfer to a high percentage of long-term repopulating stem cells and achieved long-term expression of introduced genes in appropriate lineages.[4-7] In large animal and primate models, retroviral gene transfer has been much less efficient, with reproducibly less than 1% of circulating cells containing the transferred gene long-term.[8-12] Efficient gene transfer to primitive human progenitor cells such as CFU-GEMM or long-term culture initiating cells has been reported, with gene transfer efficiencies greatly increased by exposing target cells to hematopoietic growth factors during transduction with viral vectors.[13-15] Over the past four years, investigators have begun to apply retroviral gene transfer technology directed at hematopoietic stem cells in preliminary human clinical trials.

In patients undergoing autologous transplantation as high-dose consolidation for multiple myeloma or breast cancer, we used retroviral vectors carrying the bacterial neomycin phosphotransferase gene to mark a fraction of their mobilized peripheral blood and bone marrow grafts.[16] Our protocol had four purposes. First, we wished to investigate the efficiency of retroviral gene transfer to CD34-enriched hematopoietic cells collected from adults, and transduced under culture conditions optimized on the basis of animal models and *in vitro* human preclinical assays. This critical information would be applied to designing future therapeutic trials. Second, by using two different marking vectors in each patient we could directly compare the use of mobilized peripheral blood cells versus bone marrow cells as targets for retroviral gene transfer. Third, we could determine the kinetics and other characteristics of reconstitution after autologous transplantation,

190

and the engraftment potential of mobilized peripheral blood cells as compared to bone marrow cells. Finally, if marked tumor cells were detected post transplantation, the contribution of bone marrow and mobilized peripheral blood to progression could be assessed.

We have already reported the results on eleven patients followed for at least one year after autologous transplantation of retrovirally-transduced bone marrow and peripheral blood CD34-enriched cells.[17] In this symposium we will update results on those patients, as well as describe preliminary results in a second cohort of patients transplanted using cells transduced under alternative transduction conditions. We will also briefly describe new animal model data regarding the improvement of repopulating ability and gene transfer efficiency using an ex vivo culture system in which the activity of the negative regulator of hematopoiesis TGF-ß is abrogated by inclusion of a neutralizing antibodies.[18]

Patients and Methods

Clinical Procedures: Patients received one dose of cyclophosphamide 4 gm/m^2 intravenously followed by intravenous or subcutaneous filgrastim 10 ug/kg/day. Apheresis procedures initiated when the total leukocyte count exceeded 2000 cells/ul. The first and third daily collections were cryopreserved without further processing; the second daily collection was used for genetic marking. After a rest period, the myeloma patients were treated with 5-fluorouracil (5FU), 15 mg/kg/day intravenously for three days. 10 days after the initiation of 5FU, at least one liter of bone marrow was harvested from the posterior iliac crests by standard procedures. Breast cancer patients underwent marrow harvest without 5FU pretreatment. Two-thirds of the mononuclear cells were frozen without further processing, and one third of the cells were used for the genetic marking procedure. Peripheral blood (PB) or bone marrow (BM) mononuclear cells to be used for genetic marking were processed on the Ceprate Stem Cell Concentrator to obtain a CD34-enriched population of progenitor and stem cells.[19] Myeloma patients received pretransplant conditioning therapy with melphalan 140 mg/m^2 and 1200 rads of fractionated total body irradiation. Breast cancer patients received ifosfamide 16 gm/m^2 over 4 days, carboplatin 1600 mg/m^2 over 3 days, and etoposide 1500 mg/m^2 over 3 days.

Viral vectors: Two retroviral vectors, LNL6 and G1Na.40, carrying an identical bacterial phosphotransferase gene conveying G418 (Neomycin) resistance were used.[20,21] Clinical grade supernatants harvested from producer cell lines grown to confluence in Dulbecco's modified Eagle's medium (DMEM) supplemented with 10% fetal calf serum (FCS) were obtained from Genetic Therapy Inc. The vector titer of each aliquot of supernatant used ranged from 4.2 X 10^5 to 2.1 X 10^6 biologically-active particles/ml.

Transduction with Retroviral Vectors: For the first cohort of 11 patients, CD34-enriched BM or PB cells were transduced in clinical grade supernatants at a density of 1-2 X 10^5/ml for 72 hours at 37°C in 5% CO_2. Alternating patients had LNL6 versus G1Na.40 used for the PB. If LNL6 was used for the PB, G1Na.40 was used for the BM, and vice versa. Cultures were supplemented with 4 ug/ml protamine sulfate, 20 ng/ml IL-3, and 100 ng/ml SCF. Cells from breast cancer but not myeloma patients were also transduced in 50 ng/ml IL-6. Every 24 hours, cells were centrifuged and resuspended in fresh retroviral supernatant, protamine, and growth factors. The second cohort of patients had transductions carried out on CD34-enriched cells either in the presence of retroviral supernatant but no growth factors for 6 hours, or for 72 hours in the presence of an autologous marrow stromal cell layer, without exogenous growth factors but with daily changes of retroviral supernatant.

Sample Processing and Analysis: Post-transplant PB (whole blood, mononuclear cells, and granulocytes) and BM samples were collected at 1-3-month intervals for the first year and every 6 months thereafter. 1 ug purified DNA was added to buffer, Taq polymerase and dNTPs and then divided equally between a PCR tube containing an outer pair of nested primers for the neomycin phosphotransferase gene (Neo) and one containing ß-actin primers in the presence of 10μCi/ml ^{32}PdCTP. Outer Neo primers were 5'-CAG CCG ATT GTC TGT TGT GC and 5'-GGC CAG ACT GTT ACC ACT CC. ß-actin primers were 5'-CAT TGT GAT GGA CTC CGG AGA CGG and 5'-CAT CTC CTG CTC GAA GTC TAG AGC. Amplification conditions were 95° C X 2 minutes, then 95°C X 1 minute, 60°C X 1.5 minutes, and 72°C X 2 minutes, with 20 cycles for the outer Neo amplification, and 23 cycles for the ß-actin amplification, followed by a final 10-minute 72°C extension for both reactions. The outer Neo PCR products were purified then amplified again in the presence of 10μCi/ml ^{32}PdCTP and a set of internal Neo primers: 5'-CGG ATC GCT CAC AAC CAG TC and 5'-AGC CGA ATA GCC TCT CCA CC. The inner Neo PCR conditions were 95°C X 1 minute, 60°C X 1.5 minutes, and 72°C X 2 minutes for 20 cycles, followed by extension at 72°C X 10 minutes. The final PCR products were separated on 8% polyacrylamide gels. The expected band size was 483 bp for the Neo product and 232 bp for the ß-actin product. Negative controls in every reaction set included no DNA and DNA extracted from normal peripheral blood concurrently with the test samples. Positive controls for the ß-actin were log dilutions of DNA from normal PB or BM and, for the Neo, DNA from the G1Na.40 cell line containing a single copy Neo gene diluted into normal BM DNA. PCR products positive for the Neo gene were run on a 5% denaturing gel to separate the 16 base pair difference between LNL6 versus G1Na.40-derived PCR products.

Results

Protocol Design and Clinical Outcomes: Eleven patients (6 multiple myeloma and 5 breast cancer) were entered onto the gene marking protocol in the first cohort over a one year period. In all patients, 1/3 of the mobilized PB collections were CD34-selected and transduced with either LNL6 or G1Na.40 marking vectors. In ten of eleven patients, 1/3 of the BM mononuclear cell fraction was CD34-enriched and transduced with the marking vector which was not used on the patients' respective PB cells. On average 8.80 X 10^5 and 2.58 X 10^5 transduced CD34+ cells/ kg from the PB and BM respectively were reinfused.

Patients engrafted on schedule compared to patients transplanted on the same or similar clinical protocols without gene marking. There were no toxic events attributable to the marking procedure. Because of concern over adverse consequences of replication-competent helper virus generation, post-transplantation peripheral blood mononuclear cell DNA from each patient was tested every three to six months for recombinant helper virus envelope sequences. No samples have been positive, with a sensitivity of detection of 1:10,000 gene copies by PCR for the envelope gene.

Aliquots of cells were assayed for transduction efficiency at the end of the 72-hour transduction period by two different methods. Cells were plated in methylcellulose cultures with and without G418, and the percentages of CFU-C resistant to G418 (Neo^R) were calculated. Overall mean efficiency was 21.4%. Efficiencies of transduction were similar for target cells obtained from breast cancer versus myeloma patients (18.4% versus 23.7%), but somewhat lower for peripheral blood versus bone marrow target cells (14.5% versus 29.2 %).

DNA samples prepared from bone marrow, peripheral blood, granulocyte and mononuclear peripheral blood fractions, and in some patients, sorted T and B cells were analyzed by semi-quantitative PCR for the Neo gene at the time of engraftment (day 15-30), and then every 3 months post-transplantation for up to 30 months. At the time of engraftment, the Neo gene could be detected in PB and/or BM samples from 10/10 evaluable patients, at levels estimated between 1:5,000 and 1:10 cells positive. Two myeloma patients had repeatedly positive signals at every time point assayed post-transplantation, now out to 30 months post-transplant. BM, PB, granulocyte, mononuclear cell and T cell and B cell fractions were all positive, at levels initially about 1:100-1:1000 cells +, but falling after three months to stable levels of about 1:5000-1:10,000 cells +. One breast cancer patient continued to have positive signals out over time at levels of 1:10,000 cells +. The loss of the marker gene over time in some patients suggests that in these patients only committed progenitors rather than true long-term repopulating cells were successfully transduced, or that engraftment of the manipulated cells was only transient.

In all three patients with positive Neo signals 1 year or longer post-transplantation, the granulocyte lineage has been positive for the gene. The short circulation and survival times of granulocytes mean that the positive PCR signals were not simply due to prolonged survival of transduced terminally-differentiated cells, but to continued production of daughter cells from primitive long-term repopulating cells.

One major objective of this study was to compare the gene transfer potential of mobilized PB to BM target cells. A 16 bp sequence present at the 5' end of the Neo gene in G1Na.40 but not LNL6 allowed the amplified PCR products to be distinguished on denaturing gels. In one patient with persistently + signals, both grafts contributed equally over time. The other two long-term positive patients had only the peripheral blood graft contributing to marking after the first three months.

Three breast cancer patients have relapsed post transplantation with disease in sites of their previous metastatic tumor deposits, and biopsies of tumor masses were negative for the Neo gene. One of the myeloma patients with long-term marking of PB and BM cells relapsed 28 months after transplantation, and sorted CD38-very bright plasma cells sorted from the marrow were also negative for the Neo gene.

A second cohort of myeloma and breast cancer patients have more recently been entered onto the same clinical protocol, with two new transduction conditions being tested. A total of four patients had their BM and PB CD34-enriched cells transduced for 6 hours without addition of growth factors, and two patients had their cells transduced in the presence of autologous marrow stromal cells instead of exogenous growth factors, for three days with daily changes of retroviral vector. Transduction efficiencies of CFU-C assayed at the end of the in vitro culture period were much lower than in the earlier cohort of patients. Median follow-up in this group is only nine months, but overall the results appear disappointing: only two patients have had any positive signals in the peripheral blood or bone marrow post-transplantation, at levels of 1:10,000, and these signals have been intermittent in those two patients.

In an attempt to improve gene transfer efficiency to primitive hematopoietic cells, we have been trying a number of different approaches in our animal models. TGF-ß has previously been shown to be a negative regulator of committed progenitor cells cultured ex vivo, and there was evidence for autocrine or paracrine production of this cytokine by various hematopoietic cell populations.

We asked what the effect of TGF-ß was on true long-term repopulating stem cells in the murine competitive repopulation model, and whether abrogation of autocrine/paracrine effects of this cytokine by a neutralizing antibody during ex vivo culture could improve repopulating ability as well as gene transfer efficiency in the murine model.[29] We found that TGF-ß1 had a negative effect on repopulating ability when it was added to ex vivo cultures supported by IL3, IL6, and SCF, and that, conversely, the neutralizing antibody improved repopulating ability when it was added to these cultures. Preliminary experiments suggest a positive effect on gene transfer efficiency in the murine model.

Discussion

We have shown that both mobilized peripheral blood and bone marrow CD34-enriched cells can contribute to multi-lineage engraftment long-term after autologous transplantation in adults with advanced malignancies. The question of whether peripheral blood contains true long-term repopulating stem cells with properties similar to steady-state marrow has been controversial, and is of critical import, especially if peripheral blood is to be used for allogeneic transplantation, where recovery of endogenous hematopoiesis can not occur.[30-33] The use of two different marking vectors allowed us for the first time to compare bone marrow and peripheral blood-derived engraftment in the same patient. In this study, we showed that peripheral blood grafts contributed to long-term (greater than 30 month) myeloid and lymphoid engraftment in several patients. These data support the recent enthusiasm for initial clinical trials using mobilized peripheral blood cells in allogeneic transplantation.[33,34] In our study, we found equivalent or better long-term marking from mobilized peripheral blood than from bone marrow CD34-enriched target cells. Mobilized peripheral blood is a very attractive target for gene therapy applications. A large number of primitive CD34+ cells or even more primitive LTCIC can be collected from peripheral blood after growth factor or growth factor plus chemotherapy mobilization as compared to bone marrow, allowing collection of a potentially expanded target cell population for gene transduction.[35,36] Repeated cycles of mobilization, collection, transduction, and transplantation would be feasible using peripheral blood, and is an approach to increase the number of gene-corrected cells in a patient. High cell doses have allowed engraftment without prior ablation in the murine model, and this would obviously be desirable in human applications directed at non-malignant diseases such as Gaucher disease or Fanconi anemia.[37,38]

The overall efficiency of retroviral gene transfer in this clinical trial was too low to be considered useful for therapeutic applications. Two other clinical gene transfer studies have reported higher marking efficiencies, but there were important differences in the patient populations studied. Investigators at St. Jude Children's Research Hospital transduced autologous bone marrow from children undergoing transplantation for acute leukemia or neuroblastoma.[39] Levels of marked marrow progenitors and peripheral blood mononuclear cells averaged 5% at 12-18 months post transplantation, and although some have fallen over more prolongerd periods of observation, they remain at least a log higher than what we report here. Of interest, however, is the fact that the levels of the marker gene in the peripheral blood cells was generally 1% or less lower (personal communication, Dr. Malcolm Brenner) This discrepancy has also been reported in a study of patients with SCID receiving cord blood transduced with a vector containing the ADA gene and a Neo gene.(Dr. Don Kohn, personal communication) Possible explanations include toxicity of the Neo gene product to mature cells, or immunologic reaction against mature circulating cells. These issues continue to be investigated, and we are currently reanalyzing marrow samples on our patients to see if we find the same discrepancy.

Two patient-specific factors may have contributed to the higher efficiencies these investigators observed: the younger age of St. Jude patients (range 2-19 years) and the prompt collection of autologous marrow after high dose induction chemotherapy for relapsed tumor. In contrast, our patients were middle-aged adults who had been heavily treated with multiple cycles of moderate-dose myelosuppressive therapy and may have sustained permanent stem cell depletion or damage. Higher numbers of primitive cells may have been available and in cycle in the St. Jude patients, and thus susceptible to retroviral gene transfer.[40] The other difference between the studies involved the transduction conditions: St. Jude used a brief 6 hour exposure to vector without inclusion of hematopoietic growth factors, a transduction procedure that *in vitro* and *in vivo* preclinical studies found very inefficient. [21,39,41] In our second cohort of adults whose cells were transduced under an identical procedure to the St. Jude patients, we have seen no persistent or improved marking. We are also testing the inclusion of an autologous marrow stromal support layer during transduction as another approach to improving the efficiency of gene transfer, because stromal cells or stromal matrix molecules can substitute for or enhance the effects of exogenous growth factors, and may improve gene transfer into primitive cells in animal models.[12,15,42]

We would stress the necessity of testing transduction modifications in human clinical marking trials, because no *in vitro* assays have yet proven predictive of gene transfer efficiency to human *in vivo* long-term repopulating cells. As an example, gene transfer efficiencies to CFU-C assessed at the end of transduction were much higher in our study than in the St. Jude study, yet long-term levels of the marker gene assessed in patients after transplantation were instead much greater in their patients, and did not correlate with CFU-C transduction levels.[39] Results generated over the next several years from these and other gene marking trials, as well as from preliminary trials with therapeutic intent for Gaucher Disease, Fanconi Anemia, and HIV infection will indicate whether or not retroviral gene transfer to hematopoietic stem cells will be a feasible and effective approach to therapy for these and other disorders.

References

1. Karlsson S: Treatment of genetic defects in hematopoietic cell function by gene transfer. Blood 78:2481, 1991

2. Dunbar CE, Emmons RVB: Gene transfer into hematopoietic progenitor and stem cells: progress and problems. Stem Cells 12:563, 1994

3. Mulligan RC: The basic science of gene therapy. Science 260:926, 1993

4. Miller AD: Human gene therapy comes of age. Nature 357:455, 1992

5. Bodine DM, McDonagh KT, Seidel NE, Nienhuis AW: Survival and retrovirus infection of murine hematopoietic stem cells in vitro: effects of 5-FU and method of infection. Exp Hematol 19:206, 1991

6. Sorrentino BP, Brandt SJ, Bodine D, Gottesman M, Pastan I, Cline A, Nienhuis AW: Selection of drug resistant bone marrow cells in vivo after retroviral transfer of human MDR1. Science 257:99, 1992

7. Correll PH, Colilla S, Dave HP, Karlsson S: High levels of human glucocerebrosidase activity in macrophages of long-term reconstituted mice after retroviral infection of hematopoietic stem cells. Blood 80:331, 1992

8. Schuening FG, Storb R, Stead RB, Goehle S, Nash R, Miller AD: Improved retroviral transfer of genes into canine hematopoietic progenitor cells kept in long-term marrow culture. Blood 74:152, 1989

9. Carter RF, Abrams-Ogg ACG, Dick JE, Kruth SA, Valli VE, Kamel-Reid S, Dube ID: Autologous transplantation of canine long-term marrow culture cells genetically marked by retroviral vectors. Blood 79:356, 1992

10. Schuening FG, Kawahara K, Miller AD, To R, Goehle S, Stewart D, Mullally K, Fisher L, Graham TC, Appelbaum FR, Hackman R, Osborne WRA, Storb R: Retrovirus-mediated gene transduction into long-term repopulating marrow cells of dogs. Blood 78:2568, 1991

11. Van Beusechem VW, Kukler A, Heidt PJ, Valerio D: Long-term expression of human adenosine deaminase in rhesus monkeys transplanted with retrovirus-infected bone-marrow cells. Proc Natl Acad Sci U S A 89:7640, 1992

12. Bodine DM, Moritz T, Donahue RE, Luskey BD, Kessler SW, Martin DIK, Orkin SH, Nienhuis AW, Williams DA: Long term expression of a murine adenosine deaminase (ADA) gene in rhesus hematopoietic cells of multiple lineages following retroviral mediated gene transfer into CD34+ bone marrow cells. Blood 82:1975, 1993

13. Nolta JA, Kohn DB: Comparison of the effects of growth factors on retroviral vector-mediated

gene transfer and the proliferative status of human hematopoietic progenitor cells. Human Gene Therapy 1:257, 1990

14. Hughes PFD, Thacker JD, Hogge D, Sutherland HJ, Thomas TE, Lansdorp PM, Eaves CJ, Humphries RK: Retroviral gene transfer to primitive normal and leukemic hematopoietic cells using clinically applicable procedures. J Clin Invest 89:1817, 1992

15. Moore KA, Deisseroth AB, Reading CL, Williams DE, Belmont JW: Stromal support enhances cell-free retroviral vector transduction of human bone marrow long-term culture initiating cells. Blood 79:1393, 1992

16. Dunbar CE, Nienhuis AW, Stewart FM, Quesenberry P, O'Shaughnessy J, Cowan K, Cottler-Fox M, Leitman S, Goodman S, Sorrentino BP: Amendment to clinical research projects. Genetic marking with retroviral vectors to study the feasibility of stem cell gene transfer and the biology of hematopoietic reconstitution after autologous transplantation in multiple myeloma, chronic myelogenous leukemia, or metastatic breast cancer. Hum Gene Ther 4:205, 1993

17. Dunbar CE, Cottler-Fox M, O'Shaughnessy JA, Doren S, Carter CS, Berenson R, Brown S, Moen RC, Greenblatt J, Stewart FM, Leitman SF, Wilson W, Cowan KH, Young NS, Nienhuis AW: Retrovirally-marked CD34-enriched peripheral blood and bone marrow and cells contribute to long-term engraftment after autologous transplantation. Blood 85:3048, 1995

18. Soma T, Yu JM, Dunbar C: Maintenance of murine long-term repopulating cells in ex vivo culture is affected by modulation of TGF-ß but not MIP-1⟨?⟩ activities. Blood 84:868a, 1994.

19. Berenson RJ, Bensinger WI, Hill RS, Andrews RG, Garcia-Lopez J, Kalamasz DF, Still BJ, Spitzer G, Buckner CD, Bernstein ID, Thomas ED: Engraftment after infusion of CD34+ marrow cells in patients with breast cancer or neuroblastoma. Blood 77:1717, 1991

20. Miller AD, Buttimore C: Redesign of retrovirus packaging cell lines to avoid recombination leading to helper virus production. Mol Cell Biol 6:2895, 1986

21. Cassel A, Cottler-Fox M, Doren S, Dunbar CE: Retroviral-mediated gene transfer into CD34-enriched human peripheral blood stem cells. Exp Hematol 21:585, 1993

22. Roberts A, Sporn M: Physiological actions and applications of transforming growth factor beta. Growth Factors 8:1, 1993

23. Nilsen-Hamilton M: Transforming growth factor-ß and its actions on cellular growth and differentiation. Curr Topics Develop Bio 24:95, 1990

24. Kessinger A, Armitage JO, Landmark JD, Smith DM, Weisenberger DD: Autologous peripheral hematopoietic stem cell transplantation restores hematopoietic function following marrow ablative therapy. Blood 71:723, 1988

25. Smedmyr B, Bengtsson M, Jakobsson A, Simonsson B, Oberg G, Totterman TH: Regenerationof CALLA (CD10+), TdT+ and double-positive cells in the bone marrow

and blood after autologous bone marrow transplantation. Eur J Haematol 46:146, 1991

26. Naparstek E, Or R, Nagler A, Cividalli G, Engelhard D, Aker M, Gimon Z, Manny N, Sacks T, Tochner Z, Weiss L, Samuel S, Brautbar C, Hale G, Waldmann H, Steinberg M, Slavin S: T-cell-depleted allogeneic bone marrow transplantation for acute leukemia using campath-1 antibodies and post-transplant administation of donor's peripheral blood lymphocytes for prevention of relapse. Brit J Haematol 89:506, 1995

27. Harousseau JL, Milpied N, Garand R, Bourhis JH: High dose melphelan and autologous BMT in high risk myeloma. Brit J Haematol 67:493, 1987

28. Gale RP, Armitage JO, Dicke KA: Autotransplants: now and in the future. Bone Marrow Transplant 7:153, 1991

29. Harrison DE, Jordan CT, Zhong RK, Astle CM: Primitive hemopoietic stem cells: direct assay of most productive repopulation with simple binomial, correlation and covariance calculations. Exp Hematol 21:206, 1993

30. Kessinger A: Autologous transplantation with peripheral blood stem cells: a review of clinical results. J Clin Apheresis 5:97, 1990

31. Kessinger A, Smith DM, Strandjord SE, Landmark JD, Dooley DC, Law P, Coccia PF, Warkentin PI, Weisenburger DD, Armitage JO: Allogeneic transplantation of blood-derived, T cell-depleted hemopoietic stem cells after myeloablative treatment in a patient with acute lymphoblastic leukemia. Bone Marrow Transplant 4:643, 1989

32. Brito-Babapulle F, Bowcock SJ, Marcus RE, Apperley J, Th'ng KH, Dowding C, Rassool F, Guo A-P, Catovsky D, Galton DAG, McCarthy D, Goldman JM: Autografting for patients with chronic myeloid leukaemia in chronic phase: peripheral blood stem cells may have a finite capacity for maintaining haematopoiesis. Brit J Haematol 73:76, 1989

33. Dreger P, Haferlach T, Eckstein V, Jacobs S, Suttorp M, Löffler H, Müller-Ruchholtz W, Schmitz N: G-CSF-mobilized peripheral blood progenitor cells for allogeneic transplantation: Safety, kinetics of mobilization, and composition of the graft. Brit J Haematol 87:609, 1994

34. Baumann I, Testa NG, Lange C, De Wynter E, Luft T, Dexter TM, Van Hoef MEHM, Howell A: Haemopoietic cells mobilized into the circulation by lenograstim as an alternative to bone marrow for allogeneic transplants. Lancet 341:369, 1993

35. Pettengell R, Testa NG, Swindell R, Crowther D, Dexter TM: Transplantation potential of hematopoietic cells released into the circulation during routine chemotherapy for non-Hodgkin's lymphoma. Blood 82:2239, 1993

36. Sutherland HJ, Eaves CJ, Lansdorp PM, Phillips GL, Hogge DE: Kinetics of committed and primitive blood progenitor mobilizations after chemotherapy and growth factor treatment and their use in autotransplant. Blood 83:3808, 1994

37. Stewart FM, Crittenden RB, Lowry PA, Pearson-White S, Quesenberry PJ: Long-term

engraftment of normal and post-5-fluorouracil murine marrow into normal nonmyeloablated mice. Blood 81:2544, 1993

38. Wu D-d, Keating A: Hematopoietic stem cells engraft in untreated transplant recipients. Exp Hematol 21:251, 1993

39. Brenner MK, Rill DR, Holladay MS, Heslop HE, Moen RC, Buschle M, Krance RA, Santana VM, Anderson WF, Ihle JN: Gene marking to determine whether autologous marrow infusion restores long-term haemopoiesis in cancer patients. Lancet 342:1134, 1993

40. Miller DG, Adam MA, Miller AD: Gene transfer by retrovirus vectors occurs only in cells that are actively replicating at the time of infection. Mol Cell Biol 10:4239, 1990

41. Kantoff PW, Gillio AP, McLachlin JR, Bordignnnon C, Eglitis MA, Kernan NA, Moen RC, Kohn DB, Yu SF, Karson E, Karlsson S, Zweibel J, Gilboa E, Blaese RM, Neinhuis A, O'Reilly RJ, Anderson WF: Expression of human adenosine deaminase in nonhuman primates after retrovirus-mediated gene transfer. J Exp Med 166:219, 1987

42. Moritz T, Patel VP, Williams DA: Bone marrow extracellular matrix molecules improve gene transfer into human hematopoietic cells via retroviral vectors. J Clin Invest 93:1451, 1994

Common Marmoset as a New Preclinical Animal Model for Human Gene Therapy of Hematological Disorders

Kenzaburo Tani, Hitoshi Hibino, Kenji Ikebuchi, Wu Ming-Shiuan, Yuko Nakazaki, Hidetoshi Sumimoto, Tsuyoshi Tanabe, Keisuke Takahashi, Tatsutoshi Nakahata, Shuzo Suzuki[2], Yoshikuni Tanioka[2], Richard C. Mulligan[3] and Shigetaka Asano

Department of Hematology/Oncology, The Institute of Medical Science, The University of Tokyo, Tokyo, Japan.
[2]Central Institute for Experimental Animals and Preclinical Research Laboratories Inc., Kawasaki, Kanagawa, Japan.
[3]Department of Biology, Whitehead Institute, Massachusetts Institute of Technology, Boston, U.S.A.

SUMMARY

For the purpose of secured and effective introduction of gene therapeutic approaches to human hematological disorders, we have been focusing on the common marmoset, a small non-human primates as a target preclinical animal for gene transfer. Here we characterize the common marmoset bone marrow (MBM) progenitor cells in vitro and investigate whether these cells respond to the human cytokines and are transduced by retrovirus vectors. Namely, we screened human cytokines (erythropoietin, granulocyte colony-stimulating factor (G-CSF), granulocyte macrophage colony-stimulating factor (GM-CSF), interleukin (IL)-3, IL-6, IL-11, stem cell factor (SCF), and thrombopoietin(TPO)) to examine their stimulating activities on MBM progenitor cells by colonogenic assay in methyl-cellulose. These human cytokines were demonstrated to have significant effects on MBM progenitor cells and stimulated the colony forming activity of each lineage dose-dependently. We then studied LacZ gene transfer efficiencies into MBM progenitor cells by retrovirus vector in the presence of human IL-3, IL-6 and SCF. By using the mixed cell populations of MBM stromal cells and retrovirus producer cells, the transduction efficiency to CFU-GM (CFU-GEMM) increased significantly. Our results suggest that the marmoset would be useful as a preclinical animal to evaluate the effectiveness and safety of new gene therapy vector sytems for hematological disorders.

KEY WORDS: common marmoset, retrovirus vectros, hematological disorders, hematopoietic stem cells, bone marrow stromal cells

INTRODUCTION

Although bone marrow transplantation (BMT) is today a very powerful therapeutic approach to life-threatening hematological disorders, there remain many patients who can't receive or are resistant to this therapeutic intervention because of constraints such as a lack of HLA-identical donors, high age, low performance score including severe organ damage and severe infection. It is now thought that gene therapy is a strong candidate for overcoming this situation.

There have been many published animal studies for evaluating the clinical efficacy and safety of newly developed virus or nonvirus vector systems. Most of these studies were performed with mice because they are handy to breed and have well-known biology and genetics. In developing a new gene transducing method, however, it is desirable to examine these issues in higher animals like the monkey. This is because there is a greater difference between humans and mice than between humans and monkeys in their pathophysiology as well as pharmacokinetics. From this point of view, we have recently focused on a small new world monkey, the common marmoset. This monkey has several advantages in preclinical studies because it is relatively cheap, is small, and is easy to breed. Although there are many reports concerning their physiology and pharmacokinetics, there have been no published data describing their hematopoiesis from the new viewpoints, hematopoietic cells as targets of human cytokines as well as gene transfer.

Gene transfer into human hematopoietic cells, particularly into hematopoietic stem cells, is one of the major concerns in the field of hematology, because the availability of such a technique could help cure many hematological disorders originating from abnormal hematopoietic stem cells. This technique has been developed intensively over the last 10 years and recent reports have offered some hope regarding its clinical application. Currently, the murine retroviral vector sytem is considered to be the best of several methods of gene transfer into hematopoietic cells. Previous reports, however, have suggested that the use of murine retrovirus vector for human gene therapy should be carefully performed because contaminated replication competent retroviruses (RCR) have caused malignant lymphoma in monkey experiments. Including the examination for RCR, preclinical studies using monkey are advisable to rule out side effects that would only be detected in higher animal species close to humans.

In this manuscript, we report our recent results with *in vitrro* progenitor assays of common marmoset bone marrow cells as well as gene transfer assays hematopoietic cells using murine retrovirus vector to review the suitability of the common marmoset as a preclinical animal model for human gene therapy for hematological disorders.

MATERIALS AND METHODS

Common marmoset bone marrow progenitor cell assays and their *in vitro* responses to human cytokines

Bone marrow cells were obtained from the femoral bone of a sacrificed common marmoset (3 year old female) under general anesthesia, and the mononuclear cells (MNC) were then isolated using Ficoll-Hypaque density gradient centrifuge method, as previously described. Bone marrow MNC were cultured in serum-free methyl cellulose culture condition (1.2% methylcellulose, 1% bovine serum albumin, 2×10^5 M 2-mercaptoethanol, 300μ g/ml transferrin, 160μ g/ml lecithin, 96μ g/ml cholesterol, 10-7 M sodium selenite) in the presence of various human cytokines of erythropoietin (EPO), granulocyte colony-stimulating factor (G-CSF), granulocyte macrophage colony-stimulating factor (GM-CSF), stem cell factor (SCF), interleukin (IL)-3, and IL-6. For CFU-MK assays, bone marrow MNC were cultured in methyl cellulose culture condition (1.2% methylcellulose, 1% human platelet poor albumin, 2×10^5 M 2-mercaptoethanol) in the presence of IL-6, IL-11 or TPO.

The colonies were incubated at 37°C, in 5% CO_2, 5%O_2 for 7-14 days. The number of burst-forming unit-erythroid (BFU-E), colony-forming unit-granulocyte/macrophage (CFU-GM), colony-forming unit-granulocyte/ erythroid / megakaryocyte/ macrophage (CFU-GEMM or CFU-Mix) were determined under an inversion microscope following the morphological criteria for human colonies. For the confirmation, several representative colonys were picked up, stained with standard May-Giemsa staining on glass slides, and were observed under a light microscope.

In vivo effects of human G-CSF in common marmoset

Three common marmosets (body weight 280 to 390g) were respectively irradiated at 350, 450 and 550 rads, and their peripheral blood cell number was followed up periodically. Another marmoset was also irradiated at 450 rads and was administered with human recombinant glycosylated G-CSF, at 2 μ g/kg subcutaneously for 18 days after 18 days of the irradiation. All marmosets were bred in a laminar flow.

Bacterial lacZ gene transfer into marmoset bone marrow progenitor cells with murine leukemia retrovirus vector

Amphotropic retrovirus vector of MFG-LacZ, derived from murine leukemia retrovirus containing bacterial lacZ gene, was obtained from the cultured supernatant of recombinant retrovirus producer cells of ψ CRIP-MFG-LacZ and used for supernatant transduction after the supernatant was filtered using a 0.45 μ m filter unit. The supernatant was renewed every 24 hours. The supernatant transduction for marmoset bone marrow MNC was essentially performed in the same way as coculture transduction described below, except that culture was performed without virus producer cells or marmoset bone marrow stromal cells.

For coculture transduction, bone marrow MNC(5×10^4-1×10^5 cells/ml) were cultured on the virus producer cells or mixed cellular population of the virus producer cells and the marmoset bone marrow stromal cells at a ratio of 1:1 in 1xDMEM supplemented with 10% fetal bovine serum in the presence of 8 μ g/ml polybrene, human cytokines (100ng/ml SCF, 20ng/ml IL-3, 80ng/ml IL-6). The culture medium was renewed every 48 hours and the culture was performed for 48 to 144 hours.

On completion of transduction, the bone marrow cells were cultured following the usual methylcellulose culture method in the presence of human cytokines of 10 ng/ml SCF, 10 ng/ml IL-3, 2 U/ml EPO, and 10 ng/ml G-CSF. On the 14th day of culture, the formed colonies were transferred to a 96 well culture dish, fixed with 0.5% glutaraldehyde, stained with X-gal, and counted for their positively stained colony numbers under an inversion microscope.

RESULTS

Common marmoset bone marrow progenitor cell assays and their *in vitro* responses to human cytokines

The number of marmoset bone marrow progenitor cells including BFU-E, CFU-GM, CFU-Mix, or CFU-MK were increased dose-dependently in the presence of respective human cytokines of EPO, G-CSF, GM-CSF or TPO. As shown in Figure 1, many CFU-Mix colonies were obtained in the presence of human SCF. To obtain the highest numbers of CFU-Mix colonies, the combination of

SCF, IL-3 and EPO was required. The colony size of BFU-E and CFU-GM was positively affected by the presence of SCF.

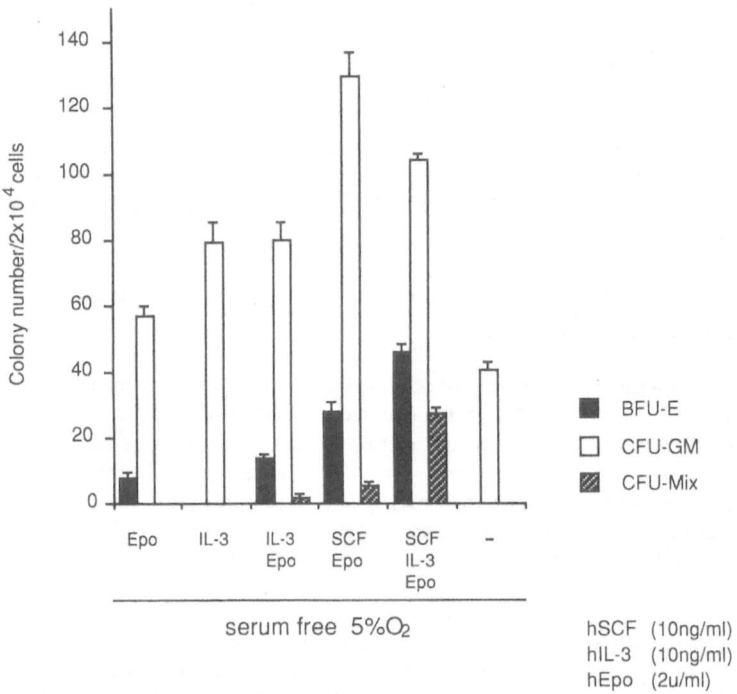

Figure 1. Effects of human cytokines for the formation of marmoset bone marrow BFU-E, CFU-GM and CFU-Mix. Human cytokines were effective for their formation. Human SCF was necessary for CFU-Mix formation as a synergistic factor.

In vivo effects of human G-CSF in common marmoset

All marmosets irradiated with 350, 450 or 550 rads showed bone marrow suppression in all cell lineages. Gradual recovery of bone marrow cell production was observed in those marmosets irradiated with 350 rads or 450 rads around day 40 after irradiation. The marmoset irradiated with 550 rads showed no bone marrow recovery until 40 days after irradiation. One marmoset administered with subcutaneous G-CSF showed significant recovery only in the myeloid series around 24 days of irradiation.

Bacterial lacZ gene transfer into marmoset bone marrow progenitor cells with murine leukemia retrovirus vector

In supernatant transduction, less than 5 % of the CFU-GM and CFU-Mix colonies were transduced by the virus supernatant. This number was not significantly affected by the addition of human cytokines. The coculture transduction using virus producer cells alone also showed very low transduction efficiency. On the other hand, repetitive coculture transduction using virus producer and marmoset bone marrow stromal cells showed significant increase of transduction efficiency up to 20% for CFU-GM and CFU-Mix. The presence of cytokines did not enhance the transduction efficiency for CFU-GM (Figure 2). For CFU-Mix, the efficiency was affected slightly by the addition of the cytokines.

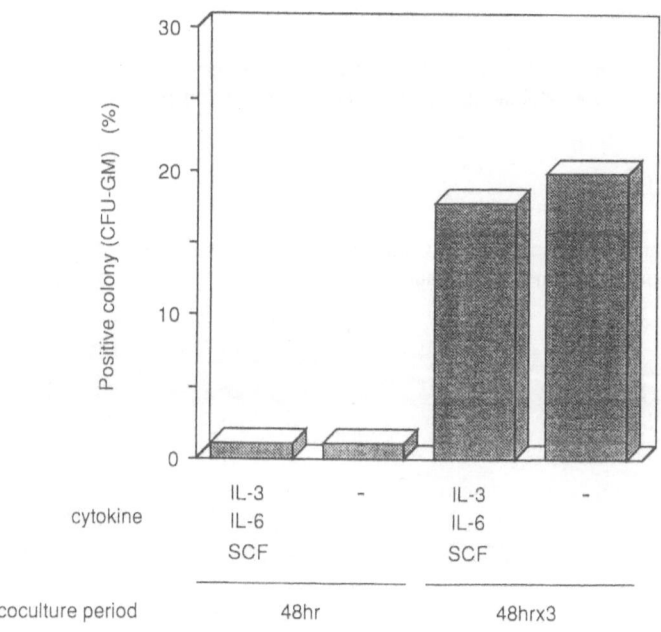

Figure 2. Transduction of LacZ gene into marmoset bone marrow CFU-GM. Repetitive transduction using coculture system using virus producer cells with marmoset bone marrow stromal cells facilitated the transduction efficiency.

DISCUSSION

Our results demonstrated that common marmoset bone marrow MNC responded to the human cytokines EPO, GM-CSF, G-CSF, IL-3, TPO dose-dependently. G-CSF also proved to be useful in accelerating *in vivo* bone marrow cell recovery after irradiation. Our results also demonstrated that about 20% of the progenitor cells could be transduced in the presence of virus producer cells and marmoset bone marrow stromal cells. The presence of human cytokines IL-3, IL-6 and SCF might help the gene transduction efficiency.

The cross reactivity of human cytokines between human and marmoset seems to favor this animal when studying human hematopoiesis *in vitro* or *in vivo*.. In mice, it is well-known that the human cytokines GM-CSF, IL-3 and SCF have no significant effect on mice hematopoietic cell growth. This difference might also accelerate the future use of common marmoset in preclinical studies of newly developed human growth factors.

The enhanced gene transduction efficiency into marmoset progenitor cells in the presence of virus producer cells and marmoset bone marrow stromal cells was compatible with the findings reported in human bone marrow progenitor cells. The cross reactivity of bone marrow stromal cells between human and marmoset requires further investigation. Also before starting *in vivo* studies using the marmoset, it is necessary to check whether this animal has its own retrovirus which can recombine with murine retrovirus to rule out the possibility of the production of replication competent retroviruses *in vivo*.

In conclusion, the common marmoset is considered to have very useful characteristics as a preclinical higher animal model for cytokine studies as well as human gene therapy.

REFERENCES

Hibino,H., Tani, K., Asano, S. et al., Common marmoset bone marrow progenitor cells: Target cells to human cytokines and gene transfer (submitted).

Development of Protein-Liposome Gene Delivery System and Its Application for the Treatment of Acquired Diseases

Yasufumi Kaneda[1], Ryuichi Morishita[2] and Victor J. Dzau[3]

[1]Institute for Molecular and Cellular Biology, Osaka University, [2]Department of Geriatrics, Osaka University School of Medicine, Suita, Osaka 565, Japan, and [3]Falk Cardiovascular Research Center, Stanford University School of Medicine, Stanford, CA94305, U.S.A.

Summary

We have developed an efficient vector system based on liposome for the delivery of oligonucleotides and genes into various organs. The liposome was decorated with fusion proteins of HVJ (Sendai virus) to introduce DNA directly into the cytoplasm and contained DNA and DNA-binding nuclear protein inside the particle to enhance its expression. Using the vector system, called the protein-liposome gene delivery system, we attempted to prevent the neointima formation of vascular walls after balloon injury. Antisense oligonucleotides against PCNA and cdc2 kinase transferred into injured arterial walls by protein-liposomes greatly reduced the message of those genes and inhibited neo-intima formation of the injured artery for 8 weeks. Moreover, double stranded oligonucleotides containing the consensus sequence for E2F binding sites inhibited the growth of smooth muscle cells and prevented neo-intima formation.

Key words: protein-liposome, gene therapy, antisense oligonucleotides, E2F decoy, prevention of restenosis

Introduction

Abnormal cell growth in vivo induces various pathological changes in organs. Among them are tumors, restenosis of blood vessels, glomerularsclerosis, lung fibrosis and so on. To date, no effective pharmacological treatment for preventing those diseases in humans has been reported. Here, we focused our efforts on the prevention of restenosis of blood vessels after angioplasty using a novel molecular delivery system.

First, effective in vivo gene transfer methods should be developed. Several problems have to be solved in transferring DNA into cells and obtaining efficient gene expression. One is the problem of introducing DNA directly into the cytoplasm without degradation. We have studied direct introduction of macromolecules into the cytoplasm by HVJ (Hemagglutinating Virus of Japan, Sendai virus). DNA encapsulated in liposomes was successfully introduced into cells by making use of the fusion activity of HVJ. Another is the efficient delivery of DNA into the nucleus even in non-dividing cells. We found that cointroduction of DNA with nuclear proteins facilitated nuclear migration of the DNA and enhanced its expression in animal organs (1,2). A method for delivering DNA with nuclear protein by protein-liposomes has been developed.

We also studied vascular remodeling using gene transfer. Multiple factors were involved in the growth stimulation of vascular smooth muscle cells (VSMCs) (3,4). It appears unlikely that selective inhibition of a particular growth factor will completely inhibit the growth of VSMC. However, cell growth results from cell division, which is regulated by cell cycle genes. Cyclins and cdks were isolated and the roles of those factors in the regulation of the cell cycle have been identified (5). We employed antisense ODNs to inhibit the expression of cell cycle genes. Cotransfection of cdc2 kinase and proliferating-cell nuclear antigen (PCNA) antisense ODNs completely inhibited the growth of VSMCs both in vitro and in vivo (6). In addition to antisense strategy, the transcription factor, E2F, for cdc2 kinase and PCNA was inhibited by introducing double stranded ODNs including the factor-binding sequence. This strategy was also useful for the prevention of neointima formation. The third approach was the transfer of NO synthase plasmid DNA into the injured blood vessels, and it was also successful in the prevention of restenosis.

Materials and Methods

(The preparation of protein-liposomes)   Protein-liposomes were prepared as described previously (7). Briefly, DNA and the nuclear protein HMG-1 were enclosed in liposomes consisting of phosphatidyl serine, phosphatidyl choline and cholesterol. The liposomes were fused with UV-inactivated HVJ and the resulting protein-liposomes were isolated through sucrose gradient centrifugation. For the delivery of oligonucleotides, cointroduction of nuclear protein was not always necessary.

(Sequences of antisense ODNs and decoy ODN for EF2)
The sequences of ODNs against human basic fibroblast growth factor (b-FGF), mouse cdc2 kinase, and rat PCNA were previously reported (8,9). The sequence of human cdk2 antisense and rat cyclin B1 were as follows: antisense cdk2 kinase (5'GAAGTTCTCCATGAAGCG-3') and   anti sense cyclin B1 (5'-GAGCGCCATGGC-TCCTCC-3'). The sequence of the phosphorothioate double stranded ODN against E2F binding site was listed elsewhere (11).

(In vitro transfection)   Rat aortic VSMCs (passage 4-8) were isolated and cultured. They were maintained in Weymouth's medium (GIBCO) with 5 % calf serum. After confluence, cells were made quiescent by placing them for 48 hrs prior to the transfection in a defined serum-free medium, as reported (10). Cells were washed with balanced salt solution (BSS : 137 mM NaCl, 5.4 mM KCl, 10 mM Tris-Cl pH 7.5), and 500ul of HVJ-liposomes (3 uM encasulated ODNs) was then added to the wells. The cells were incubated at 4 C for 5 min and then at 37 C for 30 min. Cells were maintained in fresh DSF or medium with 5 % serum. To investigate the effect of antisense phosphorothioate ODNs on the rate of DNA synthesis the cells were stimulated with angiotensin II (Ang II) and pulsed with 3H thymidine for 8 hrs period beginning 20 hrs after transfection and Ang II stimulation. When FITC labeled phosphorothioate ODN was introduced into VSMCs, cells were fixed with 4 5 paraformaldehyde at various time points after the transfer and observed by fluorescence microscopy.

(In vivo transfer of ODNs)

A No.2 French Fogarty catheter was used to induce vascular injury in male Sprague-Dawley rats (400-500g). These rats were anesthetized and a cannula was inserted into the left common carotid artery via the external carotid artery. After vascular injury of the common carotid artery, the distal injured segment was transiently isolated by temporary ligatures. The Protein-liposome complex was infused into the segment and incubated for 10 min at room temperature. After 10 min incubation, the infusion cannula was removed. Following the transfection, blood flow to the common carotid artery was restored by release of the ligatures. No adverse neurological or vascular effects were observed in any animal ungergoing this procedure. At 2, 4, and 8 weeks after transfection, rats were killed, and vessels were perfused and fixed with 4% paraformaldehyde. Three individual sections from the middle of the transfected segments were analysed. In addition, three sections from the middle section of the injured untransfected region were also analysed.

Results

In vivo gene transfer by protein-liposomes.

In protein-liposome delivery system, DNA and nuclear proteins were enclosed into the liposomes, and directly introduced into the cytoplasm from where they migrated into the nucleus. We succeeded in expressing exogenous genes in various organs by protein-liposome, as shown in Table 1. Protein-liposome is superior to other delivery systems in the following points: 1) high transfection efficiency, 2) short incubation time, 3) ability to deliver oligonucleotides, 4) no limitation of insert size, 5) no requirement for cell division, 6) no apparent toxicity, 7) no apparent antigenicity. But, the transient expression of genes in the tissues and the difticulty effecting inability for targeted delivery are limitations of protein-liposomes.

Table 1: In vivo gene transfer by protein-liposome

Organ (animal)	Gene	Duration of Gene Expression
Liver (rat, mouse)	Insulin	7-14 day
(rat)	Renin	7 days
Kidney (rat)	TGF-beta, PDGF	10 days
Heart (rat)	TGF-beta, HSP-70	> 2 weeks
Skeletal muscle (mouse)	Dystrophin	2 weeks
(rat)	Luciferase	> 4 weeks
Artery (rat)	Renin, ACE, c-NOS	> 2 weeks
Lung (rat)	TGF-beta	> 2 weeks
Patellar ligament (rat)	Lac-Z	> 4 weeks
Testis (mouse)	CAT	> 8 months

Delivery of ODN to VSMCs by protein-liposome.

When FITC-ODN was introduced into VSMCs using protein-liposome, fluorescence accumulated in the nucleus 5 min after the transfer and was detected in the nucleus at least for 72 hrs (Fig.1). In contrast, fluorescence was observed in the cellular components (probably in the endosome), not in the nucleus, by direct transfer of FITC-ODN without protein-liposome and no fluorescence was detected at 24 hrs after the transfer.

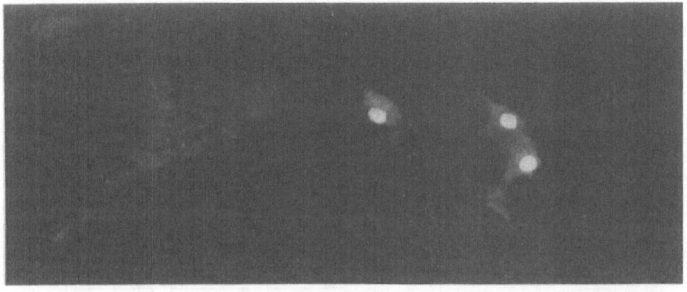

DIRECT TRANSFER   HVJ TRANSFER

Fig.1 :   Fluorescence microscopy of FITC labeled ODN using direct (DIRECT TRANSFER) versus protein-liposome (HVJ TRANSFER) method.   In direct transfer, VSMCs were incubated with 30 uM of FITC labeled phosphoriothioate antisense ODN (16 mer) (Clontech Inc.   Palo Alto, CA) for 5 min on ice and for 30 min at 37 C. In HVJ transfer, 500 ul of protein-liposome with FITC labeled ODN (3uM) was incubated for 5 min on ice and for 30 min at 37 C.   Then, after changing to fresh media, the cells were incubated in a CO_2 incubator.   Cells were fixed with 3% paraformaldehyde at 5, 30 min and 1, 3, 6, 12, 24, and 72 hrs. After mounting, cells were examined by fluorescent microscopy.   Photos show the cells at 5 min after the transfer.

Effect of antisense b-FGF on DNA synthesis.

Figure 2 shows that antisense b-FGF (AS-FGF) had no effect on cellular DNA synthesis   under basal conditions during 68-76 hrs when applied directly to VSMCs. Directly applied AS-FGF also had no effect on angiotensin II (Ang II) stimulated DNA synthesis.   When AS-FGF was delivered by protein-liposome, AS-FGF inhibited DNA synthesis either in unstimulated or Ang II treated conditions.   The reduction of cellular DNA synthesis by AS-FGF was approximately 40% compared with that by sense-FGF.   The concentrations of AS-FGF required to reduce cellular DNA synthesis to 75% were about 0.1 uM, 10 uM and 20 uM, by the protein-liposome method, lipofection and direct transfer, respectively (data not shown).   Therefore, the delivery of AS-ODN by protein-liposome was about 50 times more effective than lipofection and 100 times more effective than direct transfer.

a)

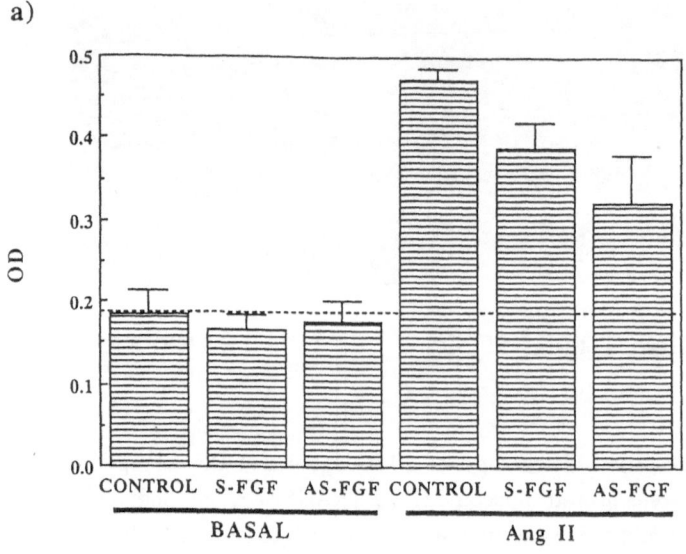

b)

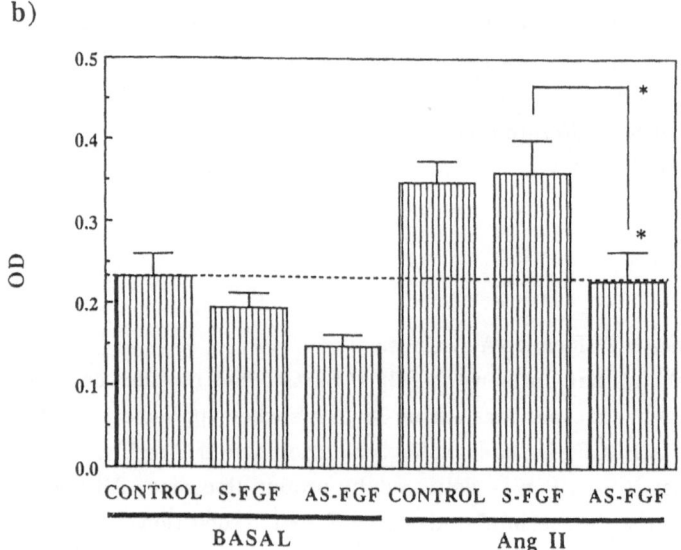

Fig.2 : Inhibitory effect of AS-FGF on DNA synthesis (^{3}H thymidine incorporation) with (a) no vector was used to deliver oligonucleotides or (b) protein-liposome method during 68-76 hrs after transfection. CONTROL: untreated VSMC, S-FGF: sense FGF transfected VSMC, AS-FGF: antisense FGF treated VSMC, BASAL: basal condition, Ang II : angiotensin II (10-6   M) stimulated condition, *P<0.05, **P<0.01 compareed to control group. Each group contains 4 samples. This experiment was repeated four times, and the figure shows representative data.

Prevention of neointima formation in carotid artery by antisense ODNs.

Since basic-FGF is one of the growth stimulants of VSMCs, other factors can stimulate the growth when AS-FGF is applied. Cell growth results from the cell division regulated by cell-cycle genes. Therefore we attempted to inhibit abnormal growth of VSMCs in vivo by suppressing the cell-cycle regulatory proteins. When both AS-PCNA and AS-cdc2 kinase were employed, VSMC proliferation in response to serum stimulation was inhibited significantly in vitro. Similarly, the combination of AS-cdc2 kinase and AS-cyclin B1 or AS-cdc2 kinase and AS-cdk2 kinase completely inhibited cellular DNA synthesis stimulated by the addition of serum. Given that neointima formation results from an initial acute phase of medial smooth muscle cell replication, we introduced both AS-PCNA and AS-cdc2 kinase or AS-cdc2 kinase and AS-cyclin B1 or AS-cdc2 kinasae and AS-cdk2 kinase into smooth muscle cells of balloon injured rat carotid artery in vivo. As shown in Fig.3, neointima formation was completely inhibited for two weeks after the transfer and the inhibitory effect was recognized up to eight weeks after a single transfection. However, when sense ODNs were introduced, no inhibitory effect was observed.

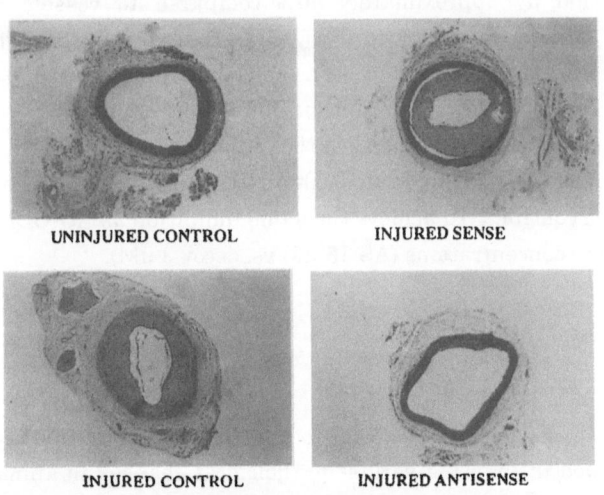

UNINJURED CONTROL   INJURED SENSE

INJURED CONTROL   INJURED ANTISENSE

Fig.3: Long-term suppression of neointima formation by AS-cdc2 kinase and AS-PCNA. Uninjured rat carotid artery (upper left), injured rat carotid artery without protein-liposome (lower left), injured rat carotid artery treated with protein-liposome containing 15 uM sense ODNs for both molecules (upper right) and injured rat carotid artery treated with protein-liposome containing 15 uM AS-ODNs (lower right) are shown. At 2 weeks after transfection, rats were sacrificed and vessels were fixed in 4% paraformaldehyde.

Novel molecular strategy "decoys" to inhibit neointima formation.

We next developed a new strategy to inhibit cell proliferation by the introduction of a single molecule. The transcription of PCNA , cdc2 kinase and some protooncogenes was activated by a common transcription factor, E2F, and the consensus DNA sequence recognized by E2F is known to be TTTCGCGC. We investigated the effect of double-stranded ODN designated as a competitor of E2F on the prevention of neointima formation.

First, decoy, double stranded-ODN homologous to E2F binding sequence, was introduced into VSMCs cultured in serum-depleted media using protein-liposome. VSMCs began to proliferate after adding 5% serum, but the serum stimulated growth was completely inhibited in the cells transfected with the decoy. Similarly, DNA synthesis followed by serum stimulation was blocked by the E2F decoy, and the mismatched sequence was not effective. Based on these in vitro results, we examined the effect of E2F decoy on the prevention of restenosis (11). E2F decoy was introduced into balloon injured rat carotid artery by protein-liposome. Our results demonstrated a marked suppression of neointima formation at 2 weeks after angioplasty by the decoy against E2F. At a dosage of 3 uM, decoy ODN inhibited neointima formation by approximately 80% compared to vessels treated with protein-liposome alone or mismatched decoy ODN-treated vessels. The decoy had no significant effect on the medial area. The selectivity of the decoy ODN effect was also confirmed. The inhibition of neointima formation was limited to the area of intraluminal transfection. In contrast, the adjacent injured carotid segments outside the area of the decoy transfection exhibited neointimal lesions similar to the sense ODN-treated control. To achieve the same inhibition as AS-ODN, decoy-ODN required much lower concentrations (AS 15 uM vs. decoy 3 uM).

Discussion

Protein-liposome seems to be a powerful tool for in vivo analysis of gene function. Indeed, we succeeded in inducing various pathological changes in animal organs by introducing responsible genes using protein-liposome (12-14). This success results from the high transfection efficiency, no apparent toxicity and no apparent antigenicity of the delivery system. In the aspect of gene therapy, antisense strategy by protein-liposome may be one of the most promising ways. There are no other methods to deliver oligonucleotides effectively. The findings that FITC-ODN delivered by protein-liposome rapidly accumulated in the nucleus (Fig.1) and that the formation of mRNAs of PCNA and cdc2 kinase was inhibited by AS-ODNs against both genes (data not shown) indicated that AS-ODN played its inhibitory role in the nucleus. Since cointroduction of AS-ODN with RNase H raised the inhibitory effect about three times more than AS-ODN alone, we suspected that AS-ODN may hybridize heterogeneous nuclear RNA in the nucleus and that the hybrid may be degraded by RNase H.

Besides the delivery system, the success of growth inhibition of VSMCs resulted from the employment of AS-ODN against cell-cycle regulators. However, several factors are responsible for the progression of each stage of the cell-cycle. That may be why the combination of different cell-cycle regulators was required for complete inhibition of cell growth. Actually, AS-ODN against a single regulator did not significantly inhibit cell growth.

The restenosis after angioplasty is a barrier to the treatment of myocardial infarction. No effective treatment has been reported. Since restenosis results from abnormal growth of VSMCs, we hypothesized that restenosis could be prevented by the blockade of genes regulating cell-cycle progression. Here we presented evidence that the complete inhibition of neointima formation could be achieved by a single administration of combined antisense ODN directed against cell cycle using protein-liposome. It appears that this antisense strategy is the most promising for the treatment of restenosis. To realize clinical use of this method, we will have to develop a catheter that will permit instillation/incubation of the protein-liposome complex and simultaneously maintain tissue perfusion. Moreover, we will have to remodel the protein-liposome complex to a simpler and more homogeneous particle.

References

1. Kaneda,Y., Iwai,K. & Uchida,T.: Increased expression of DNA cointroduced with nuclear protein in adult rat liver. Science (Wash. D.C.) 243, 375-378, 1989.
2. Kaneda,Y., Iwai,K. & Uchida,T. : Introduction and expression of the human insulin gene in adult rat liver. J. Biol. Chem. 264, 12126-12129, 1989.
3. Itoh,H., Mukoyama,M. Pratt,R.E. & Dzau,V.J. : Multiple autocrine growth factors modulate vascular smooth muscle cells growth response to angiotensin II. J. Clin. invest. 91, 2268-2274, 1993.
4. Morishita,R., Gibbons,G.H., Kaneda,Y., Ogihara,T. & Dzau,V.J. : Novel in vitro gene transfer method for study of local modulators in vascular smooth muscle cells. Hypertension 21, 894-899, 1993.
5. Meyerson,M., Faha,B., Su,L.-K, Harlow,E. & Tsai,L.-H.: The cyclin-dependent kinase family. "The cell cycle" (Cold Spring Harbor Laboratory Press) vol. 56, 177-186, 1991.
6. Morishita,R., Gibbons,G.H., Ellison,K.E., Nakajima,M., Zhang,L, Kaneda,Y., Ogihara,T. & Dzau,V.J. : Single intraluminal delivery of antisense cdc2 kinase and proliferating-cell nuclear antigen oligonucleotides results in chronic inhibition of

neointimal hyperplasia.   Proc. Natl. Acad. Sci. (USA) 90, 8474-8478, 1993.

7. Kaneda,Y. : Virus (Sendai virus envelopes)-mediated gene transfer.   Cell Biology; A Laboratory Handbook.   (Academic Press, Inc., Orland, Florida) vol3, 50-57, 1994.

8. Morrison, R.S. : Suppression of basic fibroblast growth factor expression by antisense oligonucleotides inhibits the growth of transformed human astrocytes.   J. Bio. Chem. 266, 728-734, 1991.

9. Morishita,R., Gibbons,G.H., Ellison,K.E., Nakajima,M., von ger Leyen,H., Zhang,L., Kaneda,Y., Ogihara,T. & Dzau,V.J. : Antisense oligonucleotides directed at cell cycle regulatory genes as strategy for restenosis therapy.   Transaction of the Association of American Physicians 54-61, 1993.

10. Itoh,H., Pratt,R.E., & Dzau,V.J. : Atrial natriuretic polypeptide inhibits hypertrophy of vascular smooth muscle cells.   J. Clin. Invest. 86, 1690-1697, 1990.

11. Morishita,R., Gibbons,G.H., Horiuchi,M., Ellison,K.E., Nakajima,M., Zhang,L., Kaneda,Y., Ogihara,T., & Dzau,V.J. : A gene therapy strategy using a transcription factor decoy of the E2F binding site inhibits smooth muscle proliferation in vivo. Proc. Natl. Acad. Sci. (USA) 92, 5855-5859, 1995.

12. Kato,K., Kaneda,Y., Sakirai,M., Nakanishi,M. & Okada,Y.: Direct injection of hepatitis B virus surface DNA induced hepatitis in adult rat liver.   J. Bio. Chem. 266, 22071-22074, 1991.

13. Tomita,N., Higaki,J., Kaneda,Y., Yu,H., Morishita,R., Mikami,H. & Ogihara, T. : Hypertensive rats produced by in vivo introduction of the human renin gene. Circulation. Res. 73, 898-905, 1993.

14. Isaka,Y., Fujiwara, Y., Ueda,N., Kaneda,Y., Kamada,T. & Imai,E. : Glomeruloscrerosis induced by in vivo transfection with TGF-beta or PDGF gene into rat kidney.   J. Clin. Invest. 92, 2597-2601, 1993.

Molecular Cloning Of A Human DEXH Box Gene Homologous To Yeast SKI2

Seong-Gene Lee[1], Jueun Chung[3], Inchul Lee[2], and Kyuyoung Song[3]
[1]Asan Institute for Life Sciences, Depts. [2]Pathology, [3]Biochemistry, University of Ulsan College of Medicine, 388-1 Poongnap-dong, Songpa-ku, Seoul 138-040, Korea

SUMMARY

In the course of characterizing the nuclear antigen recognized by a monoclonal antibody 170A1, we isolated a novel human cDNA homologous to yeast SKI2, reported a partial cDNA sequence, and mapped the gene to chromosome 6p21[7]. Subsequently the 5' end of the gene was obtained by rapid amplification of cDNA ends and was sequenced. Here, we report the complete nucleotide sequence of the gene. A full length cDNA contains 3,898 nucleotides in length and predicts an open reading frame of 1,245 amino acid residues with a calculated molecular weight of 137 kDa. The human gene contains seven well conserved helicase domains including DEAD/DEXH box which is an essential motif of nucleic acid-dependent NTPases and helicases; thus, it is named as Helicase Like Protein (HLP). Also, HLP has a leucine zipper motif and a putative nucleolar targeting sequence. Homology search indicates that the HLP gene is significantly homologous to the yeast SKI2 gene and a human ORF2 from male myeloblast KB-1 cell line.

KEYWORDS: human cDNA, yeast Ski2p, helicase domain, DEXH family

INTRODUCTION

We have recently cloned a novel human cDNA by screening a human fetal liver cDNA library with a monoclonal antibody, 170A1, which recognizes a human nucleolar peptide of molecular weight 90,000 [7]. It appeared to encode approximately 4- and 5-kb mRNAs, and was expressed in all the cells tested including EJ, HepG2, HeLa, and MC. The deduced amino acid sequence suggested that the gene product belonged to a growing family of proteins that share seven highly conserved amino acid regions; the DEXH family [4, 5]. The unique characteristic of this family of proteins is the presence of seven well conserved helicase domains with appropriate spacing. The DEXH family and its closely related DEAD family form the helicase superfamily II, whose members are implicated in a variety of cellular processes including splicing, translation, and development or cell growth [4, 12]. Although over 70 members of the DEAD/DEXH box family proteins have been identified, only several were isolated in humans.

217

The deduced amino acid sequence of human HLP gene had an overall homology of 63% to the recently described yeast SKI2 [13]. The SKI2 gene belongs to a system of six yeast chromosomal genes that repress the copy number of single- and double-stranded RNA viruses. The SKI2 gene encodes a polypeptide of 1,286 amino acids, and has six well conserved helicase motifs [4] and a nuclear localization sequence. The biological function of SKI2 is not yet clear, but indirect evidence suggests that Ski2p blocks translation of viral mRNAs by recognizing uncapped or poly(A)-deficient mRNAs [13]. The structural similarity between the HLP and SKI2 gene suggests that these two proteins may share common intracellular functions. However, except that the HLP gene is expressed in every cell tested so far, its precise function remains to be elucidated. As a step towards elucidation of its biological roles, the complete nucleotide sequence of the HLP gene was determined.

MATERIALS AND METHODS

5' rapid amplification of cDNA ends (RACE)

To obtain cDNA from the 5' end, human liver RNA derived single-stranded anchor ligated cDNA (5'-RACE-ReadyTM cDNA, Catalog No. 7300-1, Clontech, Palo Alto, CA) was used as a template for rapid amplification of cDNA ends. The anchor primer used in this procedure was 5'-CTGGTTCGGCCCACCTCT-GAAGGTTCCAGAATCGATAG-3' and two gene-specific primers were 5'-CGCGATTCAGGAGCTCTGAC-3' (primer 1, nt 1983-2002) and 5'-GAGGCGATAGAAATCACCAACAGGG-3' (primer 2, nt 987-1011). The cDNA was amplified in a final volume of 50 ml containing Taq polymerase buffer (10mM Tris-HCl pH 8.3, 50mM KCl, 1.5mM MgCl) supplemented with 10 pmole/ml each of anchor and primer 1, additional dNTPs to a final concentration of 0.5 mM, and 2.5 units of Taq polymerase (Perkin Elmer Cetus, USA). Thirty cycles of amplification were performed using an automated Perkin Elmer Cetus thermal cycler under the following conditions: denaturation at 94°C for 45s, annealing at 60°C for 45s, and extension at 72°C for 120s. The second PCR was performed under the same conditions using the anchor primer and the primer 2.

Subcloning and sequencing

The PCR product of 1 kb fragment was subsequently cloned into pCR™II vector (Invitrogen) according to the manufacturer's instructions and sequenced in full by a dideoxy nucleotide chain termination method [10] with Sequenase V 2.0 (USB).

Program search for sequence comparison.

Alignment of nucleotide sequences and comparisons with GenBank/EMBL databases were performed utilizing the BLAST program [1, 3]. We have used the FASTA and Clustal V program for sequence comparison between species via an E-mail server.

RESULTS

Subcloning and Sequencing of 5' cDNA clones

The human HLP gene was originally isolated by screening a human fetal liver cDNA library with a monoclonal antibody, 170A1, which recognizes a human nucleolar protein. Our previous Northern blot data suggested that the gene, 170A, encoded approximately 4- and 5-kb mRNAs [7]. The previously reported 3.1 kb cDNA sequence was obtained by assembling seven overlapping cDNA clones. Since extensive conventional screening did not yield a clone extending to the transcription start site, human liver derived single-stranded anchor ligated single stranded cDNA (Clontech, Palo Alto, CA) was used as a template for the PCR reaction involving the anchor primer and two gene specific primers. The PCR product of 1 kb fragment was shown to be contiguous to the other cDNA clones of 170A by molecular analyses (data not shown). This fragment was then cloned and sequenced.

Analysis of the HLP cDNA sequence

The complete cDNA sequence is available under GenBank Accession No.U09877. The cDNA of 3,898 nucleotides in length predicted an open reading frame of 3,735 nucleotides coding for 1,245 amino acids. Two methionines at nt 118 and 121; the latter appeared to be the first methionine because it had a purine in the -3 position and a guanine in the +4 position, characteristics common to most start codons [6]. The presence of a stop codon in the open reading frame 120 nt 5' to the first methionine proved that the open reading frame was complete. The 3 noncoding sequence was 45 bp long and a typical poly (A) addition sequence (AATAAA) [9] was not found. But an unusual varient GATAAA [11] was found only 5 nucleotides upstream of the poly (A) tail. The molecular weight of the protein calculated from the deduced sequence is about 137 kDa. Since the molecular weight of the nucleolar peptide recognized by a monoclonal antibody 170A1 was 90 kDa, it appeared that the gene we have identified did not represent the original antigen. As shown in Figure 1, the deduced amino acid sequence of 170A contains seven well conserved helicase motifs and a nucleolar localization sequence [4,5]. One of them, "DEAD/DEXH box", is an essential motif of nucleic acid-dependent NTPases and helicases, and the gene thus named tentatively as human helicase-like protein (HLP). Also a leucin zipper motif which is known to be involved in the protein-protein interaction is present between helicase domains Ia and II. (Fig.1). Considering the fact that approximately 70 genes were reported to contain DEAD/DEXH box. it was quite possible that the original nucleolar antigen of 90 kDa shared an epitope with the HLP gene. The length of 5' end of the mRNA and the position of the transcriptional start site and promoter are not known.

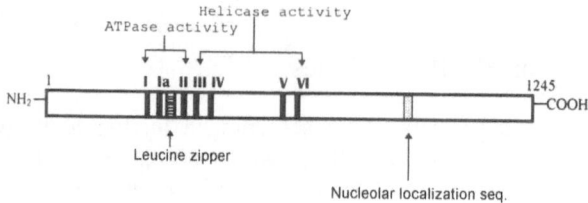

Fig. 1. Domain structure of HLP

Protein homologous to yeast Ski2p

The GenBank/EMBL Databases were searched for similarity with the HLP conceptual translation and nucleotide sequence using the BLAST program [1,3]. Two highly significant matches were found, yeast SKI2 gene (GenBank P35207) and a partial human ORF2 from human male myeloblast KB-1 cell line (GenBank D29641). Comparison of the HLP open reading frame with the amino acid sequence of yeast Ski2p and the human ORF 2 revealed overall structural similarities (Fig. 2).

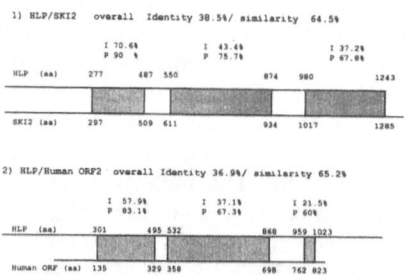

Fig. 2. Alignment of HLP with SKI2, and ORF2.
Shaded boxes indicate the regions of significant homology.

Especially the helicase motifs were highly conserved. The extent of overall homology between HLP and SKI2 was similar to the homology between HLP and the human ORF 2 except that only HLP and SKI2 had extended 3' end. While the Ski2p contained all six helicase motifs in the correct order with proper spacings and a glycine-arginine-rich domain characteristic of nucleolar RNA-binding proteins [2], the human HLP gene did not contain the glycine-arginine-rich region between helicase domains IV and V. Given the sequence homology between the HLP and human ORF 2, it seems that multiple genes of this subfamily may be present in humans. The extensive homology among HLP, yeast SKI2, and human

ORF2 suggested their evolutionary conservation between yeast and mammals, and important functions for the gene. Biochemical analyses and gene transfer experiments are underway to elucidate the biological functions of the gene and to determine the functional differences among other DEAD/DEXH family proteins.

ACKNOWLEDGMENTS

This work was supported by grants from the Asan Foundation through the Asan Institute for Life Sciences to I.L and K.S.

REFERENCES

1. Altschul SF, Gish W, Miller W, Myers EW, Lipman DJ (1990) Basic local alignment search tool. J.Mol.Biol. 215: 403-410
2. Dreyfuss G, Matunis MJ, Pinol-Roma S, Burd CG (1993) hnRNA proteins and the biogenesis of mRNA. Annu. Rev. Biochem. 62: 289-321
3. Gish W, States DJ (1993) Identification of protein coding regions by database similarity search. Nature Genetics 3: 266-272
4. Gorbalenya AE, Koonin EV, Donchenko AP, Blinov VM (1989) Two related superfamilies of putative helicases involved in replication, recombination, repair and expression of DNA and RNA genomes. Nucleic Acids Res. 17: 4713-4730
5. Hodgman TC (1988) A new superfamily of replicative proteins. Nature 333: 22-23
6. Kozak M (1989) The scanning model for translation: An update. J. Cell Biol. 108: 229-241
7. Lee S-G, Lee I, Park S-H, Kang C, Song K (1995) Identification and characterization of a human cDNA homologous yeast SKI2. Genomics 25: 660-666.
8. Linder P, Lasko PF, Leroy P, Nielsen PJ, Nish K, Schnier J, Slonimski PP (1992) Birth of D-E-A-D box. Nature 337: 121-122
9. Proudfoot NJ, Brownlee GG (1976) 3' non-coding region sequences in eukaryotic messenger RNA. Nature 263: 211-214
10. Sanger F, Nicklen S, Coulson AR (1977) DNA sequencing with chain-termination inhibitors. Proc.Natl.Acad.Sci. USA 74: 5463-5467
11. Sheets ME, Ogg SC, Wickens MP (1990) Point mutations in AATAAA and the poly(A) addition site: effects on the accuracy and efficiency of cleavage and polyadenylation in vitro. Nucleic Acids Res. 18: 5799-5805
12. Wassarman DA, Steitz JA (1991) Alive with DEAD proteins. Nature 349: 463-464
13. Widner WR, Wickner RB (1993) Evidence that the SKI antiviral system of Saccharomyces cerevisiae acts by blocking expression of viral mRNA. Mol.Cell.Biol.13: 4331-4341

Induction of Immune Response to Lymphoid Leukemia Cells by M-CSF Expression

Fumihiko Kimura[1], Miyuki Douzono[2], Jun Ohta[2], Toshiro Morita[3], Kazuma Ikeda[4], Yukitsugu Nakamura[1], Naoki Wakimoto[1], Ken Sato[1], Muneo Yamada[2], Naokazu Nagata[1], and Kazuo Motoyoshi[1]

[1]The Third Department of Internal Medicine, National Defense Medical College, 3-2 Namiki, Tokorozawa, Saitama 359, Japan; [2]Biochemical Research Laboratory, Morinaga Milk Industry Co. Ltd., Kanagawa, Japan; [3]Health Science Center, Kagawa University, Kagawa; and [4]Department of Transfusion Medicine, Kagawa Medical School, Kagawa, Japan.

SUMMARY

Macrophage colony-stimulating factor (M-CSF) enhances tumoricidal activities of macrophages. We transduced M-CSF cDNA into mouse lymphoid cell line, L1210, and investigated the anti-tumor effect of the locally expressed M-CSF. Mice injected with M-CSF-producing subline showed improved survival in comparison with mock-transfected cell line or parental cell line plus M-CSF administration. Moreover, M-CSF-expressing cells could induce immunity to the parental cells. The same improvement of survival was observed in mouse M-CSF-expressing cell lines. These observations imply that M-CSF cDNA is a candidate gene to use in gene therapy in lymphoid leukemia.

KEY WORDS: M-CSF, immunotherapy, gene therapy, leukemia

INTRODUCTION

Macrophage colony-stimulating factor (M-CSF), which was originally identified as a growth factor to induce proliferation and differentiation of monocyte progenitors, also enhances tumoricidal activity of mature monocyte/macrophages. This anti-tumor activity involves antibody-dependent monocyte-mediated cytotoxicity (ADCC), reactive nitrogen oxide intermediates, and production of tumoricidal cytokines such as tumor necrosis factor (TNF), interferon (IFN), and interleukin-1 (IL-1). Indeed, M-CSF showed the tumoricidal activity for several tumors in vivo. We also previously reported the murine model showing that M-CSF administration resulted in tumoricidal activity for the mouse lymphoid cell line, L1210, which is resistant to TNF [1]. Systemic application of M-CSF improved the survival rate of mice injected with a small number of L1210 cells. However, this effect disappeared with the increase in the inoculated cell number despite M-CSF administration. In this study, to increase the local concentration of M-CSF, we made M-CSF-expressing sublines, and examined the anti-tumor effect of locally expressed M-CSF and the ability of these M-CSF transduced cells to induce immunity to the parental cells [2].

MATERIALS AND METHODS

Human M-CSF cDNA, which was kindly provided by the Genetics Institute Inc. (Massachusetts), was truncated with SmaI, and inserted into an expression vector, pRc/CMV (Invitrogen, San Diego, CA). Expression plasmids were transfected into L1210 cells using lipofectin, and cells were selected in G418 followed by limiting dilution to establish cell lines. The M-CSF content in the conditioned media of the transfected cells was measured by an enzyme-linked immunosorbent assay (ELISA).

Male 7-week-old CDF1 mice (Charles River Japan Inc., Kanagawa, Japan) were maintained in a standard condition. All experiments included 10 animals in each group.

RESULTS

Characterization of M-CSF-producing cell lines

We obtained a mock-transfected cell line (RC13) and two M-CSF producing cell lines (SM6 and SM11). The amount of M-CSF produced by SM6 and SM11 were, respectively, 2.4 and 3.5 ng per 10^6 cells. Before inoculation of tumor cells, we checked that there was no difference in proliferation in vitro among these cell lines. Neither parental L1210, RC13, nor SM11 cells expressed CD80 (B7-1) when analyzed by flow cytometry. To identify the effect of M-CSF produced by these cells, we examined whether macrophages could inhibit the growth of the cells in vitro. Peritoneal macrophages suppressed the proliferation of M-CSF-producing cells more effectively than that of mock-transfected RC13. This difference disappeared by the addition of IFNγ (500 U/ml) plus LPS (100 ng/ml) to this culture.

Local production of M-CSF abrogated tumorigenicity of L1210 cells

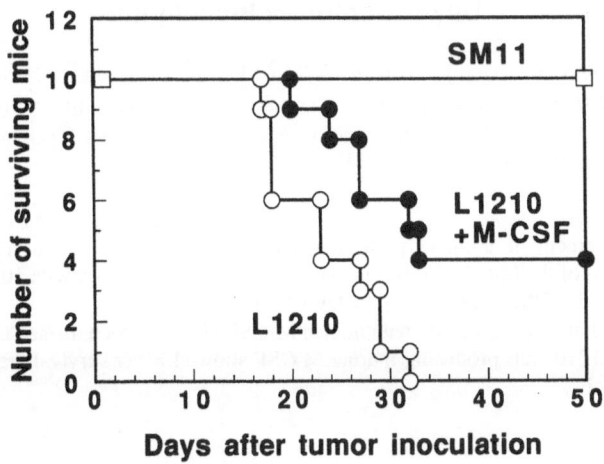

Fig. 1 Comparison of the in vivo effect of local production and systemic application of M-CSF. Mice (ten animals per group) were given an intravenous injection of 10^2 L1210 (○) or SM11 (□) cells. One group of mice (●) were followed by M-CSF administration (20 μg/kg) for 3 consecutive days.

The L1210 lymphoid leukemia cells injected intravenously proliferated in mice to invade their liver and spleen and finally replaced their hepatocytes and splenocytes just before their death. We compared the effect to increase the survival rate in M-CSF-producing sublines with the parental line plus M-CSF administration. Mice injected with 10^2 parental L1210 all died by day 32, but 40% of the mice injected with L1210 in combination with M-CSF were alive at day 50. Moreover, none of the mice injected with 10^2 SM11 cells died (Fig. 1).

An increase in the inoculated cell number to 5×10^3 decreased the survival rate of mice injected with L1210 plus M-CSF, and M-CSF administration could not increase the survival rate at 10^6 inoculation any further. However, the mice injected with 5×10^3 or 10^6 SM11 showed 80-90% survival. The survival curve after injection of 10^6 SM6 and SM11 cells is shown in Fig. 2.

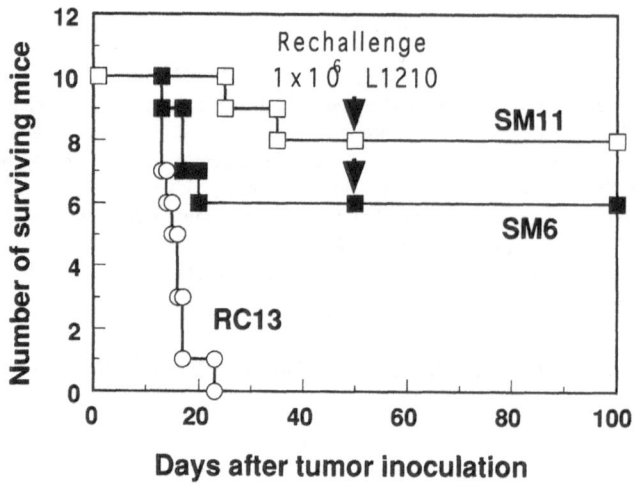

Fig. 2   Survival curve of mice injected with 10^6 M-CSF-expressing cells. Mice inoculated with SM6 (■) or SM11 (□) showed an improved survival rate in comparison with injection of mock-transfected RC13 (○) cells. All surviving mice were rechallenged with 10^6 parental L1210 cells at day 50, and they were observed up to day 100.

To test the development of immune protection against L1210 cells, all surviving mice, after intravenous injection of the M-CSF-expressing sublines, were rechallenged with 10^6 parental L1210 cells at day 50, and all of them survived up to day 100 (Fig. 2).

Although we started these experiments with human M-CSF cDNA, we confirmed later that the mice injected with 10^6 L1210 cells producing murine M-CSF showed better survival than those with the mock-transfected cells.

DISCUSSION

Immunotherapy using tumor cells modified to express cytokines is a potential therapeutic approach against cancer, and has been examined mainly in murine B16 melanoma. Although this approach is also attractive in leukemia, some cytokines such as IL-2 and GM-CSF might stimulate leukemic cell growth. In this study, we selected M-CSF as a transduced cytokine, because M-CSF-dependent leukemic progression was hardly detected after administration of M-CSF to patients as a stimulator for neutrophil recovery [3]. There was a negative correlation between M-CSF

225

expression and growth capacity of leukemic cells in suspension culture [4]. However, M-CSF-expressing myeloid leukemic cells may proliferate in an autocrine manner [5].

Our findings imply that M-CSF cDNA is a candidate gene for use in gene therapy of lymphoid leukemia. However, it may not be the best candidate for all tumors. Although M-CSF expression in the melanoma model demonstrated prolonged survival of the inoculated mice [6], transduction to the plasmacytoma cell line, J588L, induced macrophage infiltration around the tumors, but failed to reduce the tumorigenicity or increase the immunogenicity [7]. The best candidate gene may depend on the tumor type. More candidate genes need to be examined in many types of tumors to determine the best combination.

REFERENCES

1. Douzono M, Suzu S, Yamada M, Yanai N, Kawashima T, Hatake K, Motoyoshi K (1995) Augmentation of cancer chemotherapy by preinjection of human macrophage colony-stimulating factor in L1210 leukemic cell-inoculated mice. Jpn J Cancer Res 86:315-321
2. Kimura F, Douzono M, Ohta J, Morita T, Ikeda K, Nakamura Y, Sato K, Yamada M, Nagata N, Motoyoshi K (1995) Augmentation of anti-tumor immunity using genetically M-CSF-expressing L1210 cells. Exp Hematol (in press)
3. Motoyoshi K, Takaku F (1991) Human monocytic colony-stimulating factor (hM-CSF), phase I/II clinical studies. In: Mertelsmann R, Herrmann F (ed) Hematopoietic growth factors in clinical applications. New York: Marcel Dekker, Inc., pp 161-175
4. Wang C, Kelleher CA, Cheng GYM, Miyauchi J, Wong GG, Clark SC, Minden MD, McCulloch EA (1988) Expression of the CSF-1 gene in the blast cells of acute myeloblastic leukemia: association with reduced growth capacity. J Cell Physiol 135:133-138
5. Rambaldi A, Wakamiya N, Vellenga E, Horiguchi J, Warren MK, Kufe D, Griffin JD (1988) Expression of the macrophage colony-stimulating factor and c-fms genes in human acute myeloblastic leukemia cells. J Clin Invest 81:1030-1035
6. Walsh P, Dorner A, Duke RC, Su L-J, Glode LM (1995) Macrophage colony-stimulating factor complementary DNA: a candidate for gene therapy in metastatic melanoma. J Natl Cancer Inst 87:809-816
7. Dorsch M, Hock H, Kunzendorf T, Blankenstein T (1993) Macrophage colony-stimulating factor gene transfer into tumor cells induces macrophage infiltration but not tumor suppression. Eur J Immunol 23:186-190

Effects of Cytokines on the Efficiency of Gene* Transfer Into Murine Hematopoietic Progenitors

Yang Jianmin Song Xianmin Min Bihe Meng Peilin

Department of Hematology, Changhai Hospital, Second Millitary Medical University,Shanghai 200433,China

SUMMARY The purpose of this study was to evaluate the effects of cytokines on the efficiency of gene transfer into murine hematopoietic progenitors and human K562 cells mediated by retrovirus (RV) containing bacterial neomycin-resistant (neo^R) gene. Cytokines were used in bone marrow cell preincubation and retrovirus vectors —containing supernatant transfection each for 24 hours.The transfected cells were planted in semisolid culture with or without   G418.   The efficiency of gene   transfer into hematopoietic progenitors was estimated by biological assay and PCR analysis.   The most efficient combination of cytokines,IL-1α /IL-3/SCF,increased the efficiency of gene transfer into murine CFU-GM from   6.04±1.34% to 43.60±5.95%.SCF alone most efficiently facilitated the gene transfer efficiency from 19.04±1.58% to 54.46±2.13%.The results suggest that the combination of IL-1α /IL-3/SCF can increase the efficiency of gene transfer into hematopoietic stem cells (HSC) and progenitors,and in the treatment of acute myeloid leukemia (AML) by autologous bone marrow transplantion (ABMT),SCF can facilitate gene transfer into hematopoietic cells in gene-marking clinical studies.

KEY WORDS:retrovirus vector; neo gene; cytokine; gene transfer efficiency; hematopoietic progenitor

INTRODUCTION

It has been proven that the gene transfer efficiency into hematopoietic stem cells (HSCs) mediated by retrovirus vectors (RV) can be increased by raising the rate of actively proliferative HSCs. Interleukin-1α (IL-1α),interleukin-3 (IL-3) and stem cell factor (SCF) have potent stimulatory   effects   on   HSCs   and   pluripotent   hematopoietic progenitors[1,2].So we have explored the effects of IL-1α ,IL-3 and SCF on the effeciency of neo^R gene into murine hematopoietic progenitors and human K562 cells to find the most   efficient   cytokine or their combination in promoting the gene transfer into hematopoietic cells

MATERIALS AND METHODS

Retroviral plasmid LNL6 containing neo^R gene was a gift from Prof.Miller

AD,USA.The plasmid was transduced into PA317 cells by electroporation.The transduced PA317 cells were selected in medium containing G418 at 300 ug/ml(Sigma,USA).The virus titre is 7×10^5CFU/ml measured with NIH3T3 cells[3].

BALB/c murine bone marrow cells or human K562 cells at the concentration of 2×10^6/ml were preincubated in medium,to which recombinant human (rh) IL-1α (10^u/ml,Boehringer Mannheim,Germany),recombinant (r)IL-3(50^u/ml for human K562 cells, 200^u/ml for murine bone marrow cells, USA) and recombinant human (murine)(rh(m)) SCF(100ng/ml,Angen)had been added.After 24 hours, the medium was replaced by half the virus supernatant and followed by adding cytokines to concentrations as above and polybrene (Sigma,USA) to a final concentration of 4 μ g/ml. After 24 hours,the non -adherent cells were planted in semi-solid methylcellulose culture.There were two control groups without cytokines, one group was tranfected with virus supernatant and the other was not .

The semisolid culture system contains 0.3ml methylcellose, 0.2ml fetal calf serum,0.1ml conditioned medium from murine lung(not for K562 cells),0.1ml bone marrow cells (at a concentration of 2×10^6/ml for murine bone marrow cells and 1×10^5/ml for K562 cells) , and IMDM culture medium to a final volume of 1ml. The thoroughly mixed culture medium was added to 96 wells plate at 0.1ml per well. There were 6 wells with G418 and 6 wells without .The cultures were scored at 7 days for CFU-GM. neo[R] gene transfer efficiency = the number of colonies with G418 / the number of colonies without G418$\times$100%.

Two pairs of oligonucleotide primers for the neo[R] gene were chemically synthesized by the Shanghai Institute of Cytobiology.The sequences of the primers were as follow:5'CGTTGTCACTGAAGCGGGAAGG 3' (primer 1), 5 ' CCATGAATATCGGCAAGCAGGC 3' (primer 2),5' TGCTATTGGGCGAAGTGCCG 3' (primer 3)and 5' ACAAGACCGGCTTCCATCCG 3' (primer 4) . Single colonies were picked up from methylcellulose plates, lysed , incubated with proteinase K , and prepared for PCR amplification. Primer 3 and 4 were used in nested PCR by the model of 1μ l of PCR product with primer 1 and 2.neo[R] gene transfer efficiency = The number of positive colonies by PCR/the total number of colonies by PCR.Southern blot was done as a reference [4].

RESULTS

neo[R] gene transfer efficiency by biological assay

The combination of IL-1α /Il-3/SCF increased the gene transfer efficiency from 6.04$\pm$1.34% to 43.60$\pm$5.94%,which was significantly higher than the effect of IL-1α /IL-3(Tab 1). SCF alone increased the gene transfer efficiency into K562 cells from 19.04±1.58% to 54.46 ± 2.13% and was significant as compared to IL-1α /IL-3(Tab 2)

Tab .1 Results of neo^R gene transfer into murine CFU-GM

Infection conditions	Percentage of G418-resistant murine CFU-GM			Average (mean±SD)
	Experiment 1	Experiment 2	Experiment3	
IL-1α	7.39	9.21	5.59	7.40±1.81
IL-3	11.11	14.44	8.42	11.32±3.02
SCF	8.92	10.94	8.18	9.35±1.43
IL-1α /IL-3	34.48	31.67	26.05	30.73±4.29*
SCF/IL-3	18.59	21.89	16.67	19.05±2.64
IL-1α /SCF/IL-3	45.72	48.19	36.90	43.60±5.94△
no cytokines	5.53	7.56	5.03	6.04±1.34

* p<0.01 vs IL-3 group, △ p<0.05 vs IL-1α /IL-3 group

Tab 2. Efficiency of neo^R gene transfer into k562 cells

Infection conditions	Percentage of G418-resistant K562 cells		Average (mean±SD)
	Experiment 1	Experiment 2	
IL-1α	18.32	20.00	19.16±1.19
IL-3	28.81	29.97	29.39±0.82
SCF	55.99	51.96	54.46±2.13*
IL-1α /IL-3	40.13	41.93	41.03±1.27
SCF/IL-3	50.46	45.98	48.22±3.16
IL-1α /SCF/IL-3	49.89	44.04	46.97±4.14
no cytokines	20.15	17.92	19.04±1.58

* p<0.05 vs IL-1α /IL-3 group

Neo^R gene transfer efficiency by PCR analysis

Ten to twenty single colonies from the murine CFU-GM culture from the IL-1α / IL-3/SCF group without G418 in experiment 1 and of human K562 cells culture of SCF group without G418 in experiment 1 were analyzed by PCR with primer 3 and 4 and primer 1 and 2 respectively. The 157-bp band was visualized from 8 of 12 colonies of murine CFU-GM and the gene transfer efficiency was 66.67%(8/12)(Fig 1); the 325-bp band was visualized from 13 of 17 colonies of human K562 cells and the gene transfer efficiency was 76.47%(13/17).

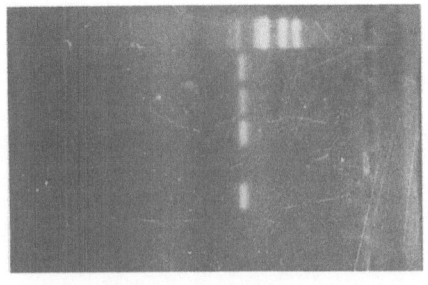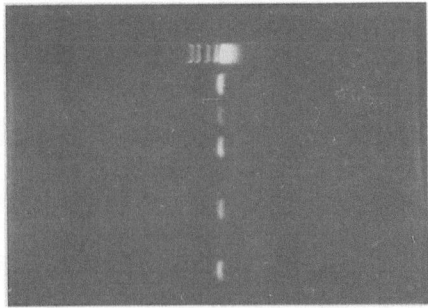

Fig.1 PCR Analysis of Murine CFU-GM
1,9:marker 2:positive control 3-7,10-16:samples 8:negative control

Nested PCR analysis and Southern blot

The Southern blot on the result of PCR and Nested PCR shows that specific hybridizing bands were visualized from all the positive G418-resistant colonies of human K562 cells.   This result further confirms specific amplification of the neo^R gene by PCR .

CONCLUSION

PCR analysis can be used to more accurately estimate the gene transfer efficiency than biological assay. The combination of IL-1α /IL-3/SCF. can increase the gene transfer efficiency of HSCs and hematopoietic progenitors.SCF can be used to increase the gene transfer efficiency into hematopoietic progenitors in gene-marking clinical studies to trace the origin of relapse of AML patients after ABMT.

REFERENCES:
1.Iscove NN, Shaw Ar, Gordon K(1989) Net increase of pluripotential hematopoietic precursors in suspension culture in response to IL-1α and IL-3.J Immunol,142:2332
2.Williams N,Bertocello I, Kavnoudias et al(1992) Recombinant rat stem cell factor stimulates the amplification and differention on fractroned mouse stem cell population. Blood 79:58
3.Miller AD,Falaw M,Verma IM(1985) Generation of helper free amphotropic retrovirus that   transduces a dominant-acting, methotrexate-resistant dihydrofolate reductase gene.Mol Cell Biol 5:431
4.Sambrook J,Fritsch EF,Maniatis T.Molecular Cloning:a laboratary manual ,2nd,New York. Cold Spring Harbor laboratory Press,1989;pp:474-491

Bone Marrow Transplantation

HEMATOPOIETIC STEM CELL TRANSPLANTS FROM UNRELATED DONORS

John A. Hansen, Jorge Sierra, Effie W. Petersdorf, Paul J. Martin and Claudio Anasetti

Fred Hutchinson Cancer Research Center, and Department of Medicine, University of Washington School of Medicine, Seattle, WA.

SUMMARY

Further improvements in the safety and efficacy of unrelated donor transplants can be expected with better GVHD prevention and facilitation of tolerance induction. New approaches such as selected depletion of distinct T cell subsets, use of purified stem cells and novel forms of immune modulation using biologicals and other engineered molecules are promising, but additional preclinical and appropriate clinical trials must be undertaken before the full potential benefits as well as limitations of these new approaches are known.

INTRODUCTION

Marrow or peripheral blood stem cell allografts are potentially life saving for patients with otherwise fatal inherited or acquired diseases such as severe combined immunodeficiency disease (SCID), thalasemia, aplastic anemia and hematological malignancies (1,2). Engraftment of normal stem cells can correct genetic abnormalities and rescue patients from high-dose cytotoxic therapy, and the mature donor T cells present in a marrow or peripheral blood stem cell graft provide an important graft-versus-leukemia (GVL) effect. The successful transplantation of marrow and hematopoietic stem cells, however, is strongly constrained by the need for HLA matching of donor and recipient, and by the necessity of controlling graft-versus-host disease (GVHD).

Fewer than 30% of patients have an HLA identical sibling, and the chance of finding this kind of an ideal match will diminish further as the size of the average family continues to decrease. Occasionally it is possible to identify a haploidentical relative who is partially HLA matched, and these cases have been informative in revealing the significance of HLA matching (3-6). However, these transplants have been successful only when mismatching is limited to one HLA-A, B, DR antigen, a situation which occurs infrequently. The remaining alternative source of normal HLA matched stem cells is an unrelated volunteer donor.

UNRELATED DONOR REGISTRIES

The extensive polymorphism of HLA has necessitated the establishment of large registries of HLA typed donors currently numbering more than 2.8 million worldwide. The U.S. marrow donor registry, known as the National Marrow Donor Program (NMDP), is a network of more than 106 donor centers and 70 transplant centers, some of which are located in other countries (7-9). A coordinating center is located in Minneapolis, MN. As of September 30, 1995, the NMDP registry has grown to more than 1.8 million HLA-A, B typed volunteers, including 608,682 donors typed for HLA-A, B and DR (Figure 1). The racial composition of the NMDP donor registry is 61.0% Caucasian, 6.9% African American, 6.2% Hispanic, 4.8% Asian, 1.2% Native American, and 19.9% other or unknown. From the beginning of NMDP operations in 1987 through September 1995, a total number of 24,844 preliminary donor searches have been submitted, 13,404 (54%) have gone on to formal searches with requests for additional HLA typing, and HLA matched donors have been identified for 3,803 transplants (15% of preliminary searches and 28% of formal searches). Donor search requests to the NMDP are submitted to the search coordinating centers in Minneapolis, Minnesota by individual member transplant centers for integration of the central database. Successful preliminary searches are followed by HLA-DR typing requests or requests for blood samples for confirmatory HLA typing and once an HLA match has been identified the transplant center submits a request for final donor consent, medical clearance and transplant scheduling. These requests are forwarded by NMDP to the appropriated donor center. The annual number of preliminary and formal donor search requests has increased steadily (Table 1).

SEARCHING FOR AN UNRELATED DONOR

The overall chance of finding an HLA-A, B and DR match at the time of an initial search has improved as the number of HLA-A, B, DR donors has increased (Table 1). Success of matching, however, varies according to the racial origin of the patient. Currently, the chance of finding at least one HLA-A, B, DR identical donor at initial search is 72% for Caucasians, 59% for Hispanics, 49% for Asians and 24% for African Americans. The time required for an unrelated donor search can be a critical problem for patients with unstable diseases such as severe aplastic anemia, or leukemia. Fortunately, the time required for an unrelated donor search through NMDP has also gradually improved as the network has become more experienced and efficient (Table 2). With the growth of the registry, particularly the number of volunteers typed for HLA-A, B and DR, the number of transplants performed has also increased (Figure 2). It is estimated that NMDP will facilitate more than 1,000 unrelated donor transplants in 1996. This represents a growth in one year of 25%. Even with the large number of volunteers available in the NMDP donor registry, all patients do not match. Reciprocal donor search agreements offer the only hope for optimizing the chance of finding an HLA match. Worldwide cooperation is increasing, and the number of HLA matched marrows exchanged between different countries has become a very significant component of the unrelated donor marrow transplant programs of several nations (Figure 3).

NATIONAL MARROW DONOR PROGRAM VOLUNTEER MARROW DONORS

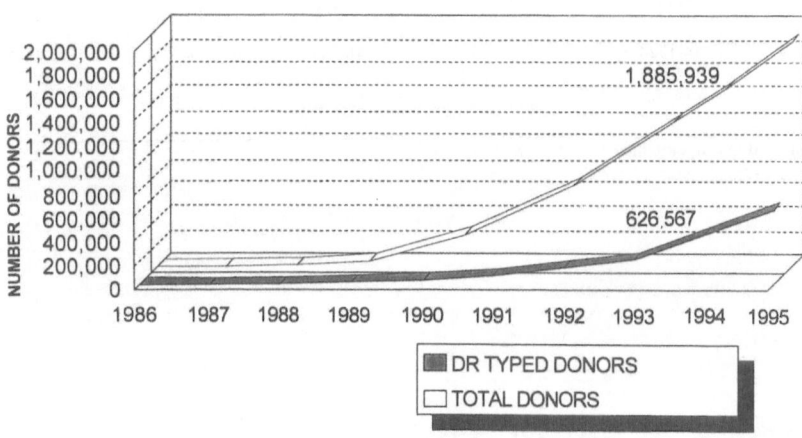

Figure 1. NMDP Donor Registry showing cumulative annual growth of HLA-A,B and HLA-A,B,DR typed volunteers.

Table 1. NMDP Donor Search Statistics. Number of HLA-A, B, DR Typed Donors, Number of New Donor Searches, and Chance of Finding an HLA-A, B, DR Identical Match at Initial Search.

Year	Number of HLA-A, B, DR Donors	Total Searches	Percent Matching
1987	2732	211	8%
1988	6970	1415	23%
1989	19905	1709	30%
1990	36410	1384	49%
1991	74301	2958	44%
1992	140623	3547	52%
1993	208723	3917	53%
1994	414122	4280	61%
1995[a]	586672	3640	66%

[a] as of July 31, 1995

Table 2. Time Interval from Start of Formal Donor Search with NMDP to Transplant[a]

	1991	1992	1993	1994	1995[b]
Median, days	182	178	149	134	129
range	44-1324	35-1723	48-2114	35-1765	38-2361
25th, 95th %	135, 290	120, 315	103, 287	93, 264	91, 228

[a]patients transplanted during time interval indicated
[b]first 6 months of 1995

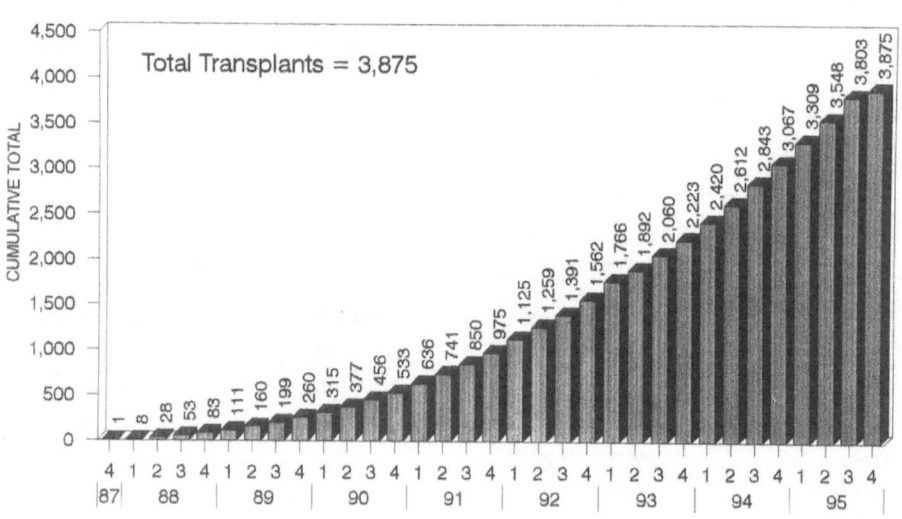

NMDP SEARCHES REACHING TRANSPLANT

Figure 2. NMDP transplants showing cumulative annual growth.

NMDP International Cooperation
October 1, 1995
443 Marrows Received From:

Netherlands	England	France	Canada	Spain
120	119	48	45	0
Germany	Israel	Australia	Switzerland	Austria
97	5	8	1	0

400 Marrows Provided To:

Canada	England	France	Sweden	Belgium
191	21	34	26	0
Israel	Japan	Italy	Germany	Australia
16	6	13	38	20
Austria	Norway	Switzerland	Hong Kong	Brazil
3	1	5	1	0
Ireland	Denmark	Spain	Netherlands	
1	5	2	17	

Figure 3. Total number of HLA matched marrow grafts that NMDP has received or provided to other countries.

HLA TYPING AND DONOR MATCHING

Recent advances in HLA typing technology have shown that standard serological methods for phenotyping are limited in detecting genetic variants, many of which can be recognized by T cells (9,10). The definitive identification of HLA alleles can be achieved using DNA-based typing methods. Many clinical laboratories have adapted DNA technology for defining DRB and DQB alleles. However, the application of high resolution typing to the class I HLA-A,B & C genes is generally feasible only in research laboratories. An HLA-A or B minor mismatch is defined as two antigens that belong to the same crossreactive group or CREG (Figure 4A). When DNA-based typing of the DRB1 locus is performed on HLA-A, B, DR matched donors there is a 40% chance that any one will be matched with the patient for the DRB1 alleles (65% if 2 donors and 95% if 5 donors are typed). When the best matched donor has been identified, 34% of patients will have at least one HLA-A, B, DRB1 identical donor; 19% a donor matched for DR, but differing for a minor mismatch at HLA-A or B; 17% a donor matched for HLA-A and B, but differing for a minor mismatch at DR (a DR serological match, but DRB1 allele mismatch); and 11% a donor differing for at least one major mismatch.

Criteria at our Center for the selection of unrelated donors are based on patient age. Patients up to the age of 55 years are eligible for an unmodified (T cell replete) marrow transplant from an unrelated donor if an HLA-A, B, DRB1 identical volunteer can be identified. If this is not possible, patients less than 36 years old are eligible for a donor incompatible for no more than one HLA-A, B or DR minor mismatch. An HLA-DR minor mismatch is defined as two haplotypes that express the same DR specificity (e.g., DR4) but that differ for DRB1 alleles (e.g., 0401 vs. 0404) (Figure 4B). Patients up to the age of 55 years for whom the best available donor is incompatible for no more than one HLA-A, B or DR mismatch are eligible for a T cell depleted marrow graft.

We have analyzed DRB1 and DQB1 allele matching, as defined by PCR/SSOP, in 364 marrow transplants serologically matched for HLA-A,B,DR (11). All patients received non-T cell depleted marrow, and cyclosporine plus methotrexate for GVHD prophylaxis. Fifty-nine (16%) were mismatched for DRB1 and 305 (84%) were matched for DRB1. The probability of clinically severe grades III-IV acute GVHD was 48% for DRB1 matched and 70% for DRB1 mismatched transplants. The relative risk of grade III-IV acute GVHD for DRB1 mismatching was 1.7 (95% CI, 1.2-2.5) and the relative risk of transplant-associated mortality was 1.5 (95% CI, 1.0-2.2). Although the number of cases mismatched for DQB1 (n=33) was relatively small, there was a trend for more GVHD in DQB1 incompatible transplants (52% and 40%). The probability of grades III-IV acute GVHD was greatest in cases mismatched for both DRB1 and DQB1 (69%). Unlike DQ, HLA-DP alleles are not usually associated with DR alleles, and thus it was not unexpected to find that more than 80% of HLA-A,B,DRB1 matched unrelated donor transplants are mismatched for DP. Our preliminary analysis of DP matching suggested that DP disparity probably does not contribute significantly to GVHD (12). A definitive comparison of the relative significance of DR, DQ and DP mismatching will require a larger number of cases fully typed for DRB, DQA, DQB, DPA and DPB.

It has been generally assumed that the mixed lymphocyte culture (MLC) assay, which primarily measures T cell activation in response to class II DR, DQ and in some cases DP disparity, should predict for GVHD. In a retrospective analysis, however we have found that MLC reactivity, in contrast to allele matching for DRB1, does not predict for clinically severe grades III-IV acute GVHD even among HLA-A,B,DR unrelated donor identical transplants (13).

We have previously shown that HLA disparity can also increase the risk of graft failure (4). Among 490 patients prepared for transplant with total body irradiation (TBI), receiving unmodified (T cell replete) marrow and methotrexate and cyclosporine for GVHD prophylaxis, 20 patients had graft failure following a first marrow transplant from an unrelated donor. In all cases, the pretransplant anti-donor cytotoxic crossmatch test of the patient's serum was negative. Review of the available HLA data demonstrated that 13 of the graft failure cases were HLA-A, B-serologically matched and DRB1-allele matched with their donor while 7 cases were

Figure 4A

A1, A3, A11, A36	B14, B64, B65
A23, A24	B8, B59
A25, A26, A34, A66, A43	B15, B17, B46, B57, B*5701, B*5702, B58, B*5801, B62, B63, B70, B71, B72, B75, B76, B77
A19, A29, A30, A31, A32, A33, A74	B16, B38, B39, B67
A2, A28, A*6801, A*6802, A*6901	B7, B27, B42, B73
	B7, B22, B54, B55, B56, B67
B5, B18, B35, B51, B52, B53, B70, B71, B72	B7, B40, B41, B48, B60, B61
B21, B44, B*4402, B*4403, B*4404, B*4405, B45, B49, B50	B13, B47

Figure 4B

DR1:	DRB1*0101-0104	DR12 (5):	DRB1*1201-1203
DR15 (2):	DRB1*1501-1504	DR13 (6):	DRB1*1301-1313
DR16 (2):	DRB1*1601-1606	DR14 (6):	DRB1*1401-1417
DR17 (3):	DRB1*0301;0304;0305	DR7:	DRB1*0701
DR18 (3):	DRB1*0302; 0303	DR8:	DRB1*0801-0811
DR4:	DRB1*0401-0421	DR9:	DRB1*0901
DR11 (5):	DRB1*1101-1113	DR10:	DRB1*1001

Figure 4. Definition of HLA minor mismatches. Panel A: Class I HLA-A and B antigens classified according to serologically-defined crossreactive groups (CREG) (adapted from the U.S. NMDP). Panel B: Class II HLA-DR major and minor mismatches. Antigens in different boxes represent major mismatches, while antigens within the same box represent minor mismatches.

mismatched for at least one HLA locus. Of the 20 patients, 18 had Ph positive CML, one had juvenile CML, and one had severe aplastic anemia. To determine the effect of HLA mismatching on risk of graft failure, a case control study was undertaken. For each case, two control patients who had successfully engrafted were matched for variables which might influence engraftment including presence or absence of serologically detectable HLA-A or B disparity, presence or absence of DRB1 disparity, disease and stage, TBI dose and fractionation, panel reactive antibody score, transplant date, donor-recipient gender, patient age and marrow cell dose. Alleles encoded at HLA-A, C, B, DRB1, DQB1 were determined by SSOP typing or direct sequencing (14,15,16). Mismatching for HLA-C alleles was found in 15 (75%) of the 20 case pairs and 12 (30%) of the 40 control pairs. The odds ratio (OR) of graft failure given an HLA-C mismatch (univariate conditional logistical regression model) was 8.3 (95% CI: 1.8, 38; p < .01). The effect of mismatching for HLA-C was also significant after accounting for the contribution of HLA-A and B allele mismatching (OR 5.2; 95% CI: 1.0-26; p = .02). This is the first clinical data we know of which demonstrate that HLA-C functions as a transplantation antigen, and that mismatching for class I genes, especially HLA-C, increases the risk of graft failure (17).

RESULTS OF UNRELATED DONOR TRANSPLANTS

Acute Leukemia.

Between September 1979 and June 1994, 174 patients with primary (or "de novo") acute leukemia or received an unrelated donor marrow transplant at our center (18,19). The diagnosis was acute myeloid leukemia (n= 74), acute lymphocytic leukemia (n= 91), or biphenotypic acute leukemia (n= 9)(14,15). Total body irradiation was used in the pretransplant conditioning regimen for 96% of cases, and GVHD prophylaxis consisted of methotrexate and cyclosporine in 85% of cases. Patient and donor were HLA-A, B and DRB1 identical in 64% of cases, mismatched for one locus in 34%, and 2 loci in 2%. The probability of grades II to IV acute GVHD was 87% and the probability of clinical extensive chronic GVHD was 64%. Kaplan-Meier probabilities of non-leukemic death, relapse and disease free survival (DFS) at 3 years are summarized in Table 3. Three variables were identified in a multivariable analysis as significant predictors of improved DFS: transplantation in complete remission as opposed to relapse or primary refractory leukemia, uncorrected marrow cell dose higher than the median of the series (3.65 x 10^8/kg), and CMV seropositive status of the patient before transplant. Marrow cell dose was the only significant factor when analysing the 66 patients transplanted in remission. A higher marrow cell dose was associated with a significant decrease in non-leukemic death and this effect was independent of age and obesity.

An analysis of patients transplanted in relapse revealed that the relative number of blasts in marrow was a significant predictor of DFS. Patients with < 30% blasts in the marrow and no blasts in the blood had 30% DFS at 5 years. Those with ≥ 30% blasts in the marrow and/or no blasts in the blood had 11% DFS. Patients with blasts in the blood had 0% DFS at 2 years. In patients with advanced and refractory

Table 3. Clinical Outcome of Unrelated Marrow Donor Transplants for Patients with Acute Leukemia[a]

Diagnosis and Stage of Disease	Number	Transplant Related Mortality	Relapse	Relapse Free Survival
CR1	11	32%	20%	55%
CR2	35	47%	41%	31%
$\geq$ CR3	20	60%	35%	26%
relapse 1	42	59%	74%	11%
refractory	14	29%	80%	14%

[a]data for transplant related mortality, relapse and event free survival are based on Kaplan-Meier statistics. "CR1" indicates first complete remission; "CR2" indicates second complete remission; "$\geq$CR3" indicates remission including third remission; and "refractory" indicates persistent primary or relapsed disease unresponsive to conventional chemotherapy.

[b]transplant related mortality (TRM) refers to death that is not associated with leukemia relapse.

disease, relapse and transplant related mortality were major causes of treatment failure. These findings emphasize the importance of comprehensive and early treatment planning for patients with acute leukemia in order to optimize the potential benefit of an unrelated donor transplant.

Chronic Myeloid Leukemia.

The anticipated 3 year survival rate for chronic myeloid leukemia (CML) patients transplanted in chronic phase from an HLA identical sibling is 80%. However, the initial studies of unrelated donor transplants for chronic phase CML reported 2 year disease-free survival rates of only 36% to 45% (16). We have analyzed the results of first unrelated donor transplants performed for 333 CML patients at our Center, 204 patients were in chronic phase, 79 in accelerated phase, 18 in second chronic phase and 32 in blast phase at the time of transplantation. The median age of the patients was 36.0 years (range, 5 to 55) and the median age of the donors was 38.5 (19.0 to 57.). The gender of the patients was 137 (41%) female and 198 (59%) male, and the gender of the donors was 104 (40%) female and 208 (60%) male. The median duration of disease prior to transplant was 21.4 months. Patients received non-T cell depleted marrow cells following cyclophosphamide and total body irradiation, and methotrexate and cyclosporine were given for GVHD prevention. A majority of the cases, 250 (75%), were identical with their donor for HLA-A,B,DRB1, 291 (9%) were incompatible for one HLA-A or B minor mismatch, 45 (14%) were incompatible for at least one HLA-DR minor mismatch, and 6 (2%) were incompatible for 2 loci (Table 6). The frequency of clinically severe grades III-IV acute GVHD was 37% for HLA identical transplants, 34% for an HLA-A or B minor mismatch, and 61% for any DRB1 mismatch (Table 4). The frequency of clinical extensive chronic GVHD was 63% for HLA identical transplants, 57% for an HLA-A or B minor mismatches, and 70% for any DRB1 mismatch. The probability of survival at 3 years was 55% for patients transplanted in chronic phase, 40% for accelerated phase, 32% for second chronic phase and 7% for blast phase. The frequency of relapse was 7% for chronic phase, 14% for accelerated phase, 17% for second chronic phase, and 56% for blast phase. A multivariable analysis of risk factors for event free survival in all patients identified as major hazards, transplantation in blast phase, patient age > 50 years, a disease duration of more than 3 years prior to transplantation and a female donor for a male patient. Mismatching for DRB1 alleles was a significant hazard for acute but not chronic GVHD. Howeve,r no effect of mismatching for DRB1 on relapse or event free survival was detected. Incompatibility for HLA-A or B minor mismatches had no measurable effect in this study. The use of a female donor was associated with a greater risk of acute GVHD, and the use of a parous female donor was associated with an increase in chronic GVHD. A higher marrow cell dose was associated with an increased risk of acute GVHD. Among patients in CP <50 years old transplanted from an HLA matched donor <1 year from diagnosis the probability of surviving 3 years was 75%, compared to 54% for patients <50 years transplanted from an HLA matched donor >3 years from diagnosis (p= .012) and 40% for patients <50 years transplanted from an HLA mismatched donor >3 years from diagnosis (p= .006). Results of these unrelated donor transplants are very good under optimal conditions when patients undergo transplantation in chronic phase within one year from diagnosis.

Table 4. HLA Matching Characteristics of Patients with Chronic Myeloid Leukemia Transplanted from an Unrelated Donor (n=333).

	Chronic Phase	Accelerated Phase	Second Chronic Phase	Blast Phase	Total
HLA-A, B, DRB1 identical	158	56	15	21	250 (75%)
HLA-A or B minor mismatch	20	8	0	2	30 (9%)
HLA-DRB1 mismatch[a]	22	12	3	8	45 (14%)
A or B minor mismatch, and DRB1 mismatch	4	1	0	1	6 (2%)

[a] matched for HLA-A, B and DR by serology, but allele mismatched for DRB1 alleles (ie, DR minor mismatch).

Table 5. Frequency of Acute and Chronic GVHD in CML Patients Transplanted from an Unrelated Donor

	HLA A, B, DRB1 identical (n=250)	A or B minor mismatch (n=30)	any DRB1 mismatch[b] (n=51)
Acute GVHD			
grade II-IV	80%	77%	94%
grade III-IV	37%	34%	61%
Chronic GVHD			
patient at risk[a]	196	21	33
none	27%	29%	15%
clinical extensive	63%	57%	70%

[a]patients alive and relapse free > 80 days.

[b]includes 6 cases also incompatible for an HLA-A or B minor mismatch.

Table 6. Relapse and Survival of Patients with Chronic Myeloid Leukemia Transplanted from an Unrelated Donor

	Chronic Phase (n=204)	Accelerated Phase (n=79)	Second Chronic Phase (n=18)	Blast Phase (n=32)
Frequency of Relapse	7%	14%	17%	56%
Survival[a]				
100 days	86%	85%	67%	69%
1 year	59%	54%	44%	28%
3 years	55%	40%	32%	7%

[a]Kaplan-Meier

Acknowledgments: This work was supported by grants AI33484, AI29518, CA18029 and HL36444 from the National Institutes of Health.

REFERENCES

1. Thomas ED: The Nobel Lectures in Immunology. The Nobel Prize for Physiology of Medicine, 1990. Bone marrow transplantation - past, present and future. Scand J Immunol 39:339-345, 1994.

2.	Good RA: Bone marrow transplantation: cellular engineering to correct primary immunodeficiency, are generative anemia and pancytopenia. Birth Defects 11:377-379, 1975

3.	Beatty PG, Clift RA, Mickelson EM, Nisperos BN, Flournoy N, Martin PJ, Sanders JE, Stewart P, Buckner CD, Storb R, Thomas ED, Hansen JA: Marrow transplantation from related donors other than HLA-identical siblings. N. Engl. J. Med. 313: 765-771, 1985.

4.	Anasetti C, Amos D, Beatty PG, Appelbaum FR, Bensinger W, Buckner CD, Clift R, Doney K, Martin PJ, Mickelson E, Nisperos BN, O'Quigley J, Ramberg R, Sanders JE, Stewart P, Storb R, Sullivan KM, Witherspoon RP, Thomas ED, Hansen JA: Effect of HLA compatibility on engraftment of bone marrow transplants in patients with leukemia or lymphoma. N. Engl. J. Med. 320: 197-204, 1989.

5.	Anasetti C, Beatty PG, Storb R, Martin PJ, Mori, M., Sanders JE, Thomas ED, Hansen JA: Effect of HLA incompatibility on graft-versus-host disease, relapse, and survival after marrow transplantation for patients with leukemia or lymphoma. Hum.Immunol. 29: 79-91, 1990.

6.	Anasetti C, Hansen J: Bone marrow transplantation from HLA-partially matched related donors and unrelated volunteer donors. In: Forman SJ, Blume KG, Thomas ED (eds) Bone Marrow Transplantation. Blackwell Scientific Publications, Cambridge, MA, pp. 665-679, 1993

7.	McCullough J, Hansen J, Perkins H, Stroncek D, Bartsch G: The National Marrow Donor Program: How it works, accomplishments to date. Oncology 3: 63-74, 1989.

8.	Stroncek D, Bartsch G, Perkins HA, Randall BL, Hansen JA, McCullough J: The National Marrow Donor Program. Transfusion 33:567-577, 1993.

9.	Stroncek, D.F., Holland, P.V., Bartch, G., Bixby, T., Simmons, R.G., Antin, J.H., Anderson, K.C., Ash, R.C., Bolwell, B.J., Hansen JA, Heal, J.M., Henslee-Downey, P.J., Jaffé, E.R., Klein, H.G., Lau, P.M., Perkins, H.A., Popovsky, M.A., Price, T.H., Rowley, S.D., Stehling, L.C., Weiden PL, Wissel, M.E., McCullough, J.: Experiences of the first 493 unrelated marrow donors in the National Marrow Donor Program. Blood 81: 1940-1946, 1993.

10.	Petersdorf EW, Smith AG, Mickelson EM, Martin PJ, Hansen JA: Ten HLA-DR4 alleles defined by sequence polymorphisms within the DRB1 first domain. Immunogenetics 33:267-275, 1991.

11.	Petersdorf EW, Longton GM, Anasetti C, Martin PJ, Mickelson EM, Smith AG, Hansen JA: The significance of HLA-DRB1 matching on clinical outcome after HLA-A, B, DR identical unrelated donor marrow transplantation. Blood 86:1606-1613, 1995.

12.	Petersdorf EW, Smith AG, Mickelson EM, Longton G, Anasetti C, Choo YC, Martin PJ, Hansen JA: The influence of HLA-DPB1 disparity on the development of acute graft-versus-host disease following unrelated donor marrow transplantation. Trans Proc 25:1230-1231, 1993.

13.	Mickelson EM, Longton G, Anasetti C, Petersdorf E, Martin PJ, Guthrie LA, Hansen JA: Evaluation of the mixed lymphocyte culture (MLC) assay as a method for selecting unrelated donors for marrow transplantation. (in press, Tissue Antigens 7/95).

14. Petersdorf EW, Setoda T, Smith AG, Hansen JA: Analysis of HLA-B*44 alleles encoded on extended HLA haplotypes by direct automated sequencing. Tissue Antigens 44:211-216, 1994.

15. Petersdorf EW, Stanley JF, Martin PJ, Hansen JA. Molecular diversity of the HLA-C locus in unrelated marrow transplantation. Tissue Antigens 1994; 44:93-9.

16. Petersdorf EW, Hansen JA. A comprehensive approach for typing the alleles of the HLA-B locus by automated sequencing. Tissue Antigens 1995; 46:73-85.

17. Petersdorf EW, Longton G, Anasetti C, Smith AG, McKinney S, Martin PJ, Hansen JA: Donor-recipient disparity for HLA-C genes is a risk factor for graft failure following marrow transplantation from unrelated donors. Blood 86:291a, 1995.

18. Balduzzi A, Gooley T, Anasetti C, Sanders JE, Martin PJ, Petersdorf EW, Appelbaum FR, Buckner CD, Matthews D, Storb R, Sullivan KM, Hansen JA: Unrelated donor marrow transplantation in children. Blood 86:3247-3256, 1995.

19. Sierra J, Storer B, Hansen J, Martin P, Petersdorf E, Appelbaum E, Buckner D, Sale G, Sanders J, Anasetti: Unrelated donor marrow transplants for acute leukemia. Blood 86:290a, 1995.

Transplantation with Purified or Unmanipulated Mobilized Blood Stem Cells in Children

Yoichi Takaue,[1] Yoshifumi Kawano,[1] Arata Watanabe,[2] Haruhiko Eguchi,[3] Takanori Abe,[1] Atsushi Makimoto,[1] Yasuhiro Okamoto,[1] and Yasuhiro Kuroda[1]

Department of Pediatrics, University of Tokushima, Kuramoto-cho, Tokushima 770[1]; University of Akita, Honmichi, Akita 010[2]; Kurume University, Asahimachi, Kurume 830, Japan[3]

SUMMARY

Experience of collection and transplant of peripheral blood stem cells (PBSC) was evaluated in children with active cancer. We found that the procedure is effective and safe. Preliminary therapeutic results of autografts with PBSC for children with acute leukemias or solid tumors are encouraging. A well-designed clinical protocol for PBSCT could provide an efficient and realistic stage for future evaluation of the potential of forthcoming cytokines in the field of cancer medicine. Moreover, an effective and relatively tumor-free form of hematopoietic support for cancer patients undergoing myeloablative chemotherapy ("indirect purging") may be possible through the use of purified CD34+ cells. We predict that its role outside of cancer therapy will continue to evolve.

KEY WORDS: blood stem cells, CD34+ cells, G-CSF, transplantation, children

INTRODUCTION

PBSC can be easily collected in children without the risk involved in anesthesia and invasive multiple marrow aspirations [1-3]. The use of G-CSF-mobilized PBSC offers the opportunity for more intensive treatment regimens for high-risk cancer, with an improved safety margin for malignant disorders for which a sharp dose-response relationship exists with chemotherapy [4,5]. The first patient to undergo peripheral blood hematopoietic stem cell transplant (PBSCT) in Japan was treated at the University Hospital of Tokushima in 1987. Since then, the field has expanded rapidly and in December 1993 we founded the world's largest cooperative trial group that solely treats children with PBSCT [6]. As of June 1995, a total of 207 children have been registered. Our preliminary data in children with relapsed acute lymphoblastic leukemia (ALL) or advanced neuroblastoma suggest that the application of PBSCT results in an increase in the salvage rate of patients, while avoiding the toxicities of high-dose therapy [7,8].

The next step in our study protocol is to consider PBSCT for a larger number of patients. The primary goal of PBSCT for children who are still within their first CR is improvement of the therapeutic ratio by decreasing the toxicities associated with intense use of toxic anticancer drugs, without jeopardizing ultimate cure rates. A prospective study is currently ongoing to address this. Selection criteria for performing PBSCT in ALL include an initial leukocyte count of greater than 100×10^9/L, the presence of leukemic cells with a bulk phenotype, infants, and CALLA(-)-ALL. Those for NHL include T-cell disease with extensive tumor invasion into vital organs and cases with involvement of the bone marrow or central nervous system at presentation.

MOBILIZATION OF PBSC IN CHILDREN

Identification of the optimal cytokines and a protocol for use in the PBSC collection procedure, with which the fewest number of apheresis procedures are required, has emerged as the major subject of future intense research in hemato-oncology. In children, a rapid increase in the blood cell count in the recovery phase of chemotherapy predicts a high cell yield by apheresis, and the optimal timing for harvesting PBSC can be determined by carefully monitoring the recovery speed of hematopoiesis alone. However, when the mobilization of PBSC by chemotherapy is coupled with the application of G-CSF, the leukocyte count alone can not be a reliable indicator for the optimal timing of PBSC harvest. Simultaneous consideration of the platelet recovery pattern or, ideally, real-time examination of CD34+ cells will be feasible. Since the cell yield decreases rapidly as collection is repeated [1], only one or two aphereses per chemotherapeutic course appears to be practical in children.

In the newly treated children with ALL, we found that the increase in progenitor yields and the enhancement of engraftment speed by G-CSF, which were clearly documented in a heavily pretreated patient population [4], were not observed [5]. We then performed a dosing study with G-CSF, which was applied after 2 to 3 courses of consolidation therapy for neuroblastoma, and which included carboplatinum, VP-16 and doxorubicin. Patients received a variable dose (50, 100, 150, 200 $mg/m^2/day$) of G-CSF. PBSC were collected by apheresis and cell yields were compared. We found a substantial interpatient variation in the yield of PBSC with each dose of G-CSF; indicating that this type of chemotherapy regimen is toxic to stem cells compared to that used for the treatment of ALL, which incorporates doxorubicin, VP-16 and cytosine arabinoside. Moreover, the interpatient variation in cell yield could not be predicted. This observation suggests a new strategy for evaluating the mobilization effect of cytokines in patients with solid tumors; i.e., initial use before the start of chemotherapy, rather than traditional use after chemotherapy. Our laboratory results suggested that cells mobilized by G-CSF alone may be more suitable for use in clinical transplants than those mobilized by the combination of chemotherapy and G-CSF. The potential risk of cancer cell contamination in this strategy can be prevented by the positive isolation of CD34+ cells ("indirect purging"). Our study indicates that, in terms of preserving engraftment potential, a simplified cryopreservation method incorporating 6% hydroxyethyl starch and 5% DMSO without a programmed freezer (PF) is at least as effective as the traditional controlled-rate freezing procedure with PF [9].

POST PBSCT G-CSF THERAPY

The current strategy for enhancing hematopoietic engraftment after BMT is the use of recombinant cytokines. There is a possibility that additional use of G-CSF may further enhance the already fast recovery rate of hematopoiesis after PBSCT. However, in our retrospective study we found that administered G-CSF did not enhance the recovery speed of granulocytes after PBSCT [10]. This appears to be confirmed by the preliminary result of subsequent prospective randomized trial, in which the number of days required to achieve an AGC of $0.5 \times 10^9/L$ and a platelet count of $50 \times 10^9/L$ were, respectively, 11.4 ± 4.3 (mean $\pm$ SD), and 19.1 ± 5.9 days in the G-CSF-treated population (n=9), while these were 11.7 ± 2.2 and 20.2 ± 10.7 days in the control group without G-CSF (n=10).

EXPANSION OF STEM CELL THERAPY STRATEGY

Since the use of G-CSF-mobilized PBSC eliminates the need for anesthesia and secures engraftment through the infusion of an overwhelming amount of stem cells, the development of an effective procedure for allogeneic transplant with PBSC to expand the stem cell donor pool and of a clinical application of a high-dose strategy is underway. PBSC collected by apheresis needs to be processed to reduce the volume of cells to be cryopreserved, thereby decreasing the toxicity at graft infusion [11], and to decrease the number of contaminated T-cells in mismatched transplant settings. A carefully constructed isolation procedure for CD34+ cells may reduce the number of T lymphocytes below the critical threshold for developing severe GVHD [12]. Separated lymphocytes can be cryopreserved and used later in the transplant course to induce a graft-versus-leukemia reaction and to prevent posttransplant lymphoproliferative disorders.

The therapeutic potential of autografts has been limited due to the lack of graft-versus-leukemia activity and possible contamination of tumor cells in the graft. An effective depletion of cancer cells or T lymphocytes may be possible through the use of purified CD34+ cells. To make the procedure clinically effective, the purity of CD34+ cells needs to be high to ensure effective depletion of tumor cells.   Studies currently in progress at the University of Tokushima employ the Isolex system (Baxter) for selection of CD34+ cells from mobilized blood for auto- and allogeneic transplantation in pediatric patients following high dose chemotherapy.   In our procedure with the use of the Baxter Isolex 50 system, cell recovery rates after purification for mononuclear cells, CFU-GM and CD34+ cells were, respectively, 1.5%, 52%, and 32%.   To overcome this low yield, the new procedure provided by the company has been tested.   In the historical engraftment data of 31 pediatric patients who underwent autografts in our institute with unfractionated blood cells containing >3 x 10^5 CFU-GM/kg, the numbers of days to achieve an absolute granulocyte count (AGC) of >0.5 x 10^9/L and platelet count of >50 x 10^9/L were, respectively, 10 and 16 days. In 5 children who were transplanted with autologous purified CD34+ cells, these values were 9 to 13 days for an AGC and15 to 22 for platelets; thus, engraftment speed appears to be comparable (Fig. 1).

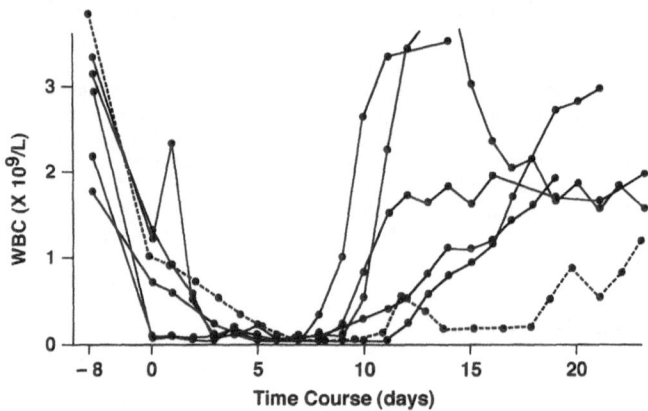

Time Course (days)

Fig. 1 Engraftment kinetics after transplantation with purified blood CD34$^+$ cells (*solid line*) and whole cord blood cells (*dashed line*).

An additional advantage of PBSC is that multiple collection procedures can be performed without invasive surgery; which may be an important consideration in gene therapy, since the target patients could be very small children.   Stem cell therapy could be extended to solid organ transplant to induce microchimerism and resultant allograft acceptance.

REFERENCES

1. Takaue Y, Watanabe T, Abe T, Hirao A, Okamoto Y, Saito S, Shimizu T, Sato J, Suzue T, Koyama T, Kawano Y, Ninomiya T, Shimokawa T, Yokobayashi A, Kuroda Y (1992) Experience with peripheral blood stem cell collection for autografts in children with active cancer.   Bone Marrow Transplant 10:241-248.

2. Takaue Y (1993) Collection of peripheral blood stem cells for autografts in children with cancer. In: Henon P, Wunder E (eds) Peripheral Blood Stem Cell Autografts. Springer-Verlag, Berlin, pp194-198.

3. Takaue Y, Kawano Y, Abe T, Okamoto Y, Suzue T, Saito S, Sato J, Watanabe T, Ito M, Kuroda Y (1995) Collection and transplant of peripheral blood stem cells in very small children weighing 20 kg or less.   Blood 86:372-380.

4. Kawano Y, Takaue Y, Watanabe T, Saito S, Hirao A, Abe T, Sato J, Ninomiya T, Shimokawa T, Yokobayashi A, Asano S, Masaoka T, Takaku F, Kuroda Y (1993) Effects of progenitor cell dose and preleukapheresis use of human recombinant granulocyte colony-stimulating factor on the recovery of hematopoiesis after blood stem cell autografting in children. Exp Hematol 21:103-108.

5. Takaue Y, Kawano Y, Kuroda Y (1995) Mobilization of peripheral blood stem cells for autografts. In: Levit DJ, Mertelsmann R (eds) Hematopoietic Stem Cells: Biology and Therapeutic Applications. Marcel Dekker, New York, pp611-630.

6. Takaue Y (1993) Peripheral blood stem cell autografts for the treatment of childhood cancer: A review of Japanese experience. J Hematother 2:513-518.

7. Takaue Y, Watanabe A, Watanabe T, Okamoto Y, Saito S, Abe T, Suzue T, Shimizu T, Sato J, Kawano Y, Kuroda Y, Murakami T, Eguchi H, Matsushita T, Kikuta A, Shimokawa T, Iwai A, Kosaka Y, Murakami R, Mimaya J, Shimizu H, Koizumi S, Fujimoto T (1994) High-dose chemotherapy and blood stem cell autografts for children with first relapsed acute lymphoblastic leukemia: A report from the Children's Cancer and Leukemia Study Group of Japan (CCLSG). Med Pediatr Oncol 23:20-25.

8. Eguchi H, Takaue Y (1994) Peripheral blood stem cell autografts in the treatment of pediatric solid tumors. In: Dicke KA, Keating A (eds) Autologous Marrow and Blood Transplantation. The Cancer Treatment Research and Educational Institute, Arlington, pp597-606.

9. Takaue Y, Abe T, Kawano Y, Suzue T, Saito S, Hirao A, Sato J, Makimoto A, Kawahito M, Watanabe T, Shimokawa T, Kuroda Y (1994) et al: Comparative analysis of engraftment after peripheral blood stem cell autografts cryopreserved by controlled vs uncontrolled-rate method. Bone Marrow Transplant 13:801-804.

10. Suzue T, Takaue Y, Watanabe A, Kawano Y, Watanabe T, Abe T, Kuroda Y, Matsushita T, Kikuta A, Iwai A, Shimokawa T, Eguchi H, Murakami T, Kosaka Y, Kudo T, Shimizu H, Koizumi S, Fujimoto T (1994) Effects of recombinant human granulocyte colony-stimulating factor (filgrastim) on the recovery of hematopoiesis after high-dose chemotherapy and autologous peripheral blood stem cell transplantation in children: a report from the Children's Cancer and Leukemia Study Group of Japan (CCLSG). Exp Hematol 22:1197-1202.

11. Okamoto Y, Takaue Y, Saito S, Hirao A, Shimizu T, Suzue T, Abe T, Sato J, Watanabe T, Kawano Y, Kuroda Y (1993) Toxicities associated with infusion of cryopreserved and thawed peripheral blood stem cell autografts in children with active cancer. Transfusion 33:578-581.

12. Suzue T, Kawano Y, Takaue Y, Kuroda Y (1994) Cell processing protocol for allogeneic peripheral blood stem cells mobilized by granulocyte colony-stimulating factor. Exp Hematol. 22:888-892.

Transplantation of Ex-Vivo Expanded Peripheral Blood Progenitor Cells After High Dose Chemotherapy in Cancer Patients

Stefan Scheding, Wolfram Brugger, and Lothar Kanz[1]

[1] Eberhardt-Karls-Universität Tübingen, Medical Clinic II, Department of Hematology, Oncology, Immunology and Rheumatology, Tübingen, Germany

SUMMARY

To minimize tumor cell contamination of peripheral blood progenitor cell (PBPC) collections, we have reduced the total volume of blood processed from the patients, followed by expansion of PBPC *ex-vivo*. We have shown that a combination of SCF, IL-1ß, IL-6, IL-3 and EPO mediated the *ex-vivo* expansion of clonogenic progenitor cells of various hematopoietic lineages and, moreover, that primitive hematopoietic stem cells, as quantitated by long-term culture initiating cells (LTC-IC), could be preserved. These preclinical studies suggested that *ex-vivo* expanded peripheral blood CD34+ cells might be able to mediate both short-term and long-term hematopoietic reconstitution following high-dose chemotherapy. In a phase I/II trial, we investigated the transplantation potential of *ex-vivo* expanded CD34+ PBPC in solid tumor patients undergoing non-myeloablative high-dose chemotherapy. Ten patients were transplanted with *ex-vivo* expanded PBPC, starting from a fixed number of 1.1×10^7 positively selected peripheral blood CD34+ cells, a cell number which corresponded to less than 1/10th of the CD34+ cells present within standard 2-hour leukapheresis preparation. The study showed that this approach is feasible and that *ex-vivo* expanded cells mediated rapid and sustained hematopoietic recovery when transplanted after high-dose VIC-E chemotherapy. The reconstitution pattern was identical to that of historical control patients who had been treated with unseparated PBPC or positively selected peripheral blood CD34+ cells. Thus, starting from a small number of peripheral blood CD34+ cells, *ex-vivo* expanded hematopoietic progenitor cells might offer new prospects for cellular therapy, including a reduced risk for tumor cell contamination, the circumvention of leukapheresis, the potential for *ex-vivo* manipulation, as well as the potential for repetitive cycles of high-dose therapy

KEYWORDS:

peripheral blood progenitor cells (PBPC), high-dose chemotherapy, autologous PBPC transplantation, ex-vivo expansion, CD34, PBPC purification

INTRODUCTION

High-dose chemotherapy (HD-CT) is potentially curative in some chemosensitive tumors and the relative dose intensity received is probably a major factor determining the outcome of chemotherapy [1]. Administration of HD-CT, however, is often limited by an unavoidable therapy-induced hematotoxicity. Here, the development of peripheral blood progenitor cell (PBPC) transplantation, which is being used increasingly for autologous stem cell transplantation after high-dose chemotherapy [2], has been shown to be a successful approach. PBPC transplantation assures complete and sustained engraftment after HD-CT in case of several disorders, such as acute leukemia (ALL and AML), lymphoma, neuroblastoma, breast cancer and other solid tumors [2 - 10]. One major concern with regard to the use of PBPC for autologous transplantation, however, is a possible graft contamination with tumor cells. Recent genetic marking studies clearly demonstrated that contaminating tumor cells in the graft contributed to disease recurrence after transplantation [11, 12]. And although PBPC preparations contain fewer contaminating tumor cells than bone marrow, circulating tumor cells have been detected in patients with disseminated neuroblastoma, lymphoma, as well as stage IV breast cancer [13, 14]. Furthermore, as demonstrated by our group, chemotherapy plus G-CSF-induced mobilization of PBPC carried a substantial risk of co-mobilizing tumor cells particularly in case of stage IV breast cancer patients [15]. Therefore, the development of effective purging strategies for PBPC preparations become imperative. This report briefly summarizes our three step approach to PBPC purging consisting of 1) PBPC recruitment linked to an effective anti-cancer treatment (in-vivo purging), 2) CD34$^+$ selection and 3) subsequent *ex-vivo* expansion (*ex-vivo* purging).

RECRUITMENT AND TRANSPLANTATION OF UNSEPARATED AND CD34$^+$-SELECTED PBPC

Three different methods are currently applied to recruit PBPC for transplantation: 1) mobilization of PBPC into the circulation is induced during the hematopoietic recovery following standard-dose chemotherapy [16 - 19]; 2) hematopoietic growth factors such as granulocyte colony stimulating factor (G-CSF) and granulocyte/macrophage (GM)-CSF lead to a recruitment of early hematopoietic cells into circulation [20 - 23]; and 3) the combination of both, growth factor application and chemotherapy considerably increases progenitor cell mobilization [9, 20, 24 -27].
Our current approach to PBPC-supported high-dose chemotherapy is to administer conventionally-dosed VIP (VP16 500 mg/m^2, ifosfamide 4,000 mg/m^2, cisplatin 50 mg/m^2) chemotherapy plus G-CSF (5μg/kg) early in the course of disease, thereby combining the harvest of transplantable PBPC with an effective anti-cancer treatment. We were able to show that the combination of standard dose VIP chemotherapy with G-CSF resulted in mobilization of sufficient numbers of PBPC for transplantation including high numbers of primitive hematopoietic cells as indicated by LTC-IC (long-term culture initiating cell) measurements [9, 27 - 30]. PBPC collection early in the course of disease is justified by the fact that the

number and quality of harvestable PBPC depends on the pretreatment status with heavily pretreated patients mobilizing only very low numbers of CD34+ cells whereas high numbers of PBPC can be harvested in case of untreated patients [27]. The quality of such VIP plus G-CSF mobilized PBPC with regard to transplantation potential is best demonstrated by our data on more than 300 patients that have received autologous transplants following various high-dose chemotherapy regimens with every one of them showing rapid and sustained engraftment and an overall treatment-related mortality of less than 2 percent.

We recently showed that tumor cells might be co-mobilized by PBPC mobilization [15] leading to a possible tumor cell contamination of PBPC transplants. Analysis of peripheral blood samples from 48 patients with advanced malignancies such as small cell lung cancer (SCLC) and non-small cell lung cancer (NSCLC), stage IV or high-risk stage II/III breast cancer showed that VIP chemotherapy followed by G-CSF increased the number of circulating tumor cells in patients that had detectable levels of contaminating tumor cells to start with as well as recruiting tumor cells in 21% of the patients with no detectable levels of circulating tumor cells prior to therapy. Clearance of circulating tumor cells was observed after one or two additional cycles of standard-dose VIP indicating an effective chemotherapy-induced in-vivo purging [15]. Based on these results we would recommend an effective cytoreductive treatment prior to PBPC harvest in order to minimize the tumor cell load.

However, transplantation of unseparated PBPC still carries the possible risk of retransplanting tumor cells. Therefore, we would prefer to further *ex-vivo* manipulate PBPC preparations to ensure an effective depletion of contaminating tumor cells. Positive CD34+ selection by immunaffinity columns, the second step of our PBPC purging approach, results in an about 2 -3 log depletion of tumor cells [31]. Recently, this approach was also tested in a phase I/II trial at our institution in patients with advanced malignancies [10]. CD34+ cells were positively selected using biotinylated anti-CD34 monoclonal antibody and the CellPro avidin-biotin immunoadsorption column device. 15 patients received a median of 2.5×10^6 positively separated CD34+ cells following high dose VIC-E (VP16 1,500 mg/m^2, ifosfamide 12 g/m^2, carboplatin 750 mg/m^2, epirubicin 150 mg/m^2) without additional unseparated PBPC or bone marrow cells. Transplantation of CD34+ cells alone resulted in identical hematological recovery patterns when compared to patients receiving unseparated PBPC transplants, thereby clearly demonstrating the feasibility of this approach.

EX-VIVO EXPANSION OF PBPC: PRECLINICAL STUDIES

The demonstration of a non-impeded functional integrity of CD34+-selected hematopoietic progenitor cells allowed us to study whether or not these cells might be expandable *ex-vivo* for possible clinical application. Successful *ex-vivo* expansion of PBPC would considerably reduce the patients' blood volume that has to be processed for transplantation, thereby further decreasing the possibility of harvesting contaminating tumor cells. Furthermore, if a differential expansion of normal PBPC versus tumor cells providing a growth advantage for normal PBPC could be achieved, this would lead to an even greater reduction of tumor cells in the graft. If clinically successful, *ex-vivo* expansion might also be used to provide sufficient numbers of PBPC for repetitive use after high-dose chemotherapy or in case of patients for whom PBPC yield is too low for transplantation even with multiple leucaphereses.

In a series of preclinical experiments, we systematically studied the requirements of hematopoietic growth factor combinations to expand PBPC in liquid culture *ex-vivo* [32] and then went on to address the question as to whether or not such a system would result in an expansion of contaminating tumor cells [33]. Positively selected CD34$^+$ cells of 18 patients mobilized by VIP chemotherapy plus G-CSF were cultured in suspension for up to 28 days. Thirty six growth factor combinations were tested for their ability to amplify hematopoietic progenitor cells. Among the combinations tested, a five-factor cocktail (S163E), containing stem cell factor (SCF), interleukin-1ß (IL-1ß), IL-**6**, Il-**3**, and erythropoietin (EPO) was found to optimally stimulate progenitor expansion. Using this growth factor combination, CFU-GM and BFU-E increased about 190-fold (range 46-930). Multipotential progenitors (CFU-GEMM) expanded 250-fold when compared to pre-expansion values and CD34$^+$/Lin$^-$ as well as mafosfamide-resistant cells also increased considerably during *ex-vivo* culture. Furthermore LTC-IC numbers were maintained during cytokine-mediated *ex-vivo* expansion [30], thus indicating that transplantation of *ex-vivo* generated cells might also provide long-term repopulating capability. Large scale expansion of CD34$^+$ cells in medium supplemented with autologous plasma and the S163E cytokine cocktail, which was performed in view of a possible clinical application, showed comparable expansion results indicating that expansion of CD34$^+$ PBPC from cancer patients *ex-vivo* for autotransplant is technically possible. To address the question whether or not contaminating tumor cells would be expanded in S163E-supported culture, we performed co-culturing experiments using primary human epithelial tumor cells (RS-85, renal cell carcinoma) as well as tumor cells from human xenografts (MCF7 breast cancer and LXFS small cell lung cancer) [33]. In serum-containing as well as serum-free S163E liquid culture, tumor cells were found not to be expanded, thus indicating a proliferative advantage of hematopoietic progenitor cells in this system. Additional trans-well experiments revealed that the growth inhibition of tumor cells was mediated by cell-to-cell interactions of tumor cells with CD34$^+$ hematopoietic cells.

EX-VIVO EXPANSION OF PBPC: CLINICAL STUDIES

The question as to whether or not such *ex-vivo* expanded cells would successfully mediate hematopoietic recovery after high-dose chemotherapy was recently addressed in a phase I clinical trial [34, 35]. Ten patients with advanced cancer received two cycles of G-CSF-supported VIP chemotherapy with PBPC being collected by leukapheresis after the second cycle. CD34$^+$ selection, which was performed using the CellPro Ceprate SC device, resulted in a 72.1 ± 9.3 percent purity with a 64 percent yield. For each patient, a total number of 1.5 x 10^7 cells corresponding to a total median of 1.1 x 10^7 CD34$^+$ cells were expanded *ex-vivo* in RPMI 1640 medium with 2 percent autologous plasma for 12 days. Analysis of *ex-vivo* expanded cells showed a median increase in cell numbers of 62.4-fold with colony-forming cells being expanded by a median of 50-fold, thus providing a median 1.23 x 10^5/kg transplantable progenitor cells. Flow cytometric analysis of the *ex-vivo* generated cells revealed that the majority of cells expressed HLA-DR and CD33 whereas less than 0.5% remained positive for CD34. During *ex-vivo* expansion, the cultured cells produced high amounts of macrophage-CSF and IL-8, whereas only low amounts of TNF-a, G-CSF, and GM-CSF were detectable. After washing in 0.9% saline before transplantation, cytokine levels for all growth factors tested dropped to undetectable levels. The transplantation potential of such *ex-vivo* expanded cells was tested after high-dose VIC-E (VP16 1500 mg/m^2, ifosfamide 12,000 mg/m^2, carboplatin 750 mg/m^2, and epirubicin 150 mg/m^2) chemotherapy. Four patients received non-expanded CD34$^+$ cells in addition to *ex-vivo* expanded cells in order to ensure hematopoietic engraftment while testing for possible toxic side effects caused by the administration of *ex-vivo* expanded cells. Six patients received *ex-vivo* expanded cells only. One patient developed neutropenic sepsis 6 days after transplantation and died on day 14 due to multi-organ failure. Every one of the nine remaining patients showed fast hematopoietic engraftment comparable to historical control patients receiving either unseparated or CD34$^+$-selected PBPC after HD-VIC-E. There were no allergic, pulmonary, or renal side effects associated with the transplantation of up to 1.6 billion cultured cells. This study demonstrated for the first time, that *ex-vivo* expanded cells can be successfully used for autografting after HD-CT. Thus, starting from a small number of peripheral blood CD34$^+$ cells *ex-vivo* expansion enables a considerable reduction of the patients' blood volume that has to be processed for transplantation. By using this *ex-vivo* expansion approach, 100 to 200 ml of blood at the time of maximum progenitor cell mobilization would yield sufficient CD34$^+$ cell numbers for transplantation, thereby minimizing the risk of a possible tumor cell contamination that is furthermore reduced by subsequent CD34$^+$ selection and the differential expansion kinetics in liquid culture.

Taken together, our studies demonstrated the feasibility of an effective three step purging approach consisting of in-vivo purging by VIP-(E) chemotherapy with subsequent PBPC harvest, CD34$^+$ selection and *ex-vivo* expansion. This multi-step procedure leads to an estimated total 6-log reduction of tumor cells in the final graft and thus might be suitable to provide a practically tumor cell-free transplant, thereby minimizing the patients' risk for a transplant-mediated relapse.

REFERENCES

1   deVita VT, Hellman S, Rosenberg SA (1990) In: Cancer: Principles and practice of oncology. 3rd edition. Lippincott, Philadelphia, pp 286-287
2   Kessinger A, Armitage JO (1991) The evolving role of autologous peripheral stem cell transplantation following high dose chemotherapy for malignancies. Blood 77:211-213
3   Stiff PJ, Koester AR, Eagleton LE, Hindman T, Braud E, Weidner, MK

(1987) Autologous stem cell transplantation using peripheral blood stem cells. Transplantation 44:585-588

4   Juttner CA, To LB, Ho JQ, Bardy PG, Dyson DN, Kimber RJ (1988) Early lympho-hematopoietic recovery after autografting using peripheral blood stem cells in acute non-lymphoblastic leukemia. Transplant Proc 20:40-42

5   Körbling M, Holle R, Haas R, Knauf W, Dörken B, Ho AD, Kuse R, Pralle H, Fliedner TM, Hunstein W (1990) Autologous blood stem-cell transplantation in patients with advanced Hodgkin s disease and prior radiation to the pelvic site. J Clin Oncol 8:978-985

6   Körbling M, Dorken B, Ho AD, Pezzutto A, Hunstein W, Fliedner TM (1986) Autologous transplantation of blood-derived hematopoietic stem cells after myeloablative therapy in a patient with Burkitt's lymphoma. Blood 67:529-532

7   Kessinger A, Armitage JO, Smith DM, Landmark JD, Bierman PJ, Weisenburger DD (1989) High-dose therapy and autologous peripheral blood stem cell transplantation for patients with lymphoma. Blood 74:1260-1266

8   Sheridan WP, Begley CG, Juttner C, Szer J, To LB, Maher D, McGrath KM, Morstyn G, Fox RM (1992) Effect of peripheral-blood progenitor cells mobilized by filgrastim (G-CSF) on platelet recovery after high-dose chemotherapy. Lancet 339:640-644

9   Brugger W, Birken R, Bertz H, Hecht T, Pressler K, Frisch J, Schulz G, Mertelsmann R, and Kanz L (1993) Peripheral blood progenitor cells mobilized by chemotherapy plus G-CSF accelerate both neutrophil and platelet recovery after high-dose VP16, ifosfamide, and cisplatin. Br J Haematol 84:402-407

10   Brugger W, Henschler R, Heimfeld S, Berenson RJ, Mertelsmann R, Kanz L (1994) Positively selected autologous blood CD34+ cells and unseparated peripheral blood progenitor cells mediate identical hematopoietic engraftment after high-dose VP16, ifosfamide, carboplatin, and epirubicin. Blood 84: 1421-1426

11   Brenner MK, Rill DR, Moen RC, Krance RA, Mirro J, Anderson WF, Ihle JN (1993) Gene-marking to trace origin of relapse after autologous bone-marrow transplantation. Lancet 341:85-86

12   Deisseroth AB, Zu Z, Claxton D, Hanania EG, Fu S, Ellerson D, Goldberg L, Thomas M, Janicek K, Anderson WF et al. (1994) Genetic marking shows that Ph+ cells present in autologous transplants of chronic myelogeneous leukemia (CML) contribute to relapse after autologous bone marrow in CML. Blood 83:3068-3076

13   Shpall EJ and Jones RB (1994) Release of tumor cells from bone marrow. Blood 83:623-625

14   Ross AA, Cooper BW, Lazarus HM, Mackay W, Moss TJ, Ciobanu N, Tallman MS, Kennedy MJ, Davidson NE, Sweet D, et al. (1993) Detection and viability of tumor cells in peripheral blood stem cell collections from breast cancer patients using immunocytochemical and clonogenic assay techniques. Blood 82:2605-2610

15   Brugger W, Bross KJ, Glatt M, Weber F, Mertelsmann R, Kanz L (1994) Mobilization of tumor cells and hematopoietic progenitor cells into

peripheral blood of patients with solid tumors. Blood 83:636-640

16   Richmann CM, Weiner RS, Yankee RA (1976) Increase in circulating stem cells following chemotherapy in man. Blood 47:1031-1039

17   Abrams RA, McCormack K, Bowles C, Deisseroth AB (1981) Cyclophosphamide treatment expands the circulating haemopoietic stem cell pool in dogs. J Clin Invest 67:1392-1399

18   To LB, Shepperd KM, Haylock DN, Dyson PG, Charles P, Thorp L, Dale BM, Dart GW. Roberts MM, Sage RE (1989). Single high doses of cyclophosphamide enable the collection of high numbers of hemopoietic stem cells from the peripheral blood. Exp Hematol 18:442-447

19   Lohrmann HP, Schreml W, Fliedner TM, Heimpel H (1979) Reaction of human granulocytopoiesis to high-dose cyclophosphamide therapy. Blut 38:9-16

20   Socinski MA, Cannistra SA, Elias A, Antman KH, Schnipper L, Griffin JD (1988) GM-CSF expands the circulating haemopoietic progenitor cell compartment in man. Lancet i:1194-1198

21   Haas R, Ho AD, Bredthauer U, Cayeux S, Egerer G, Knauf W, Hunstein W (1990) Successful autologous transplantation of blood stem cells mobilized with rhGM-CSF. Exp Hematol 18:94-98

22   Villeval JL, Dührsen U, Morstyn G, Metcalf D. Effect of recombinant human GM-CSF on progenitor cells in patients with advanced malignancies (1990) Br J Hematol 74:10-44

23   Dührsen U, Villeval JL, Boyd J, Kannourakis G, Morstyn G, Metcalf D (1988) Effects of recombinant human G-CSF on hematopoietic progenitor cells in cancer patients. Blood 72:2074-2081

24   Elias AD, Ayash L, Anderson KC, Hund M, Wheller C, Schwartz G, Telpler I, Mazanet R, Lynch C, Pap S, Pelaez J, Reich E, Critchlow J, Demetri G, Bibbo J, Schnipper L, Griffin JD, Frei E, Antman KH (1992) Mobilization of peripheral blood progenitor cells by chemotherapy and granulocyte-macrophage colony-stimulating factor for hematologic support after high-dose intensification in breast cancer. Blood 79:3010-3042

25   Pettengell R, Demuynck H, Testa NG, Dexter TM (1992) The engraftment capacity of peripheral blood progenitor cells mobilized with chemotherapy ± G-CSF. Int J Cell Cloning 10:59-61

26   Gianni AM, Siena S, Bregni M, Tarella C, Stern AC, Pileri A, Bonadonna G (1989) Granulocyte-macrophage colony-stimulating factor to harvest circulating haemopoietic stem cells for autotransplantation. Lancet ii:580-585

27   Brugger W, Bross KJ, Frisch J, Dern P, Weber B, Mertelsmann R, Kanz L (1992) Mobilization of peripheral blood progenitor cells by sequential administration of IL-3 and GM-CSF following chemotherapy with etoposide, ifosfamide, and cisplatin. Blood 79:1193-1200

28   Kanz L, Brugger W, Bross KJ, Mertelsmann R (1992) Correlation analyses between CD34+ cells and clonogenic progenitors mobilized into the peripheral blood by IL-3 + GM-CSF following polychemotherapy in cancer patients. Int J Cell Cloning 10:68-70

29   Brugger W, Frisch J, Schulz G, Pressler K, Mertelsmann R, Kanz L (1992) Sequential administration of IL-3 and GM-CSF following standard-dose

combination chemotherapy with etoposide, ifosfamide and cisplatin. J Clin Oncol 10:1452-1459

30   Henschler R, Brugger W, Luft T, Frey T, Mertelsmann R, Kanz L (1994) Maintenance of transplantation potential in ex-vivo expanded CD34+-selected human peripheral blood progenitor cells. Blood 84:2898-2903

31   Shpall EJ, Jones RB, Bearman SI, et al. (1994) Transplantation of enriched CD34-positive autologous marrow into breast cancer patients following high-dose chemotherapy: influence of CD34-positive peripheral-blood progenitors and growth factors on engraftment. J Clin Oncol 12:28-36

32   Brugger W, Möcklin W, Heimfeld S, Berenson RJ, Mertelsmann R, Kanz L (1993) Ex vivo expansion of enriched peripheral blood CD34+ progenitor cells by stem cell factor, interleukin-1ß, interleukin-6, interleukin-3, interferon-gamma, and erythropoietin. Blood 81:2579-2584

33   Brugger W, Vogel W, Scheding S, Bock T, Ziegler B, Kanz L (1995) Epithelial tumor cells are not expanded concomitantly during cytokine-mediated ex vivo expansion of peripheral blood CD34+ progenitor cells. Blood 86:295a

34   Brugger W, Scheding S, Heimfeld S, Berenson RJ, Färber L, Mertelsmann R, Kanz L (1994). Ex-vivo expanded blood CD34+ cells mediate hematopoietic recovery in patients after high-dose VP16, ifosfamide, carboplatin, and epirubicin. Blood 84:395a

35   Brugger W, Heimfeld S, Berenson RJ, Mertelsmann R, Kanz L. Reconstitution of hematopoiesis after high-dose chemotherapy by autologous progenitor cells generated ex vivo. N Engl J Med 1995, 333:283-287

Graft Versus Host Disease (GVHD) and Cryoimmunology

Shengheng Wang and Tianwen Tao
General Hospital of Navy, Beijing,100037, China

Summary

GVHD is a major, sometimes lethal, complication of bone marrow transplantation (BMT). Its development is closely related to the activities of the T lymphocytes of the donor. Many methods have been developed for its prevention and treatment, though none is wholly satisfactory. Ultra-low temperatures influence the activities of the lymphocytes. It has been reported that the development of GVHD could be inhibited if the donor's cells were pretreated at ultra-low temperatures. The correlationship between GVHD in the mouse and cryoimmunological phenomena was studied in our laboratory.

Key words: GVHD, cryoimmunology, BMT

Materials and Method

1. The in vitro pre- and post-cryopreserved (PRC and POC) yields of interleukin 2 (IL-2) and tumor necrosis factor (TNF-α) of mouse spleen cells were determined using an MTT assay.
2. The expression of CD4 and CD8 mouse spleen cells before (PRC) and after (POC) cryopreservation were estimated with specific monoclonal antibodies and flow-cytometry.
3. A GVHD model was made using the BALB/C mouse (female, recipient) and C57 B/L mouse (female, donor). BMT was performed with uncryopreserved (PRC) and cryopreserved (POC) cells of the bone marrow and spleen. The yields of IL-2, TNF-α and the expression of CD4 and CD8 spleen cells in the GVHD mouse were examined also at 1, 2 or 4 weeks post-transplant.
4. Cryopreservation of cells was performed in the liquid phase of liquid nitrogen (-196°C) for 1 to 4 weeks after a conventional two-step cooling procedure with 10% DMSO in an automatic rate-control freezer.

Results

1. Yields of IL-2 and TNF-α of mouse spleen cell (Table 1)

Tab.1   YIELDS OF IL-2(IU/ml) AND TNF-α (U/ml)

	PRC	POC
IL-2	8.0±5.2	48.2±33.4
TNF-α	32.4±7.4	23.2±9.1

The IL-2 yield was significantly higher (p<0.01) while the TNF-α yield was lower, though not significantly, in the POC group.

2. Expression of membrane antigens of mouse spleen cell (Table 2)

Tab.2 EXPRESSION OF MEMBRANE ANTIGEN OF SPLEEN CELL

		PRC	POC
CD4+	(%)	21.2±2.8	25.8±2.3
CD8+	(%)	14.7±4.2	14.0±3.1
CD4/CD8		1.47	1.71

CD4$^+$ cell population was hiigher and the CD8$^+$ population lower in the POC group. The CD4/CD8 ratio increased. No change was significant.

3. Survival duration of mouse (Table 3)

Tab.3 SURVIVAL DURATION OF MOUSE

Animal Group	n	Survival Duration Range	Mean
Transplanted			
Allogeneic			
PRC	16	14—26	20.9±3.9
POC	16	14—42	28.5±8.8
Syngeneic	4	60	
Irradiated control	16	7—15	12.0±2.6
Normal control	4	60	

Survival was longer in the mice with transplants than in those without (p < 0.01). The syngeneic transplant group survived as long as the normal control. Of the allogeneic groups, the POC group showed longer survival (p < 0.01), though all died of GVHD finally.

4. Yields of IL-2 and THF-α of GVHD mouse spleen cell (Table 4)

Tab.4 YIELDS OF IL-2 (IU/ml) AND TNF-α (U/ml) OF GVHD MOUSE

	PRC			POC		
	1st wk (n=6)	2nd wk (n=4)	4th wk (n=4)	1st wk (n=6)	2nd wk (n=4)	4th wk (n=4)
IL-2	10.5±4.7	5.9±2.6	36.9±42.0	4.0±3.9	3.1±3.0	6.7±5.3
TNF-α	28.6±5.8	53.8±31.9	35.7±10.9	23.8±3.4	49.4±34.2	31.8±6.4

The IL-2 and THF-α yields of spleen cells in mice transplantated with cryopreserved cells were both lower than those transplanted with in uncryopreserved cells at any time.

5. Expression of membrane antigens of spleen cell in GVHD mouse (Table 5)

Tab.5 EXPRESSION OF MEMBRANE ANTIGEN OF SPLEEN CELL IN GVHD MOUSE

	PRC			POC		
	1st wk (n=6)	2nd wk (n=4)	4th wk (n=4)	1st wk (n=6)	2nd wk (n=4)	4th wk (n=4)
CD4+	12.3±2.9	9.5±2.0	11.0±4.1	9.4±2.0	8.5±1.2	9.9±1.5
CD8+	9.8±1.6	10.4±1.5	11.6±1.9	7.0±1.9	9.2±1.5	8.4±2.3
CD4/CD8	1.25	0.91	0.95	1.35	0.92	1.17

The expression of CD4 and CD8 spleen cells in mice transplanted with cryopreserved cells were lower than in those transplanted with uncryopreserved cells at any time, but the ratio of CD4/CD8 was higher in the POC group.

Conclusion

1. The IL-2 yields of the post-cryopreserved mouse spleen cells increased and TNF-α decreased.
2. The expression of CD4 in the post-cryopreserved mouse spleen cells increased and CD8 decreased. The CD4/CD8 ratio increased.
3. The mice that received cryopreserved hemopoietic cell transplants survived longer than those that received uncryopreserved transplants, though GVHD developed in both groups.
4. The ability of spleen cells to produce IL-2 and TNF-α in the mice transplanted with cryopreserved cells decreased. However, the in vitro results showed the IL-2 yields increased significantly after cryopreservation.
5. The expression of CD4 and CD8 spleen cells in mice transplanted with

cryopreserved cells decreased and the CD4/CD8 ratio increased, as we found in the in vitro assay.

6. The influences of low-temperatures on the immune functions (esp. the increase in the CD4/CD8 ratio) of mouse spleen cells may be related to the longer survival time of GVHD mice.

7. All POC mice finally died of GVHD as the immune functions of the spleen cells recovered to normal levels after transplantation.

8. The in vitro higher yields of IL-2 in cryopreserved spleen cells may not be related to the post-transplant GVHD in vivo.

9. It seems that BMT with cryopreserved cells is finally unable to prevent the severe outcome of GVHD.

Transfer of Autoimmune Thyroiditis and Resolution of Palmoplantar Pustular Psoriasis following Allogeneic Bone Marrow Transplantation

Yuji Kishimoto, Yoshihisa Yamamoto, Hirokazu Taniguchi, Mutsumasa Yanabu, Shigetoshi Ohga, Takahiro Nagano, Hiroyuki Kitajima, and Shirou Fukuhara

First Department of Internal Medicine, Kansai Medical University, 10-15 Fumizonocho, Moriguchi, Osaka 570, Japan

SUMMARY

We describe the transfer of autoimmune thyroiditis and the resolution of palmoplantar pustular psoriasis (PPP) following allogeneic bone marrow transplantation (BMT). A 40-year-old man suffering from PPP underwent allogeneic BMT from his HLA-identical sister as treatment for acute myelogenous leukemia. He developed transient hyperthyroidism five months after BMT and was found to have anti-thyroglobulin antibodies. He had had normal thyroid function and no anti-thyroglobulin antibodies before BMT. The donor had no history of thyroid disease and showed normal thyroid function but was positive for anti-thyroglobulin antibodies. Thus, even when the donor has subclinical disease, thyroid dysfunction after BMT may occur due to the transfer of autoimmune thyroiditis. Immediately after BMT, the patient experienced complete clearance of his cutaneous PPP. This case may demonstrate that PPP is a partially immune-mediated disease.

KEY WORDS: autoimmune thyroiditis, palmoplantar pustular psoriasis, bone marrow transplantation, autoimmunity

INTRODUCTION

It is well accepted that donor-derived immunity is transferred with allogeneic BMT [1, 2]. Adoptive transfer of diseases related to autoimmunity have been reported during BMT [3-6]. Resolution of immune-mediated diseases following BMT has also been reported [7]. We report on a leukemic patient with both occurrences: the development of autoimmune thyroiditis and clearance of PPP following allogeneic BMT.

CASE REPORT

A 40-year-old man was diagnosed with acute myelogenous leukemia in January 1992. Bone marrow cytology revealed M6 by FAB classification with tri-lineage myelodysplasia. The patient went into complete remission following induction chemotherapy with daunorubicin, 6-mercaptopurine, and behenoyl cytosine arabinoside. After receiving three courses of consolidation chemotherapy, he developed PPP in February 1993. The skin lesions were treated with combinations of topical corticosteroids and etretinate with only partial response.

In November 1993, after myeloablation with busulphan (16 mg/kg) and cyclophosphamide (120 mg/kg), the patient received an allogeneic marrow graft from his HLA-identical younger sister (A-2, w33; B-44, 51, Bw-4; C- − , − ; DR-w15, 4, DRw-53; DQ-w1, −). The mixed lymphocyte culture was negative. Although the patient's elder sister had died of hyperthyroidism, his younger sister had no history of thyroid disease and showed normal thyroid function but was positive for anti-thyroglobulin antibodies.

Cyclosporin A (CyA) and short-term methotrexate were used for GVHD (graft-versus-host disease) prophylaxis. The hematological follow-up showed stable engraftment with complete hematopoietic recovery and sustained complete chimerism. There were no signs of acute GVHD. Immediately after BMT, the patient's skin lesions disappeared entirely.

Five months after BMT, the patient presented with 5 kg weight loss; in addition, he complained of general malaise and fever. There was no enlargement of the thyroid gland. Thyroid test results and autoantibody levels are summarized in Table 1; these showed normal thyroid function and no anti-thyroid autoantibodies prior to BMT, and hyperthyroidism and anti-thyroglobulin antibodies five months after BMT. The patient was negative for many other autoantibodies, including anti-nuclear antibodies, anti-mitochondrial antibodies and anti-TSH (thyroid-stimulating hormone) receptor antibodies. At this time, he also developed lichen planus on his buccal mucosa, with the mucosal biopsy demonstrating findings consistent with chronic GVHD. Although CyA (3 mg/kg) was given daily, additional therapy with prednisolone (40 mg/day) was administered. After immunosupression with CyA and prednisolone, the clinical symptoms improved and the thyroid functions returned to normal in a few weeks, but the elevation in anti-thyroglobulin antibodies persisted.

Table 1. Results of Thyroid Function Tests and Autoantibody Levels before and after BMT

Time of test	TSH	Free thyroxine	Thyroglobulin antibody	Microsomal antibody
	(0.42-5.80 μ U/ml)	(0.97-2.02 ng/ml)	($<$0.3 U/ml)	($<$100)*
Pre-BMT Donor	0.90	1.19	13.4	Negative
Recipient	1.04	1.71	$<$0.3	Negative
5 months post-BMT	$<$0.2	3.98	2.5	Negative
8 months post-BMT	0.94	1.38	16.1	Negative
18 months post-BMT	2.43	1.30	208.0	6400

TSH=thyroid-stimulating hormone
Parentheses indicate normal ranges.
*Titer is reciprocal serum dilution.

Eighteen months after BMT, CyA and prednisolone were discontinued. The patient remained in complete remission from his leukemia and had normal thyroid function and a high titer of anti-thyroid autoantibodies. Karyotypic examination of the bone marrow confirmed complete chimerism with donor cells. Since his transplant, the patient has had complete clearance of his cutaneous PPP despite cessation of immunosuppressive therapy.

DISCUSSION

We report a case of antoimmune thyroiditis in a recipient of allogeneic BMT; the disease was presumed to have been caused by adoptive transfer of immunocompetent cells from the donor. The full hematopoietic chimerism of the recipient after BMT was demonstrated by chromosome analyses. Thus, it was likely that the production of anti-thyroid antibodies and destruction of thyroid tissue were due to lymphoid cells from the donor. We speculate that the subclinical autoimmune disease of the donor might have been activated and accelerated to a clinical level in the milieu of the new host. Although adoptive transfer of autoimmune thyroiditis has been previously reported [3, 4], transfer of a subclinical thyroiditis of the donor has not been reported. Anti-microsomal antibodies detected eighteen months after BMT may have been newly acquired autoantibodies because of long-lasting thyroiditis. Thyroid failure may occur years after transplantation, necessitating long-term monitoring of thyroid function.

Although this report suggests transfer of autoimmune thyroiditis by bone marrow cells, other mechanisms are possible. As there was a family history of thyroid disease, the recipient may have had a genetic predisposition for thyroid disease. On the other hand, the de novo development of autoimmune disorders has been reported in chronic GVHD [8]. Although chronic GVHD may also have accelerated the autoimmune thyroiditis, occurrence of anti-thyroid autoantibodies is rare in comparison to that of other autoantibodies in chronic GVHD [9, 10]. The general immune dysregulation after BMT may have contributed to an acceleration of autoimmune thyroiditis.

This is the first reported example of resolution of PPP following allogeneic BMT. PPP is defined as a condition in which erythematous and scaly plaques studded with sterile pustules persist on the palms or soles. The usual course is prolonged and very resistant to treatment. The relationship between PPP and psoriasis vulgaris is controversial [11]. Some forms of PPP are considered distinct entities, such as metal allergy [12] or tonsillitis-related skin lesions [13]. In the pathogenesis of psoriasis vulgaris, immunological mechanisms play an important role, and clearance of the disease following allogeneic BMT has been reported [7]. Thus, this case may demonstrate that PPP is a partially immune-mediated disease as is psoriasis vulgaris, and it may give further support to the hypothesis that BMT can cure immune-mediated diseases.

REFERENCES

[1]   Lum LG (1987) The kinetics of immune reconstitution after human bone marrow transplantation. Blood 69: 369-380

[2]   Wimperis JZ, Brenner MK, Prentice HG, Reittie JE, Karayiannis P, Griffiths PD, Hoffbrand AV (1986) Transfer of a functional humoral immune system in transplantation of T-lymphocyte-depleted bone marrow. Lancet i: 339-343

[3]   Wyatt DT, Lum LG, Casper J, Hunter J, Camitta B (1990) Autoimmune thyroiditis after bone marrow transplantation. Bone Marrow Transplant 5: 357-361

[4]   Aldouri MA, Ruggier R, Epstein O, Prentice HG (1990) Adoptive transfer of hyperthyroidism and autoimmune thyroiditis following allogeneic bone marrow transplantation for chronic myeloid leukemia. Br J Haematol 74: 118-120

[5]   Lampeter EF, Homberg M, Quabeck K, Schaefer UW, Wernet P, Bertrams J, Grosse-Wilde H, Gries FA, Kolb H (1993) Transfer of insulin-dependent diabetes between HLA-identical siblings by bone marrow transplantation. Lancet 341: 1243-1244

[6]   Minchinton RM, Waters AH, Kendra J, Barrett AJ (1982) Autoimmune thrombocytopenia acquired from an allogeneic bone-marrow graft Lancet ii: 627-632

[7]   Liu Yin JA, Jowitt SN (1992) Resolution of immune-mediated diseases following allogeneic bone marrow transplantation for leukaemia. Bone Marrow Transplant 9: 31-33

[8]   Atkinson K (1990) Chronic graft-versus-host disease. Bone Marrow Transplant 5: 69-82

[9]   Rouquette-Gally AM, Boyeldieu D, Prost AG, Gluckman E (1988) Autoimmunity after allogeneic bone marrow transplantation. A study of 53 long-term-surviving patients. Transplantation 46: 238-240

[10] Holmes JA, Livesey SJ, Bedwell AE, Amos N, Whittaker JA (1989) Auto-antibody analysis in chronic graft-versus-host disease. Bone Marrow Transplant 4: 529-531

[11] Ashurst PJC (1964) Relapsing pustular eruptions of the hands and feet. Br J Dermatol 76: 169-180

[12] White SW (1982) Palmoplantar pustular psoriasis provoked by lithium therapy. J Am Acad Dermatol 7: 660-662

[13] Kuki K, Kimura T, Hayashi Y, Tabata T (1992) Focus tonsils and skin diseases with special reference to palmoplantar pustulosis. Adv Otorhinolaryngol 47: 196-202

Acute Graft Versus Host Reaction (GVHR) Against Major / Minor Histocompatibility Antigens

Toshiaki Takayanagi, Kiichi Kajino, Naoto Matsuki, Kazuya Iwabuchi, Kazumasa Ogasawara, and Kazunori Onoe[1]

[1]Section of Pathology, Institute of Immunological Science, Hokkaido University, Kita-ku, Kita 15, Nishi 7, Sapporo, 060, Japan.

SUMMARY

When irradiated minor lymphocyte stimulatory-1^a (Mls-1^a) mice were reconstituted with bone marrow cells plus mature T cells from Mls-1^b and H-2 class I incompatible mice, acute GVHR was induced in the recipients. Majority of responding cells were shown to be CD4$^+$Vβ6$^+$ T cells derived from donor mature T cells. It appeared that Mls-1^a antigen (Ag) was a major target Ag. However, when Mls-1^b donor and Mls-1^a recipient mice were H-2 matched, the severity of GVHR was mar-kedly reduced. Thus, disparity at the Mls-1 locus alone appeared not to be sufficient to induce dete-ctable GVHR. In mixed lymphocyte reaction (MLR), T cell proliferation against Mls-1^a plus H-2 class I Ag was as high as that against H-2 class I Ag alone. On the other hand, production of IL-2, IL-4 and TNF-α by the T cells responding to H-2 class I plus Mls-1^a Ag was considerably greater than that by T cells responding to class I Ag alone. The present findings suggest that CD4$^+$Vβ6$^+$ T cells responding to Mls-1^{a}Ag and producing IL-2, IL-4 and TNF-α play a significant role, which may result in augmentation of allo-responses to the host H-2 class I Ag and substantial GVHR.

KEY WORDS : GVHR, BMT, MLR, Mls-1, minor histocompatibility antigens

INTRODUCTION

Bone marrow transplantation (BMT) is now an effective and globally accepted therapy for many other-wise lethal diseases of blood including leukemia [1, 2]. In most cases of BMT, MHC is matched between donors and recipients. However, because of the serious shortage of MHC matched siblings, cases of allogeneic BMT are increasing [3]. Thus, influences of mismatch at minor histocompa-tibility loci between donors and recipients on the subsequent GVHR become increasingly a serious problem [4, 5]. In the present study, we have studied the influences of disparity at the Mls-1 locus in addition to that at MHC between donors and recipients of BMT. Herein, we report different immunological responses seen among donor T cells from various BMT chimeras where MHC and/or Mls-1 are matched or mismatched. The Mls-1 disparity appears to significantly augment GVHR generated against MHC in these chimeras probably via elevated cytokine production.

MATERIALS AND METHODS

Mouse. B10.AQR (K^q A^k E^k D^d, Thy1.2, Mls-1^b), AKR/J (K^k A^k E^k D^k, Thy1.1, Mls-1^a) and B10.BR (K^k A^k E^k D^k, Thy1.2, Mls-1^b) female mice (6-8 wk) were used throughout the study.

BMT. Recipient mice were lethally irradiated (11Gy) 24 hr before BMT. To completely deplete mature T cells, bone marrow cells from donors were treated with anti-Thy1.2 antibody and selected rabbit complement. The recipients were then inoculated with bone marrow cells (1×10^7/head) (control chimera mice). GVHR chimera mice were prepared by inoculation of the T cell depleted-bone marrow cells (1×10^7/head) plus splenic T cells (1×10^5/head) from donor mice that had been purified with nylon wool columns [6].

MLR. MLR was set up in 200 μl medium with 0.5 - 4 $\times$ 10^5 responder cells and 8 $\times$ 10^5 stimulator cells (spleen cells treated with 50 μg/ml mitomycin C) [7]. After 72 hr of incubation, cultures were pulsed with 0.5 μCi [^{3}H]TdR 18 hr before harvest. All of the data shown in the present studies indicate the mean of triplicate cultures. Δcpm = mean of experimental cpm - that of control cpm (against syngeneic stimulator).

CTLL-2 (IL-2) or CT.4S (IL-4) assay. Supernatants were collected from MLR cultures, as described. CTLL-2 or CT.4S cells were incubated with the supernatant in the presence or absence of 11B11 (anti-IL-4 mAb) for 24 hr. Cultures were pulsed with 0.5 μCi [^{3}H]TdR 24 hr before harvest. All of the data shown in the present studies indicate the mean of triplicate cultures.

Enzyme-linked-immunosorbent assay (ELISA). Amounts of tumor necrosis factor -α (TNF-α) in the supernatants was quantitatively analysed with Mouse TNF-α ELISA KIT puchased from Genzyme Corp.(Cambridge MA). All of the data shown in the present studies indicate the mean of triplicate cultures.

RESULTS AND DISCUSSION

MLR and cytokine productions

In MLR, T cells from B10.AQR mice generated considerable proliferation upon stimulation with AKR/J stimulators as well as with B10.BR stimulators (Fig.1 A). However, when productions of IL-2, IL-4 and TNF-α were compared between these MLR, AKR/J stimulators induced markedly greater responses than B10.BR stimulators (Fig.1 B, C, D)

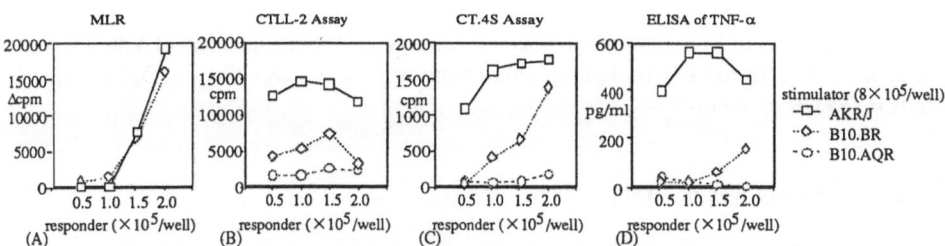

Fig.1 (A) MLR:B10.AQR against AKR/J or B10.BR. (B) CTLL-2 Assay:Culture supernatants from B10.AQR against AKR/J, B10.BR or B10.AQR MLR in the presence of anti-IL-4 mAb (11B11) . (C) CT.4S Assay:Culture supernatants from B10.AQR against AKR/J, B10.BR or B10.AQR MLR. (D) ELISA Assay of TNF-α: Culture supernatant from B10.AQR against AKR, B10.BR or B10.AQR.

Sequential changes in the proportion and number of Vβ6⁺ T cells from GVHR chimeras and functions of donor T cells

After BMT in GVHR[B10.AQR→AKR/J] chimeras, high proportions of donor derived Vβ6^{high}Thy1.2⁺ T cells which were almost CD4⁺(data not shown) were seen in the thymus. The proportion of Vβ6^{high} cells in the Thy1.2⁺ cells reached a peak 7 days after BMT, and then decre-ased (Fig.2 A). However the actual number of donor derived Vβ6^{high}Thy1.2⁺ T cells was retained in the thymus after 7 days (B). In the peripheral lymph nodes (LNs) and spleen of the chimera mice, the number of donor derived Vβ6^{high}Thy1.2⁺ T cells increased as seen in the thymus (data not shown). To study the functions of the donor derived T cells, production of IL-2 (C) and TNF-α (D) by the donor T cells, which were collected from the GVHR chimeras 7, 11 and 14 days after BMT, was measured in MLR against AKR/J. T cells from GVHR chimeras 7 days after BMT were shown to produce large amounts of IL-2 and TNF-α upon stimulation with AKR/J stimulators.

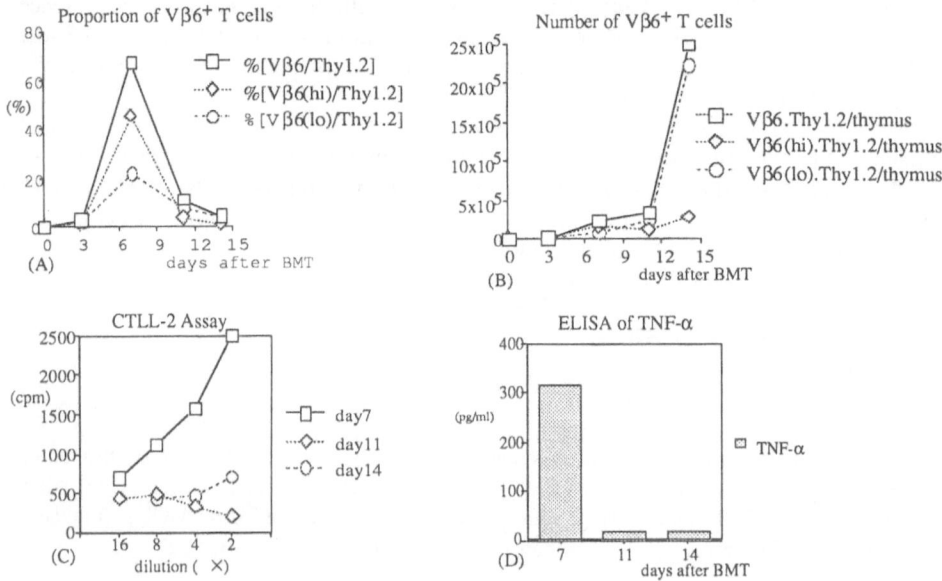

Fig.2 Proportions of Vβ6⁺ cells in the Thy1.2⁺ cells (A) and actual numbers of Vβ6⁺Thy1.2⁺ cells in the thymus of GVHR chimera. Production of IL-2 (C) and TNF-α (D) by donor T cells in GVHR chimeras.

Changes in body weight (BW)

To analyse clinical signs of GVHR caused by disparity at minor histocomapatibility loci, we compared sequential changes of BW between control and GVHR chimeras. When [B10.AQR→B10.BR]chimeras were analysed, no apparent difference was detected between control and GVHR groups (A). However in the case of [B10.AQR→AKR] chimeras where H-2 class I plus minor histocompatibility Ag are mismatched, marked reduction of BW was noted in the GVHR group as compared to that in the control group (Fig.3).

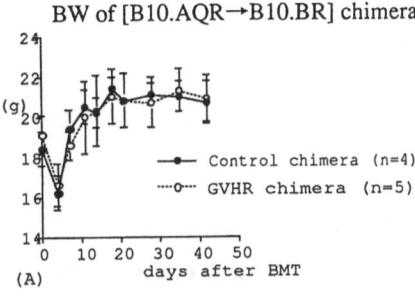
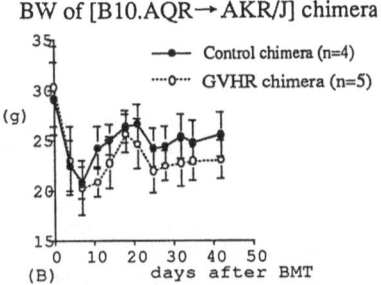

Fig.3 Changes in BW of [B10.AQR→B10.BR] (A) and [B10.AQR→AKR/J] (B).

The present findings indicate consistently that the mismatching of minor histocompatibility Ag including Mls-1a between donors and recipients induces clinically detectable GVHR in the recipients. How-ever, since the disparity at minor histocompatibility loci alone (i.e. [B10.BR→AKR/J]chimeras) did not induce detectable GVHR [8], the Mls-1 mismatch might augment GVHR generated by the host H-2 class I Ag by inducing the considerable cytokine production shown herein.

REFERENCES

1. Good RA, Kapoor N, Reisner Y (1983) Bone marrow transplantation-An expanding approach to treatment of many diseases. Cell Immunol 82:36-54
2. O'Reilly RJ (1983) Allogeneic bone marrow transplantation: Current status and future directions. Blood 62:941-964
3. Martin PJ, Hansen JA, Buckner CD, Standers JE, Deeg HJ, Stewart P, Appelbaum FR, Clift R, Fefer A, Witherspoon RP, Kennedy MS, Sullivan KM, Flournoy N, Storb R, Thomas ED (1985) Effects of in vitro depletion of T cells in HLA-identical allogeneic marrow grafts. Blood 66:664-672
4. Gleichmann E, Pals ST, Rolink AG, Radaszkiewicz T, Gleichmann H (1984) Graft-versus-host-reactions: Clues to the etiopathology of a spectrum of immunological diseases. Immunol Today 5:324-332
5. Gale AP (1985) Graft-versus-host disease. Immunol Rev 88:193-214
6. Fukushi N, Arase H, Wang B, Ogasawara K, Gotohda T, Good RA, Ono&K (1990) Thymus: A direct target tissue in graft-versus-host reaction after allogeneic bone marrow transplantation which results in abrogation of induction of self-tolerance. Proc Natl Acad Sci USA 87:6301-6305
7. Arase-Fukushi N, Arase H, Ogasawra,K, Good RA, Onoē K (1993) Production of minor lymphocyte stimulatory-1[a] antigen from activated CD4[+] or CD8[+] T cells. J Immunol 151:4445-4454
8. Hirano M, Arase H, Arase-Fukushi N, Ogasawara K, Iwabuchi K, Miyazaki T, Good RA, Onoē K (1993) Reconstitution of lymphoid tissue under the influence of a subclinical level graft versus host reaction induced by bone marrow T cells or splenic T cell subsets. Cell Immunol 151:118-132

Antileukemic Effects of Interleukin 2 after Allogeneic Bone Marrow Transplantation in AKR/J Mice

Satoshi Hashino, Masahiro Imamura, Junji Tanaka, Sumiko Kobayashi, Masaharu Kasai*, and Masahiro Asaka

Third Department of Internal Medicine, Hokkaido University School of Medicine, Kita-15 Nishi-7, Kita-ku, Sapporo, 060, Japan
*Division of Internal Medicine, Sapporo Hokuyu Hospital, 6-6 Higashi-sapporo, Shiroishi-ku, Sapporo, 003, Japan

SUMMARY

AKR/J mice show a high incidence of spontaneous virus-induced T cell leukemia at the age of 6-12 months, and a number of factors are involved in the high susceptibility to leukemia development. The present study was designed to examine whether a combination of interleukin 2 (IL-2), which has a strong immunostimulating potential, and bone marrow transplantation (BMT) from allogeneic C3H/HeJ mice sensitive to the virus and allogeneic CBA/J mice resistant to the virus could induce resistance against the development of spontaneous leukemia and exacerbate graft-versus-host disease (GVHD). Our data suggested that BMT from H-2 compatible mice that did not possess a resistant gene for virus-induced leukemia and a combined use of IL-2 after BMT could partially prevent the development of spontaneous leukemia in chimeric AKR/J mice. The GVHD observed in chimeric mice was not enhanced by the administration of IL-2.

KEY WORDS: bone marrow transplantation (BMT), interleukin 2 (IL-2), graft-versus-host disease (GVHD), graft-versus-leukemia (GVL), cytokine

INTRODUCTION

AKR/J mice display a high incidence of T cell leukemia/lymphoma at the age of 6 to 12 months, and many factors are related to the high incidence of leukemia development [1, 2]. In previous studies, several methods for preventing spontaneous leukemia in AKR/J mice have been investigated, including bone marrow transplantation (BMT) from the mice that possess resistant genes for virus-induced leukemia [2 - 5]. Recently, immunotherapy using interleukin 2 (IL-2) has been reported to lead to significant graft-versus-leukemia (GVL) effects in syngeneic BMT settings as well as allogeneic settings [6 - 8]. Thus, the present study was designed to examine whether a combination of IL-2 and BMT from allogeneic C3H/HeJ sensitive to the virus and allogeneic CBA/J mice resistant to the virus could induce resistance against the development of spontaneous leukemia and worsen graft-versus-host disease (GVHD). Our data suggested that BMT from H-2-compatible mice that did not possess a resistant gene for virus-induced leukemia and a combined use of IL-2 after BMT could partially prevent a development of spontaneous leukemia in chimeric AKR/J mice without enhancement of GVHD.

MATERIALS AND METHODS

AKR/J (H-2^k), C3H/HeJ (H-2^k), and CBA/J (H-2^k) mice which were MHC-compatible but non-MHC-incompatible were obtained from Crea Inc., Fuji, Shizuoka, Japan (AKR/J and CBA/J) and Charles River Japan Inc., Atsugi, Kanagawa, Japan (C3H/HeJ). The mice were raised under specific pathogen-free conditions in the animal facility of Hokkaido University School of Medicine. Six- to 8-wk-old male mice were used for both donors and recipients in BMT. Recipient AKR/J mice were irradiated with 860 cGy at a dose rate of approximately 70 cGy/min from MBR-1520R X-irradiator (Hitachi Medical Co., Tokyo, Japan). BM cells of C3H/HeJ or CBA/J mice were collected by flushing femurs and tibias with RPMI. Within 6 hours after irradiation, recipient mice were injected with 1x10^7 BM cells in 0.5 ml of RPMI via the lateral tail vein. All the recipients were given drinking water with antibiotics (minocycline 100 ng/ml) for 3 weeks after BMT. Recombinant IL-2 was kindly supplied by Shionogi Pharmaceutical Co., Ltd. (Osaka, Japan). No endotoxin was detected in IL-2 (< 0.25 ng/ml). The IL-2 regimen consisted of daily intraperitoneal injections of 5,000 units (in 0.1 ml of PBS) for 7 consecutive days a month. The therapy was started immediately after BMT on the first day of the month and continued until death. Control chimeras received 0.1 ml of PBS in the same manner as above.

Semiquantitative analysis of cytokine (IL-1β, IL-2, IL-4, IL-6, IFN-γ and TNF-α) mRNA was performed by the method that we have already reported [9, 10]. Briefly, spleen cells were removed aseptically from two or three mice of each group at 7 to 8 months after BMT and leukemia development. harvesting was the day after the last monthly administration. These cells were treated with Tris-NH$_4$Cl to lyse red blood cells. Each 2 μg of RNA was reverse-transcribed by 600 U murine Molony leukemia virus reverse transcriptase (BRL, Grand Island, NY, USA) with 150 pmol of random hexamer, and 1 / 20th of the resulting cDNA was used for semiquantitative polymerase chain reaction (PCR). The primers
(IL-1β A   5'ATTAGACAGCTGCACTACAGGCTC3',
IL-1β B   5'AGATTCCATGGTGAAGTCAATTAT3',
IL-2 A   5'ACATTGACACTTGTGCTCCTTGTC3',
IL-2 B   5'TTGAGGGCTTGTTGAGATGATGCT3',
IL-4 A   5'AGCTAGTTGTCATCCTGCTCTTCT3'
IL-4 B   5'CGAGTAATCCATTTGCATGATGCT3'
IL-6 A   5'GTCTATACCACTTCACAAGTCGGA3'
IL-6 B   5'TTGGATGGTCTTGGTCCTTAGCCA3'
IFN-γ A   5'CACGGCACAGTCATTGAAAGCCTA3',
IFN-γ B   5'TGAGGCTGGATTCCGGCAACAGCT3',
TNF-α A   5'ACCCTCACACTCAGATCATCTTCT3',
TNF-α B   5'CAGATTGACCTCAGCGCTGAGTTG3',
β-actin A   5'AGGGAAATCCTGCGTGACATCAAA3',
β-actin B   5'ACTCATCGTACTCCTGCTTGCTGA3')
were synthesized on a 380B DNA synthesizer (Applied Biosystems, Inc, Foster City, CA, USA). In this study, when the gene expression could be detected by electrophoresis on 2% agarose gel containing ethidium bromide after amplification of 30, 37 and 44 cycles, they were defined as +++, ++, +, +/- or - , according to increasing amounts of product detectable. All the amplified DNAs were 441 (IL-1β), 477 (IL-2), 406 (IL-4), 441 (IL-6), 376 (IFN-γ) and 423 (TNF-α) base pairs, respectively.

Each group consisted of 14 to 24 mice. The mice were checked daily to determine the survival, also including body weights and clinical signs for GVHD. Simultaneously to the in vitro assay histological examinations of skin, liver, and gut were carried out to detect any evidence of GVHD. Autopsy was also performed to examine the presence or absence of leukemia. *P* values for comparison of results in various groups were determined by Student's t-test.

RESULTS

Table 1 shows the effects of BMT and IL-2 on survival and leukemia development.
In the BMT (C3H/HeJ ⊳ AKR/J), BMT alone improved the survival but prevented leukemia development in only a few chimeras. However, the addition of IL-2 after BMT was able to

extensively prevent leukemia development. On the contrary, in the BMT (CBA/J → AKR/J), BMT alone extensively improved survival and prevented leukemia development in almost all the chimeras, as previously reported (4). In this combination, the addition of IL-2 after BMT did not further improve survival. No clinical evidence of GVHD, including weight loss, was encountered in any chimera. Also the histologic findings of skin, liver, and gut were not compatible with GVHD in all combinations of chimeras.

Table 1. Antitumor efficacy of IL-2 against spontaneous leukemia development in chimeric mice

Group	Median survival days (range)	Incidence of leukemia (%)
Normal AKR	279 (225 - 412)	100
C3H → AKR (+PBS)	386 (130 - 457)*	88
C3H → AKR (+IL-2)	428 (271 - 609)*	21
CBA → AKR (+PBS)	394 (376 - 438)**	0
CBA → AKR (+IL-2)	415 (379 - 458)**	7

*$p<0.001$, **$p<0.01$ (vs. normal AKR)

In the BMT (C3H/HeJ → AKR/J), IL-1β, IL-2, IFN-γ and TNF-α mRNA expressions of IL-2-treated mice were enhanced compared to those of PBS-treated mice (Table 2).

Table 2 Cytokine gene expressions using semiquantitative PCR

Group	IL-1β	IL-2	IL-4	IL-6	IFN-γ	TNF-α
Normal AKR	+	+	+	+	+	+
C3H → AKR (+PBS)	++	+	++	++	++	++
C3H → AKR (+IL-2)	+++	++	++	++	+++	+++
CBA → AKR (+PBS)	+	+	++	++	+/-	+/-
CBA → AKR (+IL-2)	+	+	++	++	+	+

In the allogeneic with transplantation from CBA/J to AKR/J mice, only IFN-γ and TNF-α mRNA expression of IL-2-treated mice was slightly enhanced compared to that of PBS-treated mice. However, these expressions were almost the same as those of normal AKR/J mice. Concerning to IL-4 and IL-6 mRNA expression, there were no differences between PBS-treated mice and IL-2 treated mice in the both allogeneic settings.

DISCUSSION

The present study was designed to investigate whether a combination of IL-2 and allogeneic BMT from H-2-compatible mice could induce resistance against the development of spontaneous leukemia in AKR/J mice, and to investigate the possibility that it exacerbate GVHD. Biological stimulation of the immune system in IL-2-treated chimeras was clear in allogeneic settings. It is known that IL-2 administration induces the secretion of IFN-γ and TNF-α *in vivo* [11]. On the other hand, it is also known that the onset of GVHD is related to IL-1β, IL-6, IFN-γ and TNF-α [12, 13]. However, it is not clear how soluble effector molecules are involved in GVL. The increased mRNA expressions were detected for IL-1β, IL-2, TNF-α, and IFN-γ in the IL-2-treated allogeneic chimeras transplanted from C3H/HeJ mice. These findings indicated that the IL-2 induced activation of the immune system was complicated. Recently, Takikawa et al. reported a synergistic antitumor effect between IFN-γ and IL-1α/β in the rejection of allografted tumor cells [14]. Therefore, the enhanced expression of these cytokines mRNA observed in this experimental model may indicate that these cytokines play an important role in GVL. From these experimental data we concluded that the increased cytokines were the major factor preventing leukemia development in the recipients of C3H/HeJ marrow. On the other hand, in the recipients of CBA/J marrow, not only the increased cytokines but also genetic characteristics helped to prevent the leukemia.

The observations of in the present study would contribute to a useful and effective therapeutic protocol for patients with leukemia in the HLA-matched related BMT setting. Further studies should be performed to determine the exact mechanism for the antileukemic effects induced by IL-2 after H-2-compatible BMT, and to determine the best schedule of IL-2 administration to prevent the development of spontaneous leukemia in AKR/J mice.

REFERENCES

1) McEndy DP, Boon MC, Furth J. On the role of thymus, spleen, and gonads in the development of leukemia in a high-leukemia stock of mice. Cancer Res 1944; 4: 377.
2) Yasumizu R, Hiai H, Sugiura K, et al. Development of donor-derived thymic lymphomas after allogeneic bone marrow transplantation in AKR/J mice. J Immunol 1988; 141: 2181.
3) Pollard M, Truitt RL. Allogeneic bone marrow chimerism in germfree mice. 1. Prevention of spontaneous leukemia in AKR mice. Proc Soc Exp Biol Med 1973; 144: 659.
4) Tanaka T, Obata Y, Fernandes G, Onoe K, Stockert E, Good RA. Prevention of leukemia in lethally irradiated AKR mice by CBA/H marrow transplantation. Proc Am Assoc Cancer Res 1979; 20: 114.
5) Wustrow TPU, Good RA. Expression of antigens coded in murine leukemia viruses on thymocytes of allogeneic donor origin in AKR mice following syngeneic or allogeneic bone marrow transplantation. Cancer Res 1985; 45: 6428.
6) Sykes M, Romick ML, Sachs DH. Interleukin 2 prevents graft-versus-host disease while preserving the graft-versus-leukemia effect of allogeneic T cells. Proc Natl Acad Sci USA 1990; 87: 5633.
7) Ackerstein A, Kedar E, Slavin S. Use of recombinant human interleukin-2 in conjunction with syngeneic bone marrow transplantation in mice as a model for control of minimal residual disease in malignant hematologic disorders. Blood 1991; 78: 1212.
8) Kwak LW, Campbell MJ, Levy R. Tumor resistance induced by syngeneic bone marrow transprantation and enhanced by interleukin 2 : A model for the graft versus leukemia reaction. Cancer Res 1992; 52: 4117.
9) Hashino S. (1994) Antileukemic effects of interleukin-2 on spontaneous development of leukemia after H-2-compatible allogeneic bone marrow transplantation in AKR/J mice. Hokkaido J Med Sci 69: 601-613
10) Hashino S, Imamura M, Zhu X, Imai K, Kobayashi S, Tanaka J, Fujii Y, Kasai M, Miyazaki T. (1995) Effects of interleukin 2 on leukemia development after bone marrow transplantation in AKR/J mice. Transplantation 59: 1643-1645
11) Heslop HE, Gottlieb DJ, Bianchi ACM, et al. In vivo induction of gamma interferon and tumor necrosis factor by interleukin-2 infusion following intensive chemotherapy or autologous marrow transplantation. Blood 1989; 74: 1374.
12) Tanaka J, Imamura M, Kasai M, et al. Cytokine gene expression in peripheral blood mononuclear cells during graft-verus-host disease after allogeneic bone marrow transplantation. Br J Haematol 1993; 85: 558.
13) Imamura M, Hashino S, Kobayashi H, et al. Serum cytokine levels in bone marrow transplantation: Synergistic interaction of interleukin-6, interferon-γ, and tumor necrosis factor-α in graft-versus-host disease. Bone Marrow Transplant 1994; 13: 745.
14) Takikawa O, Oku T, Yasui H, Yoshida R. Synergism between IFN-γ and IL-1α/β in growth inhibition of an allografted tumor. J Immunol 1993; 151: 2070.

DETECTION OF MINIMAL RESIDUAL DISEASE BY IMMUNOGLOBULIN HEAVY CHAIN GENE REARRANGEMENT ANALYSIS IN PATIENTS WITH B-ALL AFTER BONE MARROW TRANSPLANTATION

Qi Zhou,   Li Yu,   Fang-Ding Lou.

Department of Haematology, General Hospital of PLA, 28 Fuxing Road, Beijing, 100853, P.R.China.

SUMMARY Clonal immunoglobulin heavy chain (IgH) gene rearrangement was detected by polymerase chain reaction (PCR) and PCR conjuncting with single-strand conformational polymorphism (PCR-SSCP) in 11 bone marrow transplantation (BMT) patients with acute lymphoblastic leukemia (ALL) for detecting minimal residual disease (MRD). This study suggested that the presence of marker positive cells in complete remission pre-transplantation or persistence in the post-transplantation period is an indication of poor prognosis or long-term disease-free survival. Using clonal IgH gene rearrangement by PCR-SSCP to detect MRD pre- and post-transplantation may provide some important information for selecting a suitable time, as well as assessing the prognosis and detecting the effect of in vitro marrow purging for bone marrow transplantation.

KEY WORDS: Immunoglobulin,   Gene Rearrangement,   Leukemia,   Bone Marrow Transplantation,   Minimal Residual Disease

INTRODUCTION

As the residual leukemic cells in the bone marrow are the main cause of the relapse of leukemia after bone marrow transplantation (BMT), the detection of minimal residual disease (MRD) is highly important in assessing the possibility of relapse in leukemia after BMT, analysing the results of the conditioning regimen and evaluating the effect of in vitro marrow purging for BMT. In this study, clonal immunoglobulin heavy chain (IgH) gene rearrangement was detected by polymerase chain reaction (PCR) in 11 BMT patients with acute lymphoblastic leukemia (ALL), of whom 7 were found positive in relapse or at diagnosis. A more sensitive method, PCR-SSCP (single-strand conformational polymorphism analysis), was then used to detect MRD in the stored bone marrow films from these 7 patients in their complete remission (CR) pre- and post-transplantation.

MATERIALS AND METHODS

1. Patients and Clinical Material
Eleven patients with ALL were included in this study, They were treated with haematopoietic stem cell transplantation in our hospital between June 1987 and October 1993. Ages ranged from 12 to 44, There were 7 males and 4 females. According to FAB classification, There were two L1 cases, six L2 cases, and one L3 case. The other 2 cases had no FAB classification at diagnosis. Four cases were classified using immunophenotyping: 2 were common ALL, one was B-ALL and another was non-T-ALL. Autologous BMT (ABMT) was carried out on 8 patients, fetal liver transplantation on one patient, and allogeneic BMT (Allo-BMT) on 2 patients. First, the clonal IgH gene rearrangement was determined by PCR in bone marrow sample of each case at diagnosis or in relapse. Clonal IgH gene rearrangement was then used as a gene marker to detect MRD by PCR-SSCP in bone marrow samples taken in CR during 99 days pre-transplantation or 12 months post-transplantation. Twenty-four samples from 11 patients were examined, 4 being samples of mononuclear cells of bone marrow preserved at under -20°C and the other 20 of cells taken from Wright's stained marrow slices preserved at room temperature.

2. PCR Analysis :
DNA was extracted from the bone marrow samlpes taken from patients at diagnosis or in relapse. PCR primers used for amplifying the IgH gene were: 5'-ACG CGG TGT ATT ACT GT-3' for V region; and

274

5'-TGA GGA GAC GGT GAC C-3' and 5'-GTG ACC AGG GTC CCT TGG CCC CAG-3' for J region[1]. PCR amplification was performed twice on each sample to increase the sensitivity. The experimental condition of PCR and the method itself had been reported [2,3].

3. PCR-SSCP Analysis[4]:
This method and relative data have also been described elsewhere[3].

RESULTS

1. Clonal IgH gene rearrangement detection by PCR:
In PCR detection of bone marrow samples from 11 patients at diagnosis or in relapse, clonal rearrangement of IgH gene was found by the presence of DNA fragments of 90-130bp in 7 cases, while in 2 cases, only few diffused products were seen in the same area and nothing was found in the other 2 cases, having a total positive rate of 63.6% (7/11).

2. MRD detection by PCR-SSCP:
Using the clonal IgH gene rearrangement detected by PCR as a gene marker, MRD was tested by PCR- SSCP in bone marrow samples from the 7 cases mentione above in their CR . In 4 cases , a clonal gene rearrangement strand was found, showing the existence of minimal residual tumor cells in samples taken on the 99th, 25th, and 0 day pre-transplantation respectively. In the other 3 cases, no clonal gene arrangement strand was found, indicating negative results of minimal residual tumor cell detection. In addition, 5 of the 7 cases which had samples in their CR post-transplantation (32 daya -12 months) also had MRD detection, in which 3 were positive, and 2 negative.

3. The relationship between positive MRD and the relapse of leukemia after BMT:
In the 4 MRD positive cases in their CR pre-transplantation, one changed into negative MRD when tested on the 32th day after ABMT. Disease-free survival (DFS) is now 9 months. The other 3 patients who remain positive in the detection done on the +33th, +44th and +112th day showed relapse of leukemia on the +84th, +146th and +147th day. In the 3 MRD negative cases in their pre-transplantation, 2 had the relapse of leukemia on the +123th and +167th day respectively, and the third patient who remained negative in MRD detection one year post-transplantation has a DFS of 3.3 years up to now.

DISCUSSION

BMT is effective in leukemia to eradicate residual leukemic cell and to achieve long-term DFS. A sensitive method of detecting MRD is therefore important in giving guidance to clinical work for selecting the right time for transplantation and in marking a prognosis by judjing the eradication of leukemic cells. All B-cell origin malignancies have the same gene marker of monoclonal IgH gene rearrangement, which shows a clear strand after PCR amplification while the products of nonmal B-lymphocytes are DNA fragments of different size and have a diffusive appearance in electrophoresis. Seven of the 11 patients in this study were found to have the monoclonal gene rearrangement strand, indicating they were B-cell origin ALL. The absence of the IgH gene rearrangement strand in 2 cases without immunophenotyping at diagnosis suggested that they were possibly of non-B-cell origin, or that they might be false-negative because the PCR primers might not have covered all types of IgH gene rearrangement in the detection by PCR[5]. The other 2 cases, which were classified by immunophenotyping to be B-cell ALL (one non-T-ALL, one B-ALL), were only found to have some amplified products of different sizes distributed diffusively in the same area instead of a clonal gene rearrangement strand. These fragments of varied sizes are from the normal B cells in the malignant tissue.
positive rate of clonal IgH gene rearrangement differs with the different primers adopted. Using primers designed for the FR3 region and the J-region of the IgH gene was reported to have a positive rate of 74% in clonal IgH gene rearrangement detection in B-ALL[6], and using specific pairs of primers for the FR1 and J-regions, the positive rate was 93%[7]. We adopted the common primers for FR3 and J regions in this study, and the positive rate in IgH gene rearrangement detection was 63.6%, which was lower than that reported[6]. The reason may be that most of the patients involved

had no immunophenotyping so that there might be some T-cell origin cases which effected the positive rate.

The PCR technique detecting malignant cells at the leval of 1-5% is not sensitive enough to detect MRD in B-cell origin malignancies, and PCR-SSCP is a more suitable method and has a detection level of 1-2/1000[4]. Of the 11 patients in this study, the 7 with clonal IgH gene rearrangement by PCR in their bone marrow samples at diagnosis or in relapse were tested for MRD by PCR-SSCP in their CR pre- and post-transplantation. The results showed that the patients who were negative in MRD detection pre-transplantation had a longer DFS than those who were positive, and that those who remained positive pre- and post-transplantation were more likely to have their leukemia relapse while those who were positive pre-transplantation but turned negative post-transplantation might have a longer DFS. Three patients who were negative in MRD detection by PCR-SSCP per-transplantation had an average DFS of 249 days (123 days-3.3 years), while of the 4 patients who were positive in pre-transplantation MRD detection, three who remained positive had an average DFS of 129 days and the one who turned negative after transplantation is still alive with a DFS of more than 9 months.

Theoretically, the relapse rate of leukemia can be reduced in ABMT by in vitro marrow purging or peripheral blood stem cell transplantation (PBSCT), which may reduce the quantity of residual leukemic cells in the transfusion. Of the 4 patients in our study who were positive in MRD detection in their CR pre-transplantation, one who was transplanted with his own unpurged bone marrow but turned negative in the detection 32 days post-transplantation has a DFS of over 9 months, while the other 3 (one transplanted with purged bone marrow by tumor inhibiter and 2 transplanted with PBSC) who remained positive in the detection in 33-112 days post-transplantation had the relapse of leukemia within short periods. In spite of the insufficient number of cases studied, the results do indicate that the main cause of the relapse of leukemia after BMT may not be the residual leukemic cells in the graft tranfused but those which still remained in the host's body after BMT. So it is highly important to select an effetive conditioning regimen individually to eradicate residual leukemic cells in the body. To establish a stable and sensitive method of MRD detection is therefore also highly desirable.

REFRENCES

1. Trainor KJ, Brisco MJ, Wan JH, Neoh S. Grist S, Morley AA. (1991). Gene rearrangement in B-and T-lymphoproliferative disease detected by the polymerase chain reaction. Blood 78: 192-196

2. Wan JH,Trainor KJ,Brisco MJ, Morle AA. (1990). Monocolonality in B cell lymphoma detected in paraffin was embedded sections using the polymerase chain reaction. J Clin Pathol 43 888-890

3. Li Yu , Yan Sun, Qi Zhou, Jing-Zhong Liu, Fang-Ding Lou.(1995). Detection of minimal tumour cell in bone marrow of the patients with B-cell lineage neoplasms by PCR-SSCP. Chinese J Hematology 16 (7): 372.

4. Davis TH,Yockey CE,Balk SP. (1993) Detection of clonal immunoglobulin gene earrangement by polymerase chain reaction amplification and single strand conformational polymorphism analysis. Am J Pathol 142:1841-1847

5. Korsmeyer SJ, Arnold A, Bakhshi A.(1983) Immunoglobulin gene rearrangement and cell surface antigen expression in acute lymphocytic leukemias of T cell and B cell precursor origins. J Clin Invest 71:301-313

6. Liang R, Chan V, TK, Wong T, Chiu E. (1993) Detection of immunoglobulin gene rearrangement in lympoid malignancies of B-cell lineage by seminested polymerase chain reaction gene amplification. Am J Hematol 43: 24-28

7. Potter MN, Cross NCP, Van Dongen JJM. (1993) Molecular evidence of minimal residual disease after treatment for leukemia and lymphoma: an updated meeting report and review. Leukemia 7:1302

Marrow Transplantation and Stem Cell Transplantation in 1996
- The Developmental Perspective -

Robert A. Good

Department of Pediatrics, University of South Florida, All Children's Hospital, 801 Sixth Street South, St. Petersburg, Florida 33701-4899, USA

Today bone marrow transplantation is widely used as a life-saving approach to numerous otherwise fatal diseases. The use of marrow transplantation in the aggregate has grown rapidly indeed, almost geometrically, since the first allogeneic marrow transplantation was successfully applied in 1968 to cure otherwise fatal human disease. We can now count some 75 otherwise fatal diseases for which marrow transplantation can be employed as a life-saving measure and often to completely cure these diseases. For example, some 30 different primary immunodeficiency diseases have been treated successfully and for some of these otherwise highly lethal diseases including a wide variety of different genetically determined forms of severe combined immunodeficiency this treatment has impressively cured permanently the otherwise certainly fatal genetic disorder. Besides these many forms of primary immunodeficiency diseases, a number of different forms of aplastic anemia attributable to different pathogenetic mechanisms can be successfully treated in high frequency by BMT. In addition, allogeneic BMT has been successfully applied to the treatment and cure of several different forms of genetically determined abnormalities of hematopoietic development. These include thalassemia, sickle cell anemia, paroxysmal nocturnal hemoglobulinuria, persistent extreme forms of selective neutropenia and several other hematopoietic abnormalities that can frequently be successfully treated by marrow transplantation. These, too, may be highly lethal diseases.

However, the most frequent applications by bone marrow transplantation to save and extend healthful life has been the application of bone marrow transplantation, either allogeneic or autologous, to permit sufficiently intensive total body irradiation (TBI), plus chemotherapies to produce remissions and also sometimes to cure these highly fatal leukemias which cannot otherwise be cured by these modalities unless BMT is employed to permit long-lasting reconstruction of both hematopoietic and immunologic cellular systems. More recently, BMT has been proposed as a means to promote development of forms of immunologic tolerance which can be used to facilitate organ transplantation and because of the tolerant state to avoid the continuing or regular rejection episodes which assure that the transplanted organs will not experience immunologically-based destruction, some times over several years which underlie the fact that most organ transplants have a finite half life in 1996.

Finally, allogeneic or autologous BMT is also now being developed as a useful approach to facilitate and contribute to long-term survival and possibly cures of other kinds of malignancies which cannot be successfully treated by irradiation alone or irradiation plus chemotherapy unless BMT is used to permit such effective therapy by reconstituting the hematopoietic and immunologic systems with sufficient speed to permit use of sufficiently intense chemotherapy and irradiation therapy that eliminates or suppresses the life-threatening cancers.

It is the purpose of the current presentation to review briefly how the first clinical applications of bone marrow transplantation came about as well as to consider the preclinical and clinical scientific analyses that underlie possible application of bone marrow transplantation as a cure for immunodeficiency diseases, leukemias, abnormalities of myeloid cells, metabolic abnormalities, aplastic anemias and cancers. Of necessity, this brief review, because of limitations of time and space, cannot be exhaustive, but will focus to a major degree on personal experiences of the author and highlight the leading contributions of others to this development.

Our interest in the cells involved in immunologic functions and their relation to hematopoietic stem cells developed many years ago in Minnesota. There Fred Kolouch, a young hematologist and student of Hal Downey had been energized by the research of Bing and Plum, Danish pathologists (1), who noted that some patients with agranulocytosis exhibit bone marrow plasmacytosis while at the same time manifesting a rather striking hyperglobulinemia. These investigations drew these scientists to a rather audacious conclusion that perhaps the plasma cells by producing globulins were responsible for the hyperglobulinemia.

These findings struck a consonant note with Kolouch in Minneapolis who had at that time been following a patient with subacute bacterial endocarditis to death and upon post mortem examination discovered that in this patient both bone marrow and spleen were filled with plasma cells. This provocative observation by Kolouch added to his earlier studies with Downey in which he had also noted a striking plasmacytosis of bone marrow and other lymphoid tissues to occur in patients who suffered or died with tuberculosis and observations that in patients experiencing serum sickness plasmacytosis of bone marrow and, even some times of blood, accompanied the immunologically-based reaction (2). Consequently because of the implications of these several provocative Experiments of Nature, Kolouch designed and carried out laboratory experiments in which he showed that repeated injections of a vaccine prepared from *Streptococcus viridans* would regularly produce plasmacytosis of bone marrow especially if the young rabbits he was stimulating experienced anaphylactic shock. He drew the conclusion that his experiments might be taken to suggest that plasma cells are the cells that make antibodies which in turn are responsible for the anaphylaxis that along with plasmacytosis characterized his repeatedly stimulated rabbits (3,4). After completion of a masters degree with Downey (2), Kolouch finished his studies in medicine at the University of Minnesota and was taking fellowship training in surgery at the same time I was taking a combined PhD-MD curriculum at the University of Minnesota. Kolouch befriended me and urged me to help him prove his exciting thesis that plasma cells may represent the antibody-producing cell.

I recognized that Kolouch's linkup of plasma cells to antibody production, although most challenging, required a control for the influences of anaphylaxis (4,5). Thus, I carried out experiments in which I compared plasma cell development in bone marrow and spleen in rabbits subjected to either passive or active anaphylaxis. The design of my experiments which were among my very first experiments in immunology was to compare primary and secondary antibody production as a means of controlling for the influences of anaphylactic shock in development of plasma cells. Thus, I compared active versus passive anaphylaxis for ability to generate bone marrow and splenic plasmacytosis in rabbits. These experiments were revealing. They showed clearly that plasmacytosis in bone marrow and spleen was produced dramatically after secondary antigen exposure, whereas the response to primary exposure to the bacterial antigen did not generate readily identifiable plasmacytosis. The controls on anaphylaxis showed that anaphylaxis per se played no demonstrable role in generating plasmacytosis in either hematopoietic or lymphoid tissues (5).

These investigations were among the first independent experiments I had done. I published independently and thus launched my career in immunology. This career has been a career with a focus on functions of lymphocytes, stem cells and plasma cells. The thesis for my PhD degree at Minnesota thus was concerned with the usefulness of plasma cells in inflammatory exudates as crucial cells that signaled antibody production and hypersensitivity (6).

Following these studies, I showed that plasmacytosis could be generated regularly and quickly by a second injection or exposure to numerous different antigens following an effective primary stimulation. I showed this relationship to be true in many organs and tissues, even in the brain (6,7). I also carried out experiments in which I demonstrated in rather extensive studies that bone marrow (8), lymphoid tissue and even liver plasmacytosis (9,10) were related quite precisely to the formation and secretion of gammaglobulins and that gammaglobulin levels in the blood reflected plasmacytosis of the tissues, e.g. the bone marrow

My investigations took me to the Rockefeller Institute for study with Maclyn McCarty. There I was able to make observations on patients with Hodgkin's disease and multiple myeloma who I was investigating in other contexts (11). The observations on these patients suggested that there might be at least two different forms of immunity. The patients with Hodgkin's disease from whom I was obtaining pleural effusion fluids from which to try to crystallize C reactive protein seemed to be very susceptible to infections with TBC, fungi, e.g. cryptococci, and viruses. By contrast, when I was obtaining blood for comparative immunochemical studies of the monoclonal gammaglobulins, myeloma patients seemed to have major difficulties defending themselves against the what Rene Dubois taught me to call "high grade encapsulated bacterial pathogens" such as *Streptococcus pneumoniae, Streptococcus pyogenes, Hemophilus influenza* and also *Pseudomonas aeruginosa* (10,12).

Thus, these two groups of patients, myeloma and Hodgkin's disease patients appeared to be bisecting a microbial universe (10). In subsequent work, we found also that these two groups of patients had very different spectrums of immunodeficiencies. The Hodgkin's disease patients failed to develop what we called cell-mediated immunities including delayed type hypersensitivity and allograft rejections (12). The multiple myeloma patients promptly rejected skin grafts, whereas the Hodgkin's disease patients rejected skin grafts very slowly or not at all (10,12). The myeloma patients developed and expressed delayed allergies impressively, but associated with their serious disturbance of plasma cell development were unable to produce antibodies normally. Thus, as Experiments of Nature, these two groups of patients bisected not only the microbial universe, but also suggested an incisive dissection of the immunological universes (10-12).

Our dissection of the immunological universe had just begun when Col. Ogden Bruton (13) described the first patient with greatly increased susceptibility to infection attributable to agammaglobulinemia. Here was another Experiment of Nature which permitted further dissection of these relationships and bisection the microbial universe, the immunologic universe, and also the lymphoid universe.

At the time of Bruton's discovery, we were fortunate to have on our in patient service three boys - two of one family who also had further evidence of an X-linked genetic history. Further, during the following year we were referred five additional boys with agammaglobulinemia. Thus, all of our initial patients with agammaglobulinemia were boys and we were able to study our patients in considerable detail. From our rather extensive studies, we showed that patients with X-linked agammaglobulinemia bisected rather clearly the three separate but interrelated universes mentioned above. These patients like the myeloma patients, exhibited inordinate susceptibility to infections by high grade encapsulated extra cellular bacterial pyogenic pathogens, e.g. *Streptococcus pneumoniae, Hemophilus influenza, pseudomonas aeruginosa* and *Streptococcus pyogenes* and to a lesser extent staphylococci (14). These patients by contrast seemed capable of defending themselves against many viruses, e.g. chicken pox, measles and rubella viruses, bacteria of lower virulence, e.g. the tubercle bacilli, BCG infection or the several gram negative bacterial infections. We also discovered for the first time that the agammaglobulinemic patients could not produce plasma cells (15,16), nor could they produce germinal centers (15,16) even after repeated antigenic stimulation. Later we also recognized that the most peripheral cortical areas of lymph nodes of these patients were strikingly devoid of lymphocytes. By contrast in the deep cortical areas of lymph nodes, cells were abundant. Further, blood lymphocyte numbers were usually quite adequate in these patients (15,16). Further, these X-linked agammaglobulinemic patients regularly exhibited normal development and expression of delayed type allergy. Usually skin allograft rejection and allograft immunity were also present, even though they were unable to produce all kinds of antibodies. Thus, these patients with X-linked agammaglobulinemia like the myeloma and Hodgkin's disease patients as Experiments of Nature were bisecting sharply the immunological universes of cell-mediated immunities on the one hand and antibody production on the other (10,14,17). They also bisected the lymphoid cellular and tissue development into plasma cells, germinal centers, and Peyer's patches and the cells of far cortical regions of lymph node on the on hand, and lymphocytes of deep cortical areas of lymph nodes, later called paracortical cells, and small lymphocytes of blood on the other. They further bisected the microbial universe into two major groups of infections, one for which antibody production was crucial to the defense and one for which lymphocyte-based cell-mediated immunity was critical.

These crucial Experiments of Nature represented by patients with Hodgkin's disease and multiple myeloma and the very first population of children we studied with agammaglobulinemia, permitted development of concepts based on at least two separate populations of microorganisms and two separate cellular lymphoid systems involved in two different kinds of immunological defenses.

This dissection of the immunological defenses was further developed by the independent discovery by me and my group in Minneapolis and Miller in London that the thymus plays a crucial role in the development of bodily defense. For those of us working in Minnesota in those critical days, the initial direction of our investigations was, once again, provided by a patient who represented an important experiment of nature. The patient in question was F.H., a farmer from Western Minnesota who was called to our attention in 1952 (18,19). This patient actually thought he was addicted to the first of the tetracycline antibiotics called Terramycin. When he came to the University of Minnesota Hospitals, he had suffered repeatedly from pneumonia, at least eight episodes of pneumonia, which his doctor found could be treated with Terramycin. The patient discovered that whenever he became ill or felt poorly he could treat himself with Terramycin and he would promptly feel much better. However, when he stopped the Terramycin, his feeling of poor health promptly returned and pneumonias and/or sinus infections would recur. Because of this dependence on the antibiotic, he actually considered that he might be addicted to this new drug. We studied him with methods that reflected a developing capacity to evaluate the immune system and found, by our standards, that this patient had a very broadly based immunodeficiency indeed (14,19,20,21). It was an immunodeficiency that included all components of cell-mediated immunities, gross deficits of Ig as well as deficiency of antibody production to many different antigens. In addition, we discovered that this patient had a huge thymoma comprised of stromal-epithelial cells that occupied virtually his entire thymus. Removal of his thymus including the thymoma did not correct the severe cell-mediated and humoral immunologic deficits. The experience with immunodeficiency in this patient provoked us to inquire about what it is' the thymus does in mammalian biology.

To pursue the provocative Experiment of Nature posed by the thymoma-agammaglobulinemia patient further, we began our experimental approach by extirpating the thymus in very young rabbits -- rabbits only four weeks of age (22). These experiments carried out in 1955 and 1956 were not very revealing and with the analyses carried out in close temporal relationship to the thymectomy, no immunologic deficiency was produced by the thymectomy early in life. Because we considered our patient's thymic abnormality to be more telling than our first continued scientific experiment (19) using thymic extirpation, we continued to believe that the thymus might play a critical role in immunologic development and function. In 1957 after we had found that thymectomy in 4-week old bunnies did not produce readily demonstrable deficiencies in either humoral or cellular immunities, a personal communication from Harold Wolf in Wisconsin changed our entire view dramatically. Wolfe told me that Glick and his colleagues at Ohio State University (23,24) were right and that removal of the Bursa of Fabricius in newly hatched chickens prevented development of ability to produce antibodies. Glick had rather accidentally discovered that the thymus-like Bursa of Fabricius, which had actually been called the cloacal thymus by Jolly in 1911 (25) and 1914 (26) because of its developmental and histological similarities to the thymus, was essential to development of ability to produce antibodies. We promptly turned our entire laboratory's attention to neonatal extirpation of the thymus in several laboratory animals that included neonatal extirpation in mice, rabbits, rats and hamsters and, later, dogs.

Our experiments with mice and rabbits were promptly revealing (27,28). Neonatal thymectomy in rabbits, like bursectomy in Glick's newly hatched chickens, interfered with development of antibody-producing capacity to simple protein antigens. Neonatal thymectomy in mice prevented normal development of capacity to reject tumor or skin allografts (29). In short, neonatal thymectomy inhibited development of normal capacity for both humoral and cell-mediated immunities (30,31). About the same time we were carrying out our telling experiments, J.F.A.P. Miller in England was also experimenting with neonatal thymectomy. He had started his experiments from the perspective of Jacob Furth's discovery that leukemia in AKR mice is prevented by neonatal thymectomy. However, Miller not content only to study the influence of thymectomy in development of leukemia had also evaluated immunological function in the neonatally thymectomized mice and found that thymectomy of newborn mice of certain strains interfered dramatically with development of capacity for skin allograft rejection (32). There has been much controversy concerning whether it was Miller or me (with my associates) who discovered the key role of thymus in immunologic development. However, there is no way that we could have followed Miller's lead since our first research revealing the essential role of thymic functions in immunological development was submitted for presentation at the American Association of Immunologists Meeting in December 1960 and was presented by my fellow, Olga Archer and coauthored by one of my students, Pierce (27). Olga Archer was a visiting investigator in my laboratory and James Pierce, a young surgical fellow who was receiving his immunology training and working as a collaborator in my laboratory during 1960, 1961 and 1962. By the time of Archer's presentation to the American Association of Immunologists in April 1961, I could also summarize in the discussion of her paper our findings obtained in collaboration with Carlos Martinez and John Kersey, then a medical student (29,30,33). We had discovered that tumor immunities and skin allograft rejection, both within and across the MHC barrier were all prevented from developing in several mouse strains by neonatal thymectomy. I know that by the time all of our analyses had been presented, at least in outline, no one in the scientific community, including us, had heard any utterance from Miller. However, Miller's work presented first at a CIBA Symposium in June or July 1961 and published as a paper in Lancet (32), which came out in November 1961, has been considered by many to reflect the discovery of the role of thymus in immunologic development. Our extensive series of formal scientific papers were also appropriately published in the Proceedings of the Society for Experimental Biology and Medicine (29), Nature (28) and the Journal of Experimental Medicine (30).

That the time was right for Miller and me independently to discover the critical role played by the thymus in developmental biology is emphasized by the fact that several other scientists also had telling experiments underway on this issue at the time or shortly after we discovered the critical role of thymus in immunologic development (34,35).

Because of all of the interest in the role played by the thymus in developmental immunobiology. I organized a watershed conference on the thymus in Minneapolis in October 1962 where everyone that I could find who was working with the thymus had an opportunity to have his or her say. One highlight of that conference was a presentation by Warner, a young Australian who described his work with Szenberg (36,37). They had induced bursectomy and thymectomy or both by complex hormonal manipulations, e. g. using egg dipping into a solution of testosterone and had concluded that the thymus and bursa fulfill separate functions. They concluded that these two organs influence the development of separate lymphoid cell populations. However, in light of our perspective that had been derived from the interaction of our basic analyses and the contribution of the Experiments of Nature we had studied, we considered that the grouping of functions of the cell systems proposed by Warner and Szenberg (37) must be incorrect. They had concluded that antibodies and plasma cells, as well as delayed allergies, were all functions of the influence of the Bursa of Fabricius on lymphoid development. By contrast, the thymus they considered to be responsible for allograft immunity. However, to them graft versus host reactions were not an immune function that developed under either thymus or bursal influence (37).

Because of this disagreement, we were determined to reinvestigate in chickens the comparative functions of thymus and Bursa of Fabricius. Ray Peterson, a young associate professor of Pediatrics in Minneapolis and who was especially interested in origins of malignant cells as well as the nature of immunodeficiency diseases, led these investigations and Max Cooper, a new research fellow in our laboratory, who also was already trained as a pediatrician and qualified as an allergist, chose to work with Peterson on the analyses of the functions of thymus and Bursa on immunity and lymphoid development. After a period of planning, Peterson organized and arranged collaborative research with Ben Burmester and his coworkers at the regional poultry laboratories at East Lansing, Michigan. Employing newly hatched chickens subjected to near lethal total body irradiation and then also subjected to either bursectomy or thymectomy, or to both bursectomy and thymectomy were analyzed. With this experimental design, they showed, as suggested by our prior clinical pathologic investigations of X-linked agammaglobulinemia, that plasma cells in red pulp and germinal centers went together and their development was clearly dependent on the Bursa of Fabricius in chickens (38,39). In the irradiated newly hatched chickens, by contrast thymectomy inhibited development of other lymphoid aggregates of white pulp, which were mostly comprised small lymphocytes. Thymectomy in the newly hatched chickens also inhibited allograft rejection, capacity of the spleen cells to initiate graft versus host reactions and capacity to develop and express all forms of cell-mediated (delayed) allergy. Newly hatched x-irradiated chickens from which both thymus and bursa had been removed shortly after hatching developed neither plasma cells or germinal centers, nor did they develop the small aggregates of lymphocytes in the white pulp of spleen (38,39). Further, in the thymectomized plus bursectomized irradiated population of chickens, basically all immune functions and all lymphoid cells were prevented from developing (38,39). From these investigations, we could conclude that in chickens two distinct central lymphoid organs, the thymus that was responsible for small lymphocytes and all the cell-mediated immune functions, the bursa, which was responsible for larger lymphocytes, germinal centers, plasma cells and also antibody production.   Thus, we visualized two separate central lymphoid organs responsible for development of two separate populations of peripheral lymphoid tissues (38,39,40).

Pierson Van Alten, an embryologist from the University of Illinois who was on sabbatical leave in my laboratories, then carried out important experiments which eliminated any concern that the near fatal irradiation employed in our immunologic and lymphoid dissection may have produced crucial and differential influences.   He developed methods to thymectomize or bursectomize chick embryos *in ovo* during late embryonation and these operations employed no irradiation.   His findings showed that exactly the same dissection of lymphoid development could be achieved as with the irradiated newly hatched chickens, but in his system the dissection was possible in the complete absence of the influence of irradiation (41).

When Max Cooper presented our basic experiments in the chickens at the American Pediatric Society Meeting in 1965 (42), Angelo DiGeorge who was in the audience hastened to describe (43), in the discussion period, patients he and his associates had been studying in Pittsburgh.   In these patients, failure of thymic development and absence of thymus occurred along with failure of development of parathyroid glands and in the presence of cardiac outflow tract abnormalities in the infants.   These infants had defective cell-mediated immunities.   They had lymph nodes which showed virtually no cells in the deep cortical or paracortical regions.   However, these patients had plasma cells in the lamina propria of the gastrointestinal tract and lymph nodes, but developed germinal centers poorly.   These patients seemed to represent a striking counter point to the patients with X-linked agammaglobulinemia and they had basically normal amounts of IgM, IgG and IgA, but often had low IgA levels.   They seemed most similar to the model of immunodeficiency produced in chickens by irradiation plus   thymectomy in the newly hatched period.   They also were featured by hypocalcemia, low set abnormal ears, a characteristic small bowed mouth and micrognathia (44).   Our extensive studies of human immunodeficiency diseases in the clinic, taken together with our investigations of immunodeficiencies produced by neonatal thymectomy in rabbits and mice or in newly hatched chickens and bursectomy or thymectomy and bursectomy in irradiated newly hatched chickens, permitted us then to define human immunodeficiency diseases in the context of our new view of development of the lymphoid system and immunological functions as they now appeared to relate to the lymphoid cell populations (45).

Thus, we considered the X-linked agammaglobulinemic children to have an immunological and lymphoid cellular deficiency similar to that produced by bursectomy in irradiated newly hatched chickens.   Both exhibit deficiencies of plasma cell and germinal center development, both have a normal thymus and normal thymus-dependent lymphoid system.   The DiGeorge syndrome patients suffered from failure to develop thymus and thymus-dependent lymphoid systems. These patients had lymphoid system and immunity functional deficit-like those produced by neonatal thymectomy in mice or thymectomy in newly hatched irradiated chickens.   Finally, the several forms of severe combined immunodeficiency which I had by that time named the Swiss type agammaglobulinemia to recognize outstanding contributions concerning these diseases by Glanzmann and Riniker (46), Tobler and Cottier (47), Hitzig and Willi (48) and Barandun (49,50), were like the newly hatched irradiated chickens that had been subjected to both thymectomy and bursectomy in the newly hatched period.

With this very exciting experience of seeing both basic and clinical investigation contribute to generation of new understanding of the primary immunodeficiency diseases and also the normal development of the immune system, we constructed a scheme in which we proposed that the lymphoid cells must develop as two separate arms from pluripotent lymphoid stem cells under the guiding influence of thymus or bursal equivalent which via separate biologic amplification systems addressed fundamental effector processes. These schemes defined separate central and peripheral lymphoid system development, from putative lymphoid stem cells in marrow (51). Our new position concerning lymphoid tissues was coupled with increasing understanding of the development of the hematopoietic systems, as well as developing knowledge of transplantation immunity and immunologic tolerance. It thus became quite natural to begin to consider the possibility of treating primary immunodeficiencies by bone marrow transplantation (stem cell transplantation).

Lorenz, Uphoff et al (52). in mice had showed that the entire hematopoietic system, as well as the entire lymphoid system could be reconstructed by bone marrow transplantation of marrow from syngeneic donors. A bit later, Uphoff et al (53) showed that MHC-matched bone marrow transplants could also be effective in reconstructing hematopoiesis and lymphopoiesis in mice. Thus, in irradiated mice, BMT from a syngeneic donor, or from an H2 matched donor could reconstruct the entire hematopoietic and also the lymphopoietic system. Prehn and Main (54) showed also that bone marrow transplantation in mice could induce a tolerant state in skin allografts in the recipient mice even when the transplant was achieved across MHC barriers.

During the same period in which we were developing our concepts of the nature and development of the two major lymphoid systems, as well as the two distinct but of course interactive immunity systems, Thomas and his coworkers were doing crucial fundamental research in bone marrow transplantation working with pen bred Beagle dogs (55,56). They have showed that in relatively rare instances BMT could cure and correct the hematological and immunological responsiveness after lethal total body irradiation in their Beagle dogs. From their experiences, they concluded that it might be possible to treat and even to cure leukemias by using BMT. Experiments using BMT in leukemic patients following lethal total body irradiation followed by transplantation from identical twin donors (57,58), although not curing the leukemia at that time, showed that marrow transplantation with fully matched donors could reconstruct the entire hematopoietic system in humans as well as in experimental animals.

With this backdrop of preclinical and clinical investigation and after we had constructed our new view of lymphoid development, Fig. 1 (59), we considered that the time was ripe to attempt to cure SCID disease by BMT.

We first made an attempt to cure SCID by performing a fetal liver cell transplantation. However, this effort failed when an inadvertent blood transfusion from an unmatched donor produced a fatal graft versus host disease (60). We then wrote a theoretical paper in which we proposed that the way to cure severe combined immunodeficiency or the so called Swiss type agammaglobulinemia in humans was to employ a bone marrow transplant to provide normal stem cells which could be expected to replace abnormal or defective stem cells which had led to development of the grossly deficient development of both of the two major immunity systems. To avoid lethal graft versus host disease, I proposed we attempt to use as donor an MHC-match sibling which we might expect to be perfectly matched at the MHC one time in four (61).

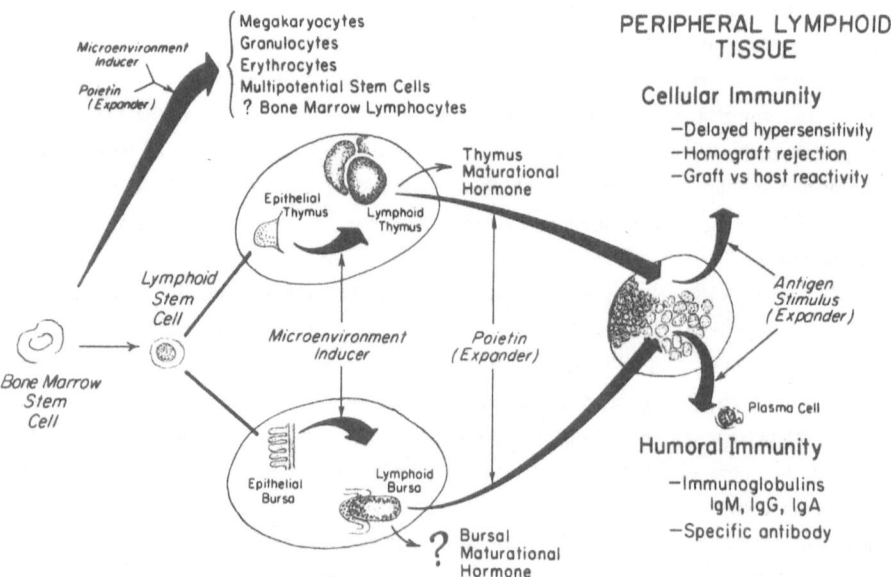

Fig. 1   Scheme defining differentiation of the bone marrow stem cell. Note that there are two lines of differentiation of the lymphoid stem cell: a thymus-dependent population, which gives rise to lymphocytes responsible for the cell-mediated immunological responses, and a thymus-independent/bursal-dependent population, which is ultimately responsible for plasma cell development and immunoglobular synthesis.

Perhaps, fortunately, for us no one accepted the challenge we had presented and we ourselves had the first opportunity to attempt to cure an otherwise certainly lethal disease by BMT. This opportunity came when Dr. L'Heureux of Meridan, Connecticut, referred to us in June 1968 a male infant with SCID who had four normal healthy female siblings.   This patient was the 12th male child over three generations to suffer from this form of SCID.   The disease had been fatal in all eleven of the male children of the family who had this disease previously. Although as was current technology of the time, our tissue typing of the patient and his sisters was not perfect we interpreted the data to reveal that our patient with X-linked SCID was well enough matched with one of his sisters to permit an attempt to cure his otherwise surely fatal disease by BMT. Thus, in early August 1968, we performed a BMT (62) from this MHC best-matched sister to our patient with SCID. Within two months, evidence of correction of the immunodeficiency disease was apparent. However, the BMT in the patient had induced a severe graft versus host disease, one feature of which was an aplastic anemia. Everyone familiar with my clinical research argued that I should attempt to eliminate the graft which had produced the rather dramatic immunologic correction but also the aplastic anemia that so dramatically had complicated this initial BMT with which we were trying to cure his SCID. I could not agree because first of all I did not know how to eliminate the BMT and, second, because at best this approach would only get us back to where our effort at treatment had begun -- namely to the certainly fatal SCID with which we had started. Instead, I proposed we should give a second BMT from the same quite well matched sibling donor in an effort to cure for the first time a form of aplastic anemia (63). This second graft of bone marrow from the same MHC-matched sister-donor was carried out and it produced in dramatic fashion full correction of the aplastic anemia. This graft also strengthened the initial lymphoid cellular graft which together corrected fully the child's SCID (63-66).

Following this second BMT, the child thrived, graft versus host reaction abated, immunologic reconstruction proceeded and the patient ended up completely cured of not one but two otherwise regularly fatal diseases using BMT. The recipient has lived a normal life for 27 years (64-66). He is a complete bone marrow chimera since all the cells which are diving or can be made to divide have a female cellular karyotype and thus are clearly derived from his sister. He has thrived in vigorous good health and now has grown up and is happily married and has fraternal twin boys who are perfectly normal in every way (66).

This patient thus experienced the first two completely curative bone marrow transplants from an MHC matched sibling donor and the two bone marrow transplantations given to him cured two otherwise lethal diseases, the genetically determined SCID and the aplastic anemia which was iatrogenic and immunologically based.

Our achievement with this patient was consolidated both by our own further experience with BMT and also by confirmatory successful BMT to cure other forms of immunodeficiency. Wiskott-Aldrich syndrome that had to be treated by lethal doses of cyclophosphamide plus BMT was partially cured. The WAS treatment represented the first instance where highly lethal cyclophosphamide plus BMT at least partially corrected the hematological and immunodeficiency disease represented by WAS (67). A confirmatory and successful BMT was then carried out in Holland in the year following our dramatic bone marrow transplantations and was like our case dramatically successful in curing a child who suffered from the otherwise regularly lethal form of BMT in tissue matched sibling dogs (69,70) of the autosomal recessive SCID of the Swiss type (68).

Following our success to cure the initial X-SCID patient by BMT, we subsequently were able to treat successfully and cure completely 5/6 children with three different forms of SCID over the subsequent four years.

Shortly following our success with the initial patient with SCID and following their demonstration of regular success also employing MHC (69,70) matched sibling donors, Thomas and his colleagues did their first allogeneic BMT transplants in an effort to treat leukemia. BMT which was shown also to contribute to curing acute myeloid leukemia cured the leukemia in only 11 of the first 100 patients. That was when BMT was used as a last resort (71). However, BMT plus irradiation and chemotherapy achieved a real advantage over any chemotherapy for these patients at that time. Thus, in further earth shaking clinical research with acute myeloid leukemia it became possible for this group in Seattle to treat acute myeloid leukemia by BMT during first remission and to cure or produce long-term remissions of the acute myeloid leukemia in nearly 60% of these patients (72).

The problem with needing to employ an MHC matched sibling donor for curative BMT was that an MHC matched sibling donor could be located in only about 30-35% of American families. This discouraging fact has been addressed now in several ways. We showed that in extended families a matched non-sibling donor could occasionally be identified who was suitable to make possible a successful and curative BMT (73). We also found that an occasional donor from the general population might be available which was a suitable for treatment of an otherwise fatal disease (74,75).

Reisner, working as a predoctoral fellow in Sharon's laboratory used serial lectin agglutination, plus differential centrifugation that employed soybean and peanut lectins to remove the T lymphoid cells from marrow or marrow plus spleen cell preparations and thus to cure animals from hematological and lymphocytic deficits produced by lethal total body irradiation (76). When I became aware of his work, I asked Reisner to come to our laboratory to help us prepare human bone marrow so that it could be used when donor and recipient were imperfectly matched to permit bone marrow transplantation when no suitably MHC matched donor was available. With the anti T cell antiserum available for humans, we could not completely remove dangerous T cells and T precursors from human marrow. The method Reisner had development for mice that removed dangerous T cells and also apparently dangerous immediate precursor of T cells from mouse marrow did not work in humans. Thus, Reisner had to develop a new lectin-based method to permit BMT in humans in which donor and recipient were not perfectly matched at MHC. Reisner's work in my laboratory was most successful. He employed the soybean lectin as agglutinin and also sheep RBC as lectins to permit removal of T cells and T precursors when a prospective marrow donor was not perfectly matched at MHC (77).

In short, after much hard work, Reisner showed that the hazardous T cells and T cell precursors could be removed by agglutination and differential centrifugation using soy bean agglutinin and SRBC lectin (77). This made possible haploidentical BMT from mother or father to child which permitted us to cure SCID when by a maternal or paternal BMT was available but no MHC matched sibling was available (78). This method has now been applied to cure large numbers of children with different forms of SCID when no matched sibling is available (79,80).

However, initially the selective removal of T cells and T cell precursors with soybean and sheep RBC lectins did not always work well to permit curing of leukemia (81,82). Instead recurrence of leukemia took place in too high a frequency after haploidentical T cell purged marrow transplants were used (82). However, more recently bone marrow transplantation or T cell purged bone marrow from haploidentical donors coupled with peripheral blood preparations of stem cells following stimulation of donor with growth factors to harvesting stem cells and, then again, removal of T cells from these preparations have led to more encouraging results with hematopoietic cells from haploidentical donors. Such relatively complex cell preparations might also prove of value if one is attempting to extend current treatment for diseases other than leukemias as well as the leukemias with which Reisner has been working (82).

It is encouraging that preclinical experimental analyses of T cell purged haploidentical marrow transplantation in mice has permitted full immunologic and hematologic reconstruction after lethal total body irradiation plus dimethylmyleran treatment that was used for immunosuppression plus myeloablation. The mice transplanted from haploidentical donors experience vigorous life in conventional environments and exhibit full vigor of many cell-mediated immunities and normal full capacity for production of all forms of antibody without demonstrable immunologic deficits.

The reconstruction of the two lymphoid systems plus all immunologic functions using marrow from haploidentical donors have regularly been most impressive as a means of treatment of all forms of SCID. If abnormal B lymphocytes are abundant in the patient with SCID and are not or cannot be removed from the recipient donor as is the case in some children, deficits of Ig and antibody production may remain while T cell-mediated immunities are fully reconstructed. Such patients may require treatment with IVIG following the otherwise life-saving BMT which thus far has been very long lasting.

National Marrow Donor Program

Further to solution of the problem of availability of donors for stem cell transplantations when a matched sibling donor is not available a registry of tissue typed or partially tissue typed donors which may be further matched with the recipient according to most advanced typing methods are now available in several countries, including the United States (83-86). Most of these registries are interactive with one another. Thus, the number of volunteers in the American Marrow Donor Program now exceeds 1.75 million volunteer donors and nearly 2.5 million volunteer donors are available in all the registries put together. The use of volunteer marrow donor is an extremely valuable approach and will be discussed elsewhere in this volume by John Hanson of the Seattle Bone Marrow Transplant Program who is a leader in this field (85,86).

Fetal Stem Cell Transplantations

Finally, recent investigations have shown that cellular engineering as with BMT can also often be achieved and some times with impressive advantage over the usual BMT by employing cells of fetal origin (87-93). Such cells are found in sufficient numbers in cord blood obtained from human placenta to achieve full reconstruction of both hematopoiesis, lymphopoiesis and also full immunologic reconstitution. To date well over one hundred cord blood transplants have already been used to treat numerous different diseases that include leukemias treated with TBI plus cyclophosphamide and/or other myeloablative and/or immunosuppressive regimens. Further, numerous aplastic anemias, Fanconi syndrome, X-SCID, SCID of several other types and cellular hematopoietic disturbances (88-91). It is already indicated from these studies that fetal blood obtained from the placentas at delivery possess stem cells that may have significant advantages over bone marrow as a source of stem cells (91-93). For example, a smaller number of cord blood cells may be sufficient to achieve full reconstruction of the hematopoietic systems and lymphoid systems. Graft versus host reactions and GVH disease may be less of a problem with cord blood cells than with transplants of marrow. Further, graft versus host reactions may also respond better to treatment when the GVHD has been produced by cord blood cells than when they are caused by bone marrow cells (94).

Only time will give a complete answer as to the value of cord blood for cellular engineering. Cord blood banks are being developed for treatment of many patients with primary immunodeficiencies, aplastic anemias, Fanconi syndrome, leukemias, cancers, developmental abnormalities of hematopoietic system and numerous other diseases. For the present, it is encouraging to note that full immunologic and hematologic reconstitution can be achieved by fetal stem cells contained in the cord blood. Although originally it seemed likely that the number of cells and the number of stem cells obtainable from cord blood might not be sufficient to achieve hematopoietic and lymphopoietic reconstitution of patients which are larger than infants or young children (95). That view has now been shown to be fallacious since older children (96) fully mature normal sized females and even patients as large as a 74 kg male have been successfully reconstituted following total body irradiation using only a single cord blood transplant (94). During reconstitution, granulocytic lineage and of megakaryocyte lineage and platelet counts seems to be reconstituted slightly slower after cord blood transplants than is observed following bone marrow transplantation. By contrast, reconstitution of immunologic functions may occur even more rapidly following transplantation with a single cord blood preparation than following bone marrow transplantation (94). Hal Broxmeyer of Indianapolis (89), Pablo Rubinstein of New York (93,94), Kurtzberg of Durham, Gluckman (90) in France and Wagner of Minneapolis (91), have had the most experience with cord blood transplantation. Indeed, each of these scientists have monitored the experiences with cord blood transplants quite precisely. From their reports and personal communications to us, it would appear that the future of cord blood transplantation will be very bright.

Several advantages over bone marrow transplants have already been indicated in research on treatment with cord blood from cord blood banks over bone marrow transplants. Among these are the following:

1. The cord blood is a cell population that is usually discarded as waste along with the placental membranes after all normal pregnancies.

2. At least 4 million deliveries are carried out each year from which this valuable resource has not been used.

3. With proper organization, a high proportion of these cord blood samples might be available in the form of cord blood banks to provide cord blood for transplantation as it is needed.

4.   Infections and infestations in the fetus are very few. As an example, cytomegalovirus (CMV) infection which may potentially and frequently compromise bone marrow transplants and thus represents a threat to the transplant recipients in 60-100% of bone marrow donors. By contrast, with cord blood less than 1% of cord blood appear to contain cells infected by CMV. Similar relationships may hold for a number of other infections that are common in adults but uncommon in the fetus.

5.   It appears to be a real possibility, perhaps because of the relative immaturity of the transplanted cells, that greater MHC disparity may be tolerated when cord blood cells are transplanted than when marrow cells are used. Perhaps mechanisms involved in development of immunologic tolerance are more likely to be engaged when cord blood transplants are employed than when bone marrow cells are used. At any rate, matching at 5/6 MHC determinants seems quite adequate for cord blood transplants and current evaluation of 4 of 6 MHC matched cord blood transplants are underway and being evaluated.

6.   The ready availability of the typed frozen cord blood cells for transplant makes possible prompt treatment of disease as is often necessary. The typed cord blood cells are ready to go and can be transplanted promptly after being appropriately matched, e.g., by DNA typing.

7.   With only 5,000 cord blood preparations in Rubinstein's Bank in New York City, it appears that as high a frequency of satisfactory matches is being achieved as can be accomplished with the 1.7 million volunteers in the National Marrow Donor Program (94).

8.   Cord blood banks might work even better than with complex populations like that of the United States when the population is more homogenous as in Japan. African Americans population of the United States exhibits an incredibly broad MHC heterogeneity.

History is Still Very Short

One must keep in mind that the clinical application of cord blood banks as a highly functional source of hematopoietic and lymphopoietic stem cells and adaptable hematopoietic and lymphopoietic precursors is at a very early stage of development and long-term results of cord blood transplants are not yet available. However, for most scientists working in this area, the prospects for cord blood transplantation look encouraging.

Summary

In summary, the perspective we have tried to provide in this brief review is simple. For us it started from contributions to understanding the nature and development of the lymphoid and hematopoietic systems which raised the possibility of the full reconstitution from stem cells after failure of development or following their complete destruction as with irradiation and chemotherapy. These contributions plus developing understanding from certain human patients as experiments of nature permitted development of sufficient insight into the pathogenesis of human immunodeficiency diseases and histological diseases including leukemias to permit initial efforts at bone marrow transplantation and also of fetal tissue transplantation. The art and science of bone marrow transplantation to permit treatment of human diseases has developed rapoidly and the possibility of using cells of fetal origin has been introduced and this field too is developing at a great rate. Indeed, fetal cord blood cell transplantation may have real advantages over bone marrow transplantation. Possible additional applications of these resources, already addressing more than 75 fatal diseases for approaching treatment of additional hazardous or fatal diseases is being pursued. Stem cell resources are also being defined precisely because these may become targets of molecular engineering which can extend this development much further (97).

KEY WORDS:bone marrow transplantation (BMT), stem cell transplantation

Acknowledgement

I thank Ms. Tazim Verjee for manuscript preparation.

References

1. Bing, J. and Plum, P.: Serum proteins in leucopenia. (Contribution on question about place of formation of serum proteins), Acta Med. Scaninav. 92:415-428, 1937;1 also, Ugesk. f. laeger 99:738-743, 1937.

2. Kolouch, F.: A study of the bone marrow plasma cell of mammals with special reference to its origin in the rabbit under normal and experimental conditions. Thesis, University of Minnesota, pp. 1-84, 1938.

3. Kolouch, F.: Origin of bone marrow plasma cell associated with allergic and immune states in rabbits. Proc. Soc. Exper. Biol. & Med., 39:147-148, 1938.

4. Kolouch, F., Good, R.A. and Campbell, B.: The reticulo-endothelial origin of the bone marrow plasma cells in hypersensitive states. J. Lab. Clin. Med. 32:749-755, June, 1947.

5. Good, R.A.: Effect of passive sensitization and anaphylactic shock on rabbit bone marrow. Proc. Soc. Exp. Biol. Med. 67:203-205, 1948.

6. Good, R.A.: The morphologic mechanisms of hyperergic inflammation in the brain; with special reference to the significance of local plasma cell formation. Ph.D. dissertation, the Graduate School of the University of Minnesota, November, 1947.

7. Good, R.A.: Experimental allergic brain inflammation, a morphological study. J. Neuropathol. Exp. Neurol. 9:78-92, January, 1950.

8. Good, R.A. and Campbell, B.: Relationship of bone marrow plasmacytosis to the changes in serum gamma globulin in rheumatic fever. Am. J. Med. 9:330-342, September, 1950.

9. Page, A.R. and Good, R.A.: Plasma cell hepatitis, with special attention to steroid therapy. A.M.A. J. Dis. Child. 99:288-314, March, 1960.

10. Good, R.A.: Morphological basis of the immune response and hypersensitivity. In: Host-Parasite Relationships in Living Cells (H.M. Felton, et al., eds.). Springfield, Illinois, Charles C. Thomas, pp. 78-160, 1957.

11. Kunkel, H.G., Slater, R.J. and Good, R.A.: Relation between certain myeloma proteins and normal gamma globulin. Proc. Soc. Exp. Biol. Med. 76:190-193, 1951.

12. Kelly, W.D., Good, R.A.and Varco, R.L.: Anergy and skin homograft survival in Hodgkin's disease. Surg. Gynecol. Obstet. 107:565-570, November 1958.

13. Bruton, O.C.: Agammaglobulinemia. Pediatrics 9:722, 1952.

14. Good, R.A. and Zak, S.J.: Disturbances in gamma globulin synthesis as "experiments of nature". Pediatric 18:109-149, July, 1956.

15. Good, R.A.: Studies of agammaglobulinemia. II. Failure of plasma cell formation in the bone marrow and lymph nodes of patients with agammaglobulinemia. J. Lab. Clin. Med. 56:167-181, 1955.

16. Good, R.A.: Absence of plasma cells from bone marrow and lymph nodes following antigenic stimulation in patients with agammaglobulinemia. Revue d' Hematol. 9:502-503, 1954.

17. Good, R.A. and Varco, R.L.: A clinical and experimental study of agammaglobulinemia. In: Essays on Pediatrics, in Honor of Irvine McQuarrie (R.A.

Good and E.S. Platou, Eds.), Minneapolis, Lancet Publications, pp. 103-129, 1955.

18.   Good, R.A.: Agammaglobulinemia -- a provocative experiment of nature.   Bull. Univ. Minn. Hosp. Minn. Med. Found. 26:1-19, October, 1954.

19.   MacLean, L.D., Zak, S.J., Varco, R.L. and Good, R.A.:   Thymic tumor and acquired agammaglobulinemia: a clinical and experimental study of the immune response. *Surgery* 40:1010-1017, 1956.

20.   Good, R.A. and Varco, R.L.:   A clinical and experimental study of agammaglobulinemia.   J. Lancet 75:245-271, June, 1955.

21.   Mazzitello, W.F. and Good, R.A.:   Agammaglobulinemia.   Minn. Med. 39:308, May, 1956.

22.   MacLean, L.D., Zak, S.J., Varco, R.L. and Good, R.A.:   The role of the thymus in antibody production: an experimental study of the immune response in thymectomized rabbits.   Transplant. Bull. 4:21, 1957.

23.   Glick, B., Chang, T.S. and Jaap, R.G.:   The bursa of Fabricius and antibody production. Poult. Sci. 35:224, 1956.

24.   Glick, B.:   Further evidence for the role of the bursa of Fabricius in antibody production. Poultry Sci. 37:240, 1958.

25.   Jolly, J.:   Sur la function hematopoietique de la burse de fabricius.   Comple. Rend. Soc. Biol.   70:498, 1911.

26.   Jolly, J.: Sur les mouvements amiboides des petites cellules de la bourse de Fabricius et du thymus.   C.R. Soc. Biol. 77:148, 1914.

27.   Archer, O.K. and Pierce, J.C.:   Role of the thymus in development of the immune response. Fed. Proc. 20:26, 1961.

28.   Archer, O.K., Pierce, J.C., Papermaster, B.W. and Good, R.A.:   Reduced antibody response in thymectomized rabbits.   Nature 191:191-192, July 14, 1962.

29.   Martinez, C., Kersey, J., Papermaster, B.W. and Good, R.A.:   Skin homograft survival in thymectomized mice.   Proc. Soc. Exp. Biol. Med.   109:193-196, 1962.

30.   Good, R.A., Dalmasso, A.P., Martinez, C., Archer, O.K., Pierce, J.C. and
      Papermaster, B.W.:   The role of the thymus in development of immunologic
      capacity in rabbits and mice.   J. Exp. Med. 116:773-796, November, 1962.

31.   Archer, O.K., Papermaster, B.W. and Good, R.A.:   Thymectomy in rabbit and
      mouse: consideration of time and lymphoid peripheralization.   In: The
      Thymus in Immunobiology: Structure, Function, and Role in Disease (R.A. Good and
      A.E. Gabrielsen, Eds.), New York, Hoeber-Harper, pp. 414-435 1964.

32.   Miller, J.F.A.P.:   Immunological function of the thymus.   Lancet 2:748, 1961

33.   Good, R.A.:   Discussion of Archer-Pierce presentation at The Federation of American
      Society of Experimental Biology, April 1961.

34.   Waksman, B.H., Arnason, B.G. and Jankovic, B.D.:   Role of the thymus in immune
      reactions in rats. IV. Changes in lymphoid organs of thymectomized rats.   J. Exp. Med.
      116:187, 1962.

35.   Parrott, J.M., DeSoussa, M.a.B. and East, J.:   Thymus-dependent areas in the lymphoid
      organs of neonatally thymectomized mice.   J. Exp. Med. 123:191, 1966.36.

36.   Warner, N.L., Szenberg, A. and Burnet, F.M.:   The immunological role of different
      lymphoid organs in the chicken.   I.   Dissociation of immunological responsiveness.
      Australian J. Exper. Biol. & M. Sc. 40:373, 1962.

37.   Warner, N.L. and Szenberg, A.:   Immunologic studies on hormonally bursectomized and
      surgically thymectomized chickens: dissociation of immunologic responsiveness.   In: *The
      Thymus in Immunobiology* (R.A. Good and A.E. Gabrielsen, Eds.), Harper and Row
      Publishers, New York. pp. 395-435, 1964.

38.   Cooper, M.D., Peterson, R.D.A. and Good, R.A.:   Delineation of the thymic and bursal
      lymphoid systems in the chicken.   Nature 205:143-146, January 9, 1965.

39.   Cooper, M.D., Peterson, R.D.A., South, M.A. and Good, R.A.:   The functions of the
      thymus system and the bursa system in the chicken.   J. Exp. Med. 123:75-102, January,
      1966.

40.   Good, R.A., Gabrielsen, A.E., Cooper, M.D. and Peterson, R.D.A.: The role of the
      thymus and bursa of Fabricius in the development of effector mechanisms. Ann. N.Y.

Acad. Sci. 129:130, 1966.

41.   van Alten, P.J., Cain, W.A., Good, R.A. and Cooper, M.D.:   Gamma globulin production and antibody synthesis in chickens bursectomized as embryos.   Nature 217:358, 1968

42.   Cooper, M.D., Peterson, R.D.A. and Good, R.A.:   A new concept of the cellular basis of immunity.   J. Ped. 67:907, 1965b.

43.   DiGeorge, A.M.:   Discussion (following presentation by M.D. Cooper).   Perlman and Good, J. Ped. 67:908, 1965.

44.   DiGeorge, A.M.:   Congenital absence of the thymus and its immunologic consequences: concurrence with congenital hypoparathyroidism.   In *Immunologic Deficiency Diseases in Man*. (D. Bergsma and R.A. Good, Eds.), New York, National Foundation Press, (Birth Defects: Original Article Series, Vol. IV, No. 1), pp. 116-150, 1968.

45.   Peterson, R.D.A., Cooper, M.D. and Good, R.A.:   The pathogenesis of immunologic deficiency diseases.   Am J. Med. 38:579-604, April, 1965.

46.   Glanzmann, E. and Riniker, P.:   Essentielle lymphocytophthise. Ein neues Krankheitsbild aus der Sauglingspathologie.   Ann. Paediat. (Basel) 17:1, 1950.

47.   Tobler, R. and Cottier, H.:   Familiare lymphopenie mit agammaglobulinamie und schwerer moniliasis.   Helvet. Pediatr. Acta 13:313, 1958.

48.   Hitzig, W.H. and Willi, H.: Hereditare lymphoplasmocytare Dysgenesie ("Alymphocytose mit Agammaglobulinamie").   Schweiz. med. Wschr. 91:1625, 1961.

49.   Barandun, S., Huser, J.J. and Hassig, A.:   Klinishce erscheinungsformen des antikorpermangelsyndroms.   Schweiz. med. Wschr. 88:78, 1958.

50.   Cottier,   H.   and   Barandun,   S.:   Morphologische   Poathologie   des Antikorpermangelsyndroms.   In: Das Antikopermangelsyndrom Benno Schwabe and Co., Verlag, Basel-Stuttgart, p. 461, 1959.

51.   Cooper, M.D., Perey, D.Y., Peterson, R.D.A., Gabrielsen, A.E. and Good, R.A.:   The two-component concept of the lymphoid system.   In: Immunologic Deficiency Diseases in Man (D. Bergsma and R.A. Good, eds.), New York, The National Foundation, 1968, pp. 7-16 (Birth Defects: Original Article Series, Vol. IV, No. 1, 1968).

52.   Lorenz, E, Uphoff, D., Reid, T.R. and Shelton, E.:   Modification of irradiation injury in
       mice and guinea pigs by bone marrow injections. J. Natl. Cancer Inst. 12:197-201, 1951.

53.   Uphoff, D.E.:   Alteration of homograft reaction by Amethoptein in lethally irradiated mice
       treated with homologous marrow,.   Proc. Soc. Exp. Biol. Med. 99:651, 1958.

54.   Main, J.M. and Prehn, R.T.:   Successful skin homografts after the administration of high
       dosage X radiation and homologous bone marrow.   J. Natl. Cancer Inst. 15:1023, 1955.

55.   Thomas, E.D., LeBlond, R., Graham, T.C. and Storb, R.:   Marrow infusions in dogs
       given midlethal or lethal irradiation.   Radiat. Res. 41:113-124, 1970.

56.   Storb, R. and Thomas, E.D.:   Bone marrow transplantation in randomly bred animal
       species and in man.   In proceedings of the Sixth Leucocyte Culture Conference (M.R.
       Schwarz, ed.), pp. 805-840.   Academic Press, New York, 1972.

57.   Thomas, E.D., Rudolph, R.H., Fefer, A., Storb, R., Slichter, S. and Buckner, C.D.:
       Isogeneic marrow grafting in man.   Exp. Hematol. 21:16-18, 1971.

58.   Fefer, A., Buckner, C.D., Clift, R.A., Fass, L., Lerner, K.G., Mickelson, E.M., Nieman,
       P., Rudolph, R., Storb, R. and Thomas, E.D.:   Marrow grafting in identical twins with
       hematologic malignancies.   Transpl. Proc. 5:927-931, 1973.

59.   Good, R.A., Peterson, R.D.A., Perey, D.Y., Finstad, J. and Cooper, M.D.:   The
       immunological deficiency diseases of man: consideration of some questions asked by
       these patients with an attempt at classification.   In: Immunologic Deficiency Diseases in
       Man (D. Bergsma and R.A. Good, eds.), New York, The National Foundation, 1968, pp.
       17-39 (Birth Defects: Original Article Series, Vol. IV, No. 1, 1968).

60.   Hong, R., Kay, H.E.M., Cooper, M.D., Meuwissen, H., Allan, M.J.G. and Good, R.A.:
       Immunological restitution in lymphopenic immunologic deficiency syndrome. Lancet
       1:503-506, March 9, 1968.

61.   Hong, R., Gatti, R.A. and Good, R.A.:   Hazards and potential benefits of
       blood-transfusion in immunological deficiency.   Lancet 2:388-389, August 17, 1968.

62.   Gatti, R.A., Meuwissen, H.F., Allen, H.D., Hong, R. and Good, R.A.:
       Immunological reconstitution of sex-linked lymphopenic immunological deficiency
       Lancet 2:1366-1369, December 28, 1968.

63. Good, R.A., Gatti, R.A., Hong, R. and Meuwissen, H.J.: Graft treatment of immunological deficiency. Lancet 1:1162, June 7, 1969. (Letters to the Editor)

64. Good, R.A., Gatti, R.A., Hong, R. and Meuwissen, H.J.: Successful marrow transplantation for correction of immunological deficit in lymphopenic agammaglobulinemia and treatment of immunologically induced pancytopenia. Exp. Hematol. 19:4-10, 1969.

65. Good, R.A.: Immunologic reconstitution: the achievement and its meaning. Hosp. Pract. 4:41-47, April, 1969.

66. Bortin, M.M., Bach, F.H., van Bekkum, D.W., Good, R.A. and van Rood, J.J.: 25th anniversary of the first successful allogeneic bone marrow transplants. Bone Marrow Transplantation 14:211-212, 1994.

67. Bach, F.H., Albertini, R.J., Joo, P., Anderson, J.L.Y. and Bortin, M.M.: Bone marrow transplantation in a patient with the Wiskott-Aldrich syndrome. Lancet I:1364, 1968.

68. deKonig, J., L.J. Dooren, D.W. van Bekkum, J.J. van Rood, K.A. Dicke and J. Radl. Transplantation of bone marrow cells and fetal thymus in an infant with lymphopenic immunological deficiency. Lancet i:1223, 1969.

69. Epstein, R.B., Storb, R., Ragde, H. and Thomas, E.D.: Cytotoxic typing antisera for marrow grafting in littermate dogs. Transplantation 6:45-58, 1968.

70. Storb, R., Epstein, R.B., Rudolph, R.H. and Thomas, E.D.: The effect of prior transfusion on marrow grafts between histocompatible canine siblings. J. Immunol.105:627-633, 1970b.

71. Thomas, E.D., Buckner, C.D., Banaji, M. et al.: One hundred patients with acute leukemia treated by chemotherapy, total body irradiation, and allogeneic marrow transplantation. Blood 49:511-533, 1977.

72. Thomas, E.D., Storb, R., Clift, R.A., Fefer, A., Johnson, F.L., Neiman, P.E., Lerner, K.G., Glucksberg, H. and Buckner C.D.: Bone marrow transplantation (First of Two Parts). N. Eng. J. Med. 292:832-43, 895-902, 1975.

73. Hansen, J.A., O'Reilly, R.J., Good, R.A. and Dupont, B.: Relevance of major human histocompatibility determinants in clinical bone marrow transplantation. Transplant. Proc. 8:581-589, December, 1976.

74. O'Reilly, R.J., Dupont, B., Pahwa, S., Grimes, E., Smithwick, E.M., Pahwa, R., Schwartz, S., Hansen, J.A., Siegal, F.P., Sorell, M., Svejgaard, A., Jersild, C., Thomsen, M., Platz, P., L'Esperance, P. and Good, R.A.: Reconstitution in severe combined immunodeficiency by transplantation of marrow from an unrelated donor. N. Engl. J. Med. 297:1311-1318, December 15, 1977.

75. O'Reilly, R.J., Pahwa, R., Dupont, B. and Good, R.A.: Severe combined immuno-deficiency: transplantation approaches for patients lacking an HLA genotypically identical sibling. Transplant. Proc. 10:187-199, March, 1978.

76. Reisner, Y., Itzicovitch, L., Meshorer, A. and Sharon, N.: Hemopoietic stem cell transplantation using mouse bone marrow and spleen cells fractionated by lectins. Proc. Natl. Acad. Sci. USA 75:2933, 1978.

77. Reisner, Y., Kapoor, N., Hodes, M.Z., O'Reilly, R.J. and Good, R.A.: Enrichment for CFU-C from murine and human bone marrow using soybean agglutinin. Blood 59:360, 1982.

78. Reisner, Y., Kapoor, N., Kirkpatrick, D., Pollack, M.S., Cunningham-Rundles, S., Dupont, B., Hodes, M.Z., Good, R.A. and O'Reilly, R.J.: Transplantation for severe combined immunodeficiency with HLA-A, B, D. Dr incompatible parental marrow cells fractionated by soybean agglutinin and sheep red blood cells. Blood 61:341, 1983.

79. Buckley, R.H., Schiff, S.E., Sampson, H.A., Schiff, R.I., Markert, M.L., Knutsen, A.P., Hershfield, M.S., Huang, A.T., Mickey, G.H. and Ward, F.E.: Development of immunity in human severe primary T cell deficiency following haploidentical bone marrow stem cell transplantation. J. Immunol. 136:2398-2407, 1986.

80. O'Reilly, R.J., Kernan, N.A., Cunningham, I., Brochstein, J., Castro-Malaspina, H., Laver, J., Flomenberg, N., Emanuel, D., Gulati, S., Keever, C., Small, T., Collins, N.H. and Bordignon, C.: Allogeneic transplants depleted of T cells by soybean lectin agglutination and E-rosette depletion. Bone Marrow Transplant 3:3, 1988.

81. Reisner, Y., Kapoor, N., Kirkpatrick, D., Pollack, M.S., Dupont, B., Good, R.A. and O'Reilly, R.J.: Transplantation for acute leukaemia using HLA-A and B non-identical parental marrow cells fractionated with soybean agglutinin and sheep red blood cells. Lancet, 2:327-331, 1981.

82. Aversa, F., Tabilio, A., Terenzi, A., Verlardi, A., Falzetti, F., Giannoni, C., Iacucci, R.,

Zei, T., Martelli, M.P., Gambelunghe, C., Rosetti, M., Caputo, P., Latini, P., Aristei, C., Raymondi, C., Reisner, Y. and Martelli, M.F.: Successful engraftment of T-cell depleted haploidentical "three loci" incompatible transplants in leukemia patients by addition of recombinant human granulocyte colony-stimulating factor - mobilized peripheral blood progenitor cells to bone marrow inoculum. Blood 84:3948-3955, 1994.

83. Beatty, P.G., Hansen, J.A., Longton, G.M., Thomas, E.D., Sanders, J.E., Martin, P.J., Bearman, S.I., Anasetti, C., Petrsdorf, E.W., Mickelson, E.M., Pepe, M.S., Appelbaum, F.R., Buckner, C.D., Clift, R.A., Petersen, F.B., Stewart, P.S., Storb, R.F., Sullivan, K.M., Tesler, M.C. and Witherspoon, R.P.: Marrow transplantation from HLA-matched unrelated donors for treatment of hematologic malignancies. Transplantation 51:443, 1991.

84. McGlave, P., Bartsch, G., Anasetti, C., Ash, R., Beatty, P., Gajewski, J. and Kernan, N.A.: Unrelated donor marrow transplantation therapy for chronic myelogenous leukemia: Initial experience of the National Marrow Donor Program. Blood 81:543-550, 1993.

85. Hansen, J.A., Anasetti, C., Petersdorf, E., Clift, R.A. and Martin, P.J.: Marrow transplants from unrelated donors. Transplant Proc. 26:1710-1712, 1994.

86. Anasetti, C., Etzioni, R., Petersdorf, E.W., Martin, P.J. and Hansen, J.A.: Marrow transplantation from unrelated volunteer donors. Annu. Rev. Med. 46:169-179, 1995.

87. O'Reilly, R.J., Pahwa, R., Sorrell, M., Kapoor, N., Kapadia, A., Kirkpatrick, D., Pollack, M., Dupont, B., Incefy, G., Iwata, T. and Good, R.A.: Transplantation of fetal liver and thymus in patients with severe combined immunodeficiencies. In: *The Immune System: Functions and Therapy of Dysfunction: Proceedings* of the Seronon Symposia, Vol. 27 (G. Doria and A. Eshkol, eds.), New York, Academic Press, 1980, pp. 241-253.

88. Broxmeyer, H.E., Kurtzberg, J., Gluckman, E., Auerbach, A.D., Douglas, G., Cooper, S., Falkenburg, J.H.F., Bard, J. and Boyse, E.A.: Umbilical cord blood hematopoietic stem and repopulating cells in human clinical transplantation. Blood Cells 17:313-329, 1991.

89. Broxmeyer, H.E., Cooper, S., Yoder, M. and Hangoc, G.: Human umbilical cord blood as a source of transplantable hematopoietic stem and progenitor cells. Current Topics in Microbiology and Immunobiology 177:195-204, 1992.

90. Gluckman, E., Broxmyer, H.E., Auerbach, A.D., Friedman, H.S., Douglas, G.W.,

Devergie, A., Esperou, H., Thierry, D., Socie, G., Lehn, P., Cooper, S., English, D., Kurtzberg, J., Bard, J. and Boyse, E.A.: Hematopoietic reconstitution in a patient with Fanconi's anemia by means of umbilical-cord blood from an HLA-identical sibling. New Eng. J. Med. 321:1174-1178, 1989.

91. Wagner, J.E., Kernan, N.A., Steinbuch, M., Broxmeyer, H.E. and Gluckman, E.: Allogeneic sibling umbilical-cord-blood transplantation in children with malignant and non-malignant disease. Lancet 346:214-219, 1995.

92. Rubinstein, P., Dobrila, L., Rosenfield, R.E., Adamson, J.W., Adamson, J.W., Migliaccio, G., Migliaccio, A.R., Taylor, P.E. and Stevens, C.E.: Processing and cryopreservation of placental/umbilical cord blood for unrelated bone marrow reconstitution. Proc. Natl. Acad. Sci. USA 92:10119-10122, 1995.

93. Rubinstein, P., Taylor, P.E., Scaradavou, A., Adamson, J.W., Migliaccio, G., Emanuel, D., Berkowitz, R.L., Alvarez, E. and Stevens, C.E.: Unrelated placental blood for bone marrow reconstitution: organization of the placental blood program.
Blood Cells 20:587-600, 1994.

94. Rubinstein - Personal communication

95. Nathan, D.E.: The beneficence of neonatal hematopoiesis (editorial). New Eng. J. Med. 321:1190-1191, 1989.

96. Pahwa, R.N., Fleischer, A., Than, So and Good, R.A.: Successful hematopoietic reconstitution with transplantation of erythrocyte-depleted allogeneic human umbilical cord blood cells in a child with leukemia. Proc. Natl. Acad. Sci. USA 91:4485-4488, 1994.

97. Blaese, M.: Steps toward gene therapy: 1. The initial trials. Hospital Practice 33-40, 1995

The Prospects for BMT — from Mouse to Human

Susumu Ikehara

First Department of Pathology, Kansai Medical University, 10-15 Fumizono-cho, Moriguchi City, Osaka, 570 Japan

SUMMARY

Using animal models for autoimmune diseases, we have found that bone marrow transplantation (BMT) can be used to treat not only systemic autoimmune diseases but also organ-specific autoimmune diseases. We have also found that transplantation of hemopoietic stem cell (HSC)-enriched populations from autoimmune-prone mice to normal mice induces autoimmune diseases in the recipients. These findings have recently been confirmed in humans; BMT can be used to treat autoimmune diseases, whereas autoimmune diseases have been transferred from donors to recipients by BMT. Based on these findings, we have proposed a new concept of stem cell disorders to include aplastic anemia, leukemia and autoimmune diseases. To elucidate the differences between normal and abnormal HSCs, we have established a method for purifying HSCs and have found qualitative differences between them both in vivo and in vitro. Although normal HSCs do not readily proliferate in major histocompatibility complex (MHC)-incompatible microenvironments, abnormal HSCs show a marked proliferative response. Abnormal HSCs are thus more resilient than normal HSCs. Based on these findings, we have attempted to recruit donor-derived stromal cells by grafting non-irradiated bones subcutaneously in the case of BMT across MHC barriers. The bone grafts have, in fact, led to successful long-term reconstitution even in chimeric resistant combinations such as [Normal → MRL/lpr] and [DBA/2 → C57BL/6] chimeric mice. T cell functions are completely restored by bone grafts; this is due to the migration of stromal cells into the thymus, where they are engaged in positive selection as thymic nurse cells. Stromal cells thus play a crucial role in successful BMT across MHC barriers. Intractable diseases are defined as diseases of unknown etiopathogenesis, and for which therapeutic strategies remain to be established. Of the 36 diseases recognized as intractable by the Ministry of Health and Welfare of Japan, we show that approximately half will become curable by BMT.

KEY WORDS: bone marrow transplantation (BMT), autoimmune diseases, hemopoietic stem cells (HSCs), stromal cells, stem cell disorders

302

INTRODUCTION

In the last decade, remarkable advances have been made in BMT. However, because of the difficulty of obtaining HLA-matched donors, BMT in humans has continued to suffer problems such as graft-versus-host disease (GVHD) and graft rejection.

Various mouse strains that spontaneously develop autoimmune diseases have contributed not only to better understanding of the fundamental nature of autoimmune diseases but also to the analysis of their etiopathogenesis. The etiopathogenesis of systemic autoimmune diseases has previously been attributed to T cell deficiencies, polyclonal B-cell activation, macrophage dysfunction and environmental factors such as hormonal disturbances [1]. However, there has recently been an increase in information suggesting that autoimmune diseases originate from defects in hemopoietic stem cells (HSCs) [2-10].

In this paper, we show that autoimmune diseases are stem cell disorders, and provide evidence that BMT may become a useful tool for deciding if a certain intractable disease is a stem cell disorder.

Thymic abnormalities in autoimmune diseases

The thymus contains more than 95% thymocytes and small numbers of macrophages, epithelial cells and nurse cells. Only very few plasma cells and B cells can be detected in the normal thymus [11]. However, it is reported that lymphoid follicles have been detected in the thymuses of patients with autoimmune diseases such as myasthenia gravis (MG) and systemic lupus erythematosus (SLE) [12,13]. We have found that plasma cell infiltration into the thymus is a common feature in autoimmune-prone mice, and that the destruction of the blood-thymus barrier results in premature thymic involution in autoimmune-prone mice [14]. However, it is not known why thymic abnormalities develop in autoimmune-prone mice.

To answer this question, we transplanted the thymus or bone marrow from normal mice to autoimmune-prone mice, and vice versa. The data are summarized in Fig. 1; thymic abnormalities originate from defects in the bone marrow of autoimmune-prone mice, and the transplantation of bone marrow cells from normal mice to autoimmune-prone mice prevents both thymic abnormalities and autoimmune diseases [15]. We have recently found that abnormal HSCs (but neither the presence of extrinsic factors such as autoantibodies nor intrinsic thymic abnormalities) induce thymic abnormalities [16]; autoreactive T cells that have developed from abnormal HSCs destroy the blood thymus barrier, resulting in plasma cells and B cells infiltrating the thymus.

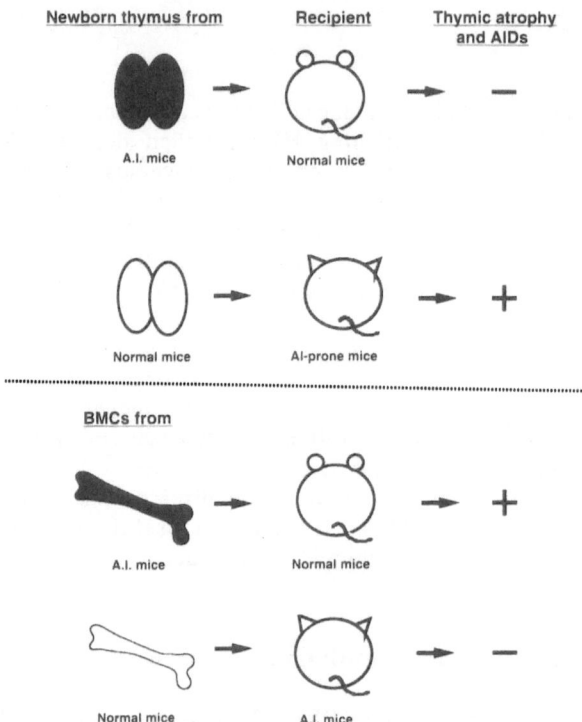

Fig. 1 The cause of thymic abnormalities in autoimmune (A.I.)-prone mice. When the newborn thymuses of A.I.-prone mice are engrafted under the renal capsule of normal mice (BALB/c nu/nu), the thymuses do not show abnormalities (premature involution or plasma cell infiltration, etc.), and the nu/nu mice do not show autoimmune diseases (AIDs). In contrast, when bone marrow cells (BMCs) from A.I.-prone mice are transferred into normal mice, the mice show thymic abnormalities.

Treatment of systemic autoimmune diseases by BMT

The next step was to examine whether BMT could be used to treat systemic autoimmune diseases.

When female (NZB × NZW)F1 (B/W F1) (> 6 months), female MRL/lpr (> 2 months), and male BXSB (> 6 months) mice that had already shown clear evidence of autoimmune diseases were lethally irradiated and then reconstituted with either allogeneic bone marrow cells of young (< 2 months) BALB/c nu/nu (H-2^d) mice or T-cell depleted bone marrow cells of BALB/c mice, the recipients survived in good health for more than 3 months after BMT [5].

In BXSB and B/W F1 mice, BMT had completely curative effects. Glomerular damage was ameliorated, and the levels of autoantibodies (anti-DNA and anti-Sm antibodies (Abs)) and circulating immune complexes (CICs) ---- particularly gp-70 anti-gp-70 CICs ---- were reduced.

The repair of glomerular damage was noted by performing renal biopsies before and after BMT, as shown in Fig. 2. In addition, immunological functions were normalized; T-cell functions including IL-2 production were restored, and hyperfunctions of macrophages and B cells decreased. Assays for both mixed-lymphocyte reaction (MLR) and generation of cytotoxic T-lymphocytes (CTLs) revealed that newly-developed T cells from BMT-treated mice were tolerant of both bone marrow donor-type and host-type MHC determinants, but responded vigorously to third-party cells. In vitro primary anti-sheep red blood cell (SRBC) plaque-forming cell (PFC) assay also showed that some degree of cooperation was achieved among antigen-presenting cells (APCs), helper T cells, and B cells. Long-term observation following BMT revealed that auoimmune diseeases of BXSB and B/W F1 mice remain successfully corrected for more than one year following BMT [7].

In contrast to BXSB and B/W F1 mice, MRL/lpr mice regularly suffered a relapse approximately 5 months after BMT. H-2 typing revealed that all the immunocompetent cells of the chimeras had been replaced by host (MRL/lpr)-derived cells by that time. The T cells of the chimeras showed responsiveness to donor BALB/c (H-2^d)-type but not to recipient MRL/lpr (H-2^k)-type MHC determinants in both assays for MLR and the generation of CTLs. In addition, abnormal B220$^+$ Ly-1$^+$ cells reappeared in such mice. These results indicate that MRL/lpr mice possess abnormal radioresistant (9.5Gy) hemopoietic stem cells (HSCs), and also provide additional evidence that the etiopathogenesis of autoimmune diseases resides in defects or characteristics located at the HSC level [7].

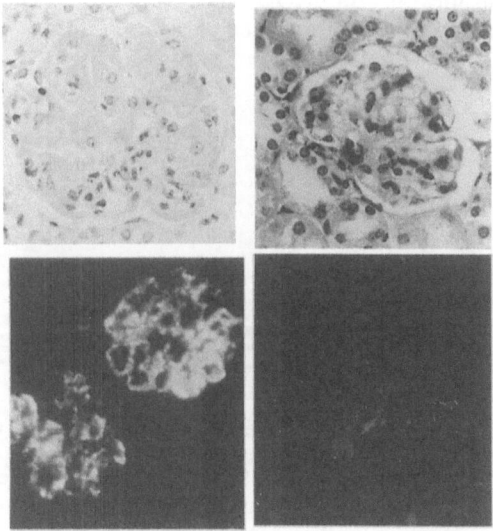

Fig. 2 Histopathologic and immunofluorescent findings in the glomeruli of B/W F1 mice before and after BMT. Typical wire-loop lesions (top left) and IgG deposits (bottom left) are present in the glomeruli of the 8 - month -old B/W F1 mouse before BMT. Five months after BMT, IgG deposits are markedly reduced (bottom right), and the glomeruli of the mouse exhibit a normal appearance on hematoxylin-eosin staining (top right).

Prevention and treatment of insulin-dependent diabetes mellitus (IDDM), an organ-specific autoimmune disease

Based on the above observations, we attempted to determine whether organ-specific autoimmune diseases could be treated by BMT using an animal model for IDDM, the NOD mouse.

First, we attempted to prevent insulitis and overt diabetes by BMT. NOD mice (> 4 months) were lethally irradiated and then reconstituted with T cell-depleted BALB/c bone marrow cells. The mice were sacrificed more than 3 months after BMT. No lymphocyte infiltration was observed in the islets of the BMT-treated NOD mice. Immunohistochemical studies revealed the presence of intact beta cells as well as alpha and delta cells. Glucose tolerance tests (GTTs) indicated that BMT-treated NOD mice exhibit a normal glucose response. Diabetic nephropathy was also corrected by BMT. Thus, BMT can prevent insulitis and overt diabetes [6]. However, we could not treat overt diabetes in NOD mice by BMT, because mice with overt diabetes have no beta cells.

We next performed a combined transplantation of fetal or newborn pancreas plus allogeneic bone marrow, since we know that organ allografts are accepted if the organ is transplanted from the same donor as the bone marrow at the same time [17]. NOD mice that had already developed overt diabetes were lethally irradiated and then reconstituted with allogeneic BALB/c bone marrow cells. The pancreatic tissues from fetal or newborn BALB/c mice were then engrafted under the renal capsules of NOD diabetic mice. Three months after the transplantation, the mice exhibited a normal GTT pattern, and insulin levels in the sera were also normalized. Immunohistochemical studies revealed the presence of beta cells in the islets engrafted under the renal capsules of the NOD mice (Fig. 3). Thus, we succeeded in treating diabetes by a combined transplantation of pancreas and bone marrow [9].

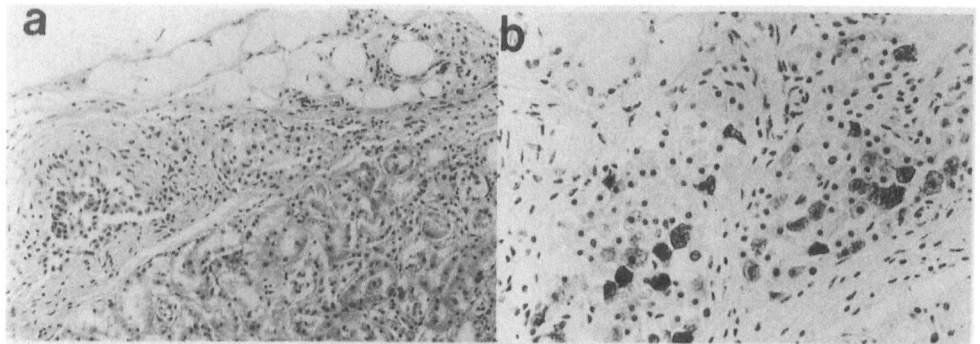

Fig. 3 Histology of engrafted pancreas. Clusters of islet cells are observed under the renal capsule by hematoxylin-eosin staining (**a**). These cells are shown to contain insulin by means of immunohistological staining (**b**).

Prevention and treatment of both organ-specific and systemic autoimmune diseases

We have recently found that (NZW x BXSB)F1 (W/BF1) mice, which develop lupus nephritis with myocardial infarction [18], s h o w thrombocytopenia with age, and that the thrombocytopenia is attributable to the presence of both platelet-associated and circulating anti-platelet antibodies [10]. In addition, we have very recently found that myocardial infarction in W/BF1 mice is due to the presence of anti-cardiolipin Abs, and that the mouse is an animal model for anti-phospholipin Ab syndrome [19].

Transplantation of bone marrow cells from normal mice to W/BF1 mice was found to exert preventative and curative effects on lupus nephritis, thrombocytopenia and anti-phospholipid Ab syndrome; the platelet counts were normalized, and circulating anti-platelet Ab levels as well as anti-phospholipid Ab levels were reduced [10,19].

Transfer of insulitis and diabetes into normal mice by transplantation of bone marrow cells from NOD mice

We attempted to transfer IDDM to normal mice by transplanting NOD bone marrow cells to C3H/HeN mice. Mice of this strain express I-Eα molecules and have an aspartic acid at residue 57 (Asp-57) of the I-Aβ chain [20,21]. We selected this strain because it has been postulated that failure to express the Eα gene is the abnormality that permits NOD mice to develop insulitis, leading to diabetes [22,23]. Also, it is thought that replacement of Asp-57 with Ser (non-Asp) in NOD mice [24] and with non-Asp in humans [25] may be the molecular anomaly responsible for the development of IDDM.

Female C3H/HeN (H-2^K) mice were lethally irradiated (9.5Gy) at the age of 8 weeks and then reconstituted with T cell-depleted bone marrow cells of young (<8 weeks) female NOD (K^d, 1-A^{g7}, D^b) mice. As controls, more than 50 C3H/HeN (H-2^K) mice were lethally irradiated and then reconstituted with T cell-depleted bone marrow cells of C3H/HeN, C57BL/6J (H-2^b), or BALB/c (H-2^d) mice. Even though these survived more than 1 year (survival rate, >90%), neither insulitis nor overt diabetes developed. However, two of four [NOD→ C3H/HeN] chimeric mice developed both insulitis and overt diabetes more than 40 weeks after BMT. These mice exhibited elevated glucose levels and abnormal glucose tolerance curves, as shown in Fig. 4 [8].

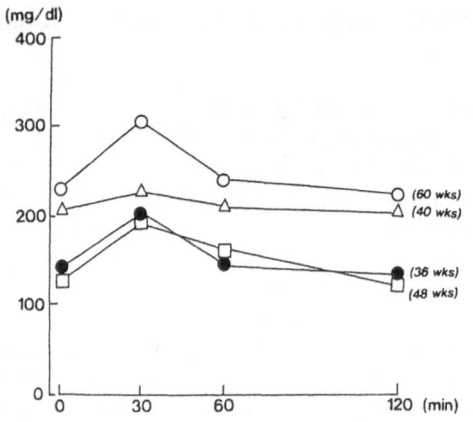

Fig. 4 Glucose tolerance tests (GTTs) in [NOD → C3H/HeN] mice. Two [NOD → C3H/HeN] mice show impaired GTTs (O and Δ).

Transfer of ITP and SLE into normal mice by transplantation of bone marrow cells from W/BF1 mice

The next step was to investigate whether both systemic (SLE) and organ-specific (ITP) autoimmune diseases could be transferred to normal mice by BMT. Since the male W/BF1 mouse, which develops lupus nephritis and myocardial infarction, is an impressive animal model of ITP, we used W/BF1 (H-2^Z/H-2^b) mice as donors and C3H/HeN (H-2^K) or C57BL/6J (H-2^b) mice as recipients.

C3H/HeN or C57BL/6J mice were lethally irradiated (9.5Gy) and then reconstituted with T cell-depleted bone marrow cells of young (<8 weeks) male W/BF1 mice. [W/BF1→C57BL/6J] mice showed thrombocytopenia (<10^5 platelets per mm^3; normal mice >10 x 10^5) in 5 of 11 mice (45%) 3 months after BMT, and in 5 more of the same 11 mice (total 10/11: 91%) by 5 months after BMT. [W/BF1→ C3H/HeN] mice also developed thrombocytopenia in 4 of 8 mice (50%) by 3 months after BMT and in 6 of 8 mice (75%) by 6 months after BMT.

Cytofluorometric analyses demonstrated the presence of both platelet-associated antibodies and circulating anti-platelet antibodies in the thrombocytopenic mice. Immunohistopathological analyses revealed typical wire-loop lesions in the glomeruli of the [W/BF1→C57BL/6J] or [W/BF1→C3H/HeN] mice, as shown in Fig. 5.

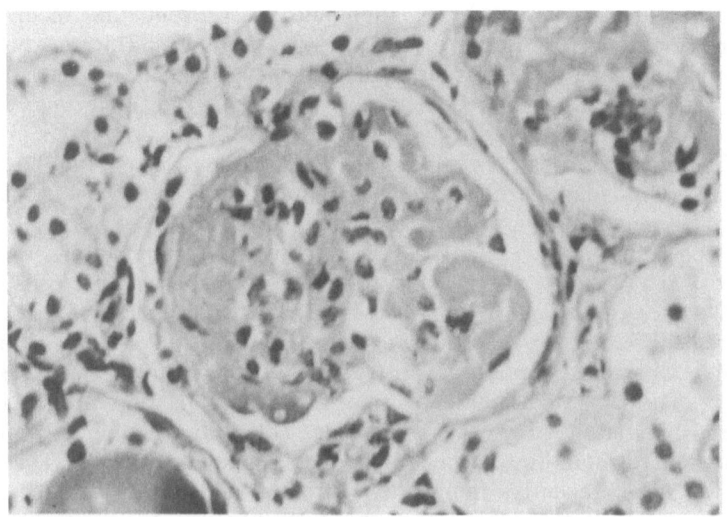

Fig. 5 Histology of a glomerulus of a [W/B F1 → C3H/HeN] mouse 5 months after BMT. Note the deposits of PAS-positive materials in both capillary and mesangial areas.

To confirm that the defective HSCs were indeed the elements responsible for the development of the autoimmune diseases, we transferred cells in a HSC-enriched fraction (fraction II) of W/BF1 bone marrow cells to C3H/HeN mice, since both Visser et al [26] and we [27] have reported that, after T cells, B cells and macrophages have been depleted from bone marrow cells, spleen colony-forming units (CFU-S) are enriched in a low-density fraction (fraction II) obtained by a Percoll discontinuous-density centrifugation method. Lethally irradiated (9.5Gy) C3H/HeN mice that had been injected with W/BF1 HSC-enriched bone marrow cells were also found to develop thrombocytopenia and lupus nephritis [8].

We therefore conclude from these experiments that the etiopathogenesis of both systemic and organ-specific autoimmune diseases can be attributed to abnormalities in the HSC population.

Successful BMT by bone grafts in chimeric-resistant combinations

Since MRL/lpr mice possess abnormal radioresistant HSCs, they suffer a relapse 5 months after conventional BMT [7], as mentioned above. We have recently found that there is an MHC restriction between HSCs and stromal cells; when bones are engrafted, donor-derived stromal cells present in the engrafted bones can migrate into the recipient bone marrow, which is replaced by both donor-derived stromal cells and hematopoietic cells.

Based on these findings, we attempted to prevent the recurrence of autoimmune diseases in MRL/lpr mice by the transplantation of both bone marrow cells and bones (as a source of stromal cells). MRL/lpr mice were irradiated (8.5Gy) and then reconstituted with C57BL/6 bone marrow cells plus bone grafts. The mice survived more than 48 wks after this treatment. Immunohistologic studies revealed that the mice were completely free from both lymphadenopathy and autoimmune diseases such as lupus nephritis and rheumatoid arthritis, as shown in Fig. 6. Sera from these mice showed normal levels of CICs and rheumatoid factors. Normal functions of both T cells and B cells were noted. Abnormal T cells such as Thy-1+ B220+ cells present in nontreated MRL/lpr mice could not be seen in the thus-treated mice. In addition, to our surprise, spleen cells from thus-treated mice showed completely normal in vitro primary anti-SRBC PFC responses. These results indicate that stromal cells in allogeneic bone marrow transplantation play a crucial role not only in the prevention of graft failure but also in the successful cooperation among APCs, T cells, and B cells; we have recently found that stromal cells in the bone marrow migrate into the thymus, where they become engaged in positive selection (manuscript in preparation). Although MRL/lpr mice are radiosensitive (while HSCs are radioresistant) and usually die of interstitial pneumonia or fatty liver due to the side effects of radiation, it should be noted that this strategy allows a reduction in the radiation dose (9.5Gy → 8.5Gy), and that these mice can survive more than 48 wks without showing any symptoms of autoimmune diseases [28].

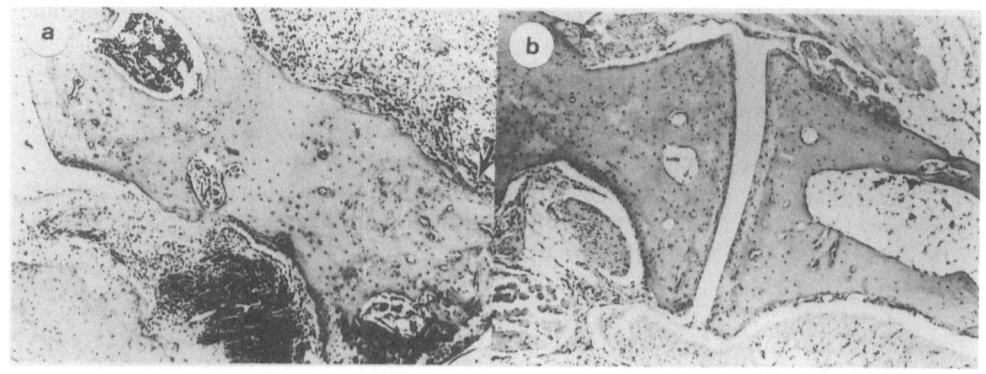

Fig. 6 Histopathologic findings in the hindpaw joint of a nontreated MRL/lpr mouse (a) and MRL/lpr mouse with BMT plus bone graft (b). The joint of the nontreated mouse shows marked lymphoid cell infiltration and pannus formation (a) whereas the joint of the treated mouse shows neither lymphoid cell infiltration nor pannus formation (b).

Using another chimeric-resistant combination [DBA → C57BL/6], we have confirmed that chimeric resistance can be overcome by BMT plus bone grafts [29]. These results indicate that BMT plus bone grafts (stromal cell recruitment) will be a valuable strategy in the treatment of various diseases, including immunologic, hematologic, and metabolic disorders.

Treatment of non-insulin-dependent diabetes mellitus (NIDDM) by BMT

The effects of allogeneic BMT on NIDDM were examined using KK-Ay mice. KK-Ay mice reconstituted with KK-Ay bone marrow cells showed glycosuria, hyperinsulinemia, and hyperlipidemia. However, KK-Ay mice (H-2^b) that had been lethally irradiated (9.0Gy) and then reconstituted with T cell-depleted bone marrow cells from normal BALB/c mice (H-2^d) showed not only a normal glucose response with negative urine sugar (Fig.7) but also decreased serum insulin and lipid levels 4 mo after BMT. Morphological recovery of islets and glomeruli was also noted after allogeneic BMT. These findings suggest that BMT can be used to treat not only a certain type of NIDDM but also its complications such as hyperlipidemia and diabetic nephropathy [30].

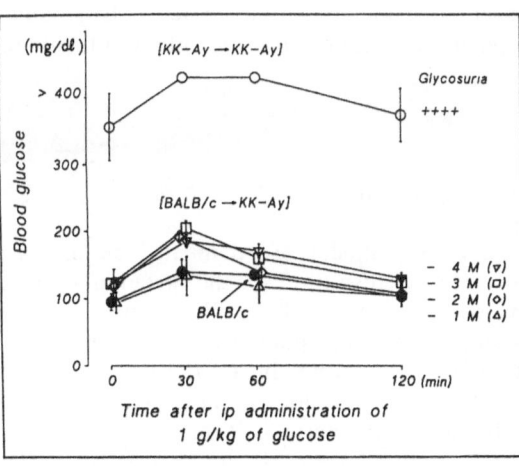

Fig. 7 GTTs in [KK-Ay → KK-Ay] and [BALB/c→KK-Ay] mice : syngeneic group (○), allogeneic group (1 mo (Δ), 2 mo (◊), 3 mo (□), and 4 mo (∇) after BMT), and non-treated BALB/c mice (•).

Focal segmental glomerular sclerosis (FGS) as a stem cell disorder

The etiopathogenesis of FGS remains unknown. Using a new animal model for FGS (FGS mouse), we have demonstrated that bone marrow transplantation from normal mice to FGS mice with a high grade of proteinuria (+++) ameliorates FGS, and that the transplantation of bone marrow cells or partially purified HSCs from FGS mice induces FGS in normal mice, as shown in Fig. 8. These findings strongly suggest that FGS is a stem cell disorder; the abnormalities may be genetically programmed at the level of the HSCs [31].

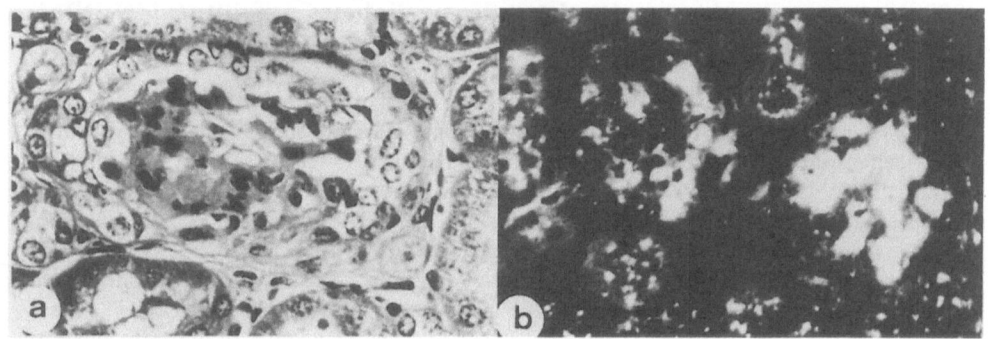

Fig. 8 Histopathologic findings in the kidney of a [FGS → B6] chimeric mouse. (**a**) Glomerulosclerosis is seen in a kidney of the [FGS → B6] mouse 17 wks after BMT. (**b**) IgG deposits are noted in two glomeruli of the mouse.

BMT for treatment of metabolic disorders

The C57BL/Ksj spm/spm mouse, an animal model of Niemann-Pick diseases, shows defective sphingomyelinase activity resulting in the accumulation of sphingomyelin (foam cells) in various organs.   To replace the defective enzyme, allogeneic bone marrow-plus-liver transplantation was performed. BMT with or without concomitant liver grafting in C57BL/KsJ spm/spm mice at the age of 2-9 weeks led to an amelioration of the hepatosplenomegaly.   The treatment, however, neither prevented the development of neurological signs nor increased the life-span.   The sphingomyelin and cholesterol contents of the liver decreased, while sphingomyelinase activity in the liver increased after BMT, as shown in Fig. 9.   Foam cells disappeared from the bone marrow, liver, spleen, thymus, and lymph nodes, but depletion of Purkinje cells was not completely prevented.

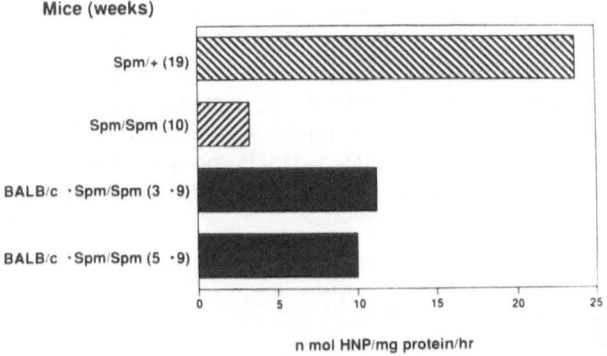

Mice (weeks)

Fig. 9 Restoration of sphingomyelinase activity in the liver of C57BL/KsJ spm/spm mice by transplantation of the bone marrow cells and liver from BALB/c mice.

These results suggest that BMT either alone or with liver transplantation may become a useful strategy for the treatment of a certain type of Niemann-Pick disease in which the central nervous system is not involved [32]; in fact, BMT has already been used successfully to treat a patient with Niemann-Pick disease without neurological manifestations [33].

Necessity of three types of cell for successful BMT across MHC barriers

We have thus succeeded in treating various intractable diseases. For human application, we have been clarifying what cells are essential to successful BMT across MHC barriers, and found that three types of cell are necessary: pluripotent hemopoietic stem cells (P-HSCs), natural suppressor cells (NSCs), and stromal cells present in the bone marrow.

P-HSCs are defined as cells with the capacity to self-renew eternally and to differentiate into cells in all lineages including lymphoid cells. We have previously demonstrated that P-HSCs can be purified by both in vivo and in vitro 5-fluorouracil (5-FU) treatments, followed by sorting wheat germ agglutinin-binding (WGA$^+$) cells [27]. However, the 5-FU treatments (both in vivo and in vitro) have cytotoxic effects even on P-HSCs. We have therefore modified the method to include only in vivo 5-FU treatment followed by sorting CD71$^-$Class I^{high} cells from lineage- negative (Lin$^-$) cells. The sorted cells (only 4 cells) have the long-term repopulating ability in the assay of (male → female) chimeras [34]. It has been reported that HSCs are c-kit$^+$ or c-kit^{low} [35,36]. We have, however, found that the P-HSCs are c-kit$^-$, as shown in Fig. 10. In vitro studies revealed that this population cannot proliferate in the presence of putative cytokines such as GM-CSF, stem cell factor (SCF) and IL-3, whereas it can do by direct interaction with stromal cells without adding any cytokines (Fig. 11). The morphology of P-HSCs was examined using an electron microscope. As shown in Fig. 12, the cells had a large nucleus with narrow cytoplasm. Their chromatin pattern was dispersed, but small aggregates appeared at nuclear margins. There were few cytoplasmic organellas but abundant free ribosomes. It should be noted that P-HSCs possess microvilli; they show active movement like neutrophils, as observed on video tape.

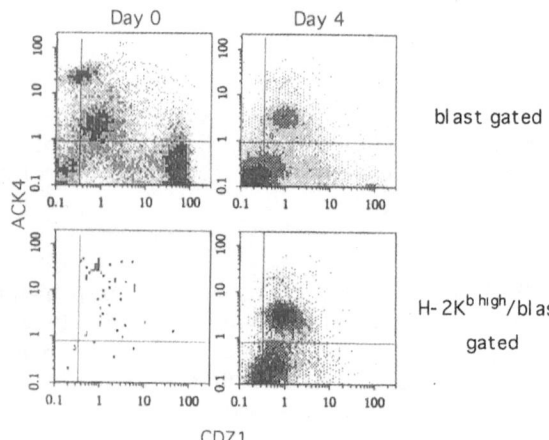

Fig. 10 Analysis of c-kit expression on P-HSCs. FACS analysis shows that P-HSCs (Class I^{high} CD71$^-$ blasts) are c-kit$^-$.

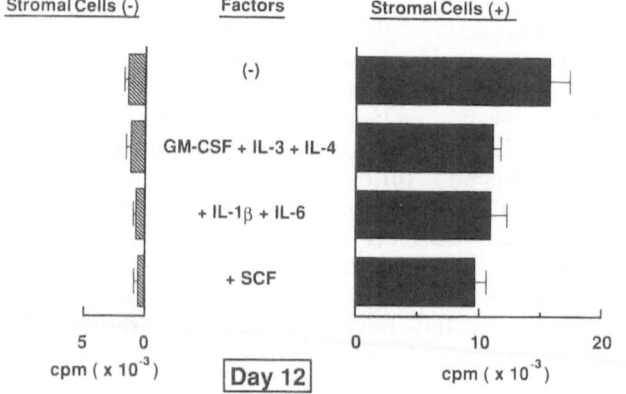

Fig. 11 Necessity of stromal cells for P-HSCs to proliferate. When P-HSCs were cocultured with stromal cells, the P-HSCs proliferated without the addition of cytokines, whereas they did not without stromal cells.

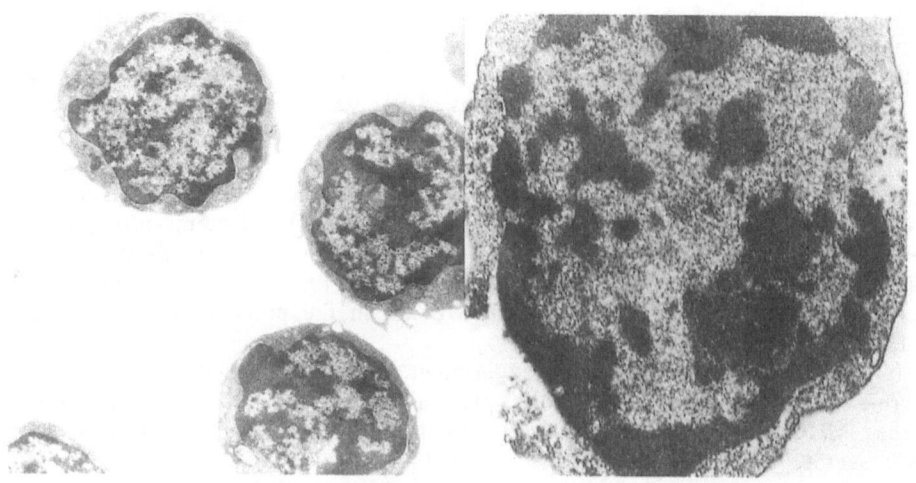

Fig. 12 Electron microscopic findings of P-HSCs. P-HSCs show large nuclei with narrow cytoplasm and microvilli.

   The second type of cells are NSCs. It has been reported that NSCs have the capacity to suppress various immunological functions including GVHR and graft rejection. However, the precise lineage and the markers of NSCs remain unclear. We have found that NSCs belong to a population of HSCs (WGA+IL-3R+) in the cycling phase [37,38]. We postulate that NSCs are engaged in negative feedback regulation in hemopoiesis, as shown in Fig. 13.

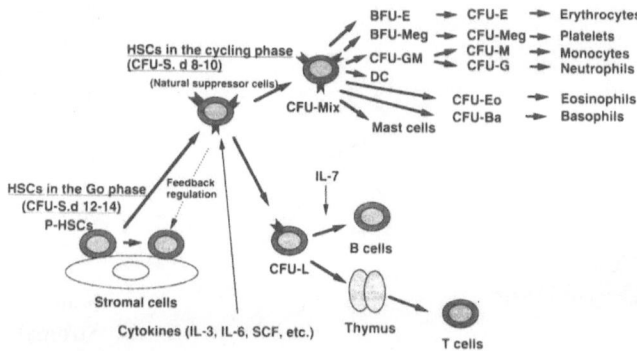

Fig.13 Hierarchy of hemopoietic cells. P-HSCs are stromal cell-dependent, whereas HSCs in the cycling phase can respond to cytokines such as IL-3, IL-6 and SCF. The latter are engaged in negative feedback regulation in hemopoiesis as natural suppressor cells.

The third type of cells are stromal cells. We have produced monoclonal antibodies (mAbs) against stromal cells using a PA-6 cell line. An mAb was found to react with stromal cells present only in the bone marrow but not in the spleen, lymph node, or thymus [39]. Endosteal cells in the bone marrow were found to be stained by this mAb. Observation of the interaction of P-HSCs with stromal cells using a video tape revealed that P-HSCs migrate into the stromal cells and crawl under them: stromal cells embrace the P-HSCs as mothers do their children. This finding prompted us to examine whether stromal cells secrete a factor that attracts P-HSCs. We have, indeed, found that stromal cells secrete two or more factors that attract P-HSCs and granulocytes [40]. We are in the process of purifying the P-HSC-chemotactic factor.

As shown in the MRL/lpr experiment, it is likely that bone grafts to recruit donor-derived stromal cells play a crucial role in successful BMT across MHC barriers, since stromal cells present in the engrafted bones not only secrete a P-HSC-chemotactic factor [40] (Fig. 14), but also protect P-HSCs from the attack of radioresistant host CTLs, NK cells, macrophages, K cells, etc. (Fig. 15). We have very recently found that bone marrow stromal cells migrate into the thymus, where they engage in positive selection as thymic nurse cells (Fig. 16) (manuscript in preparation). Therefore, newly-developed T cells can cooperate with B cells and APCs across MHC barriers, which results in the complete restoration of T-dependent antibody responses, as already mentioned in MRL/lpr experiments.

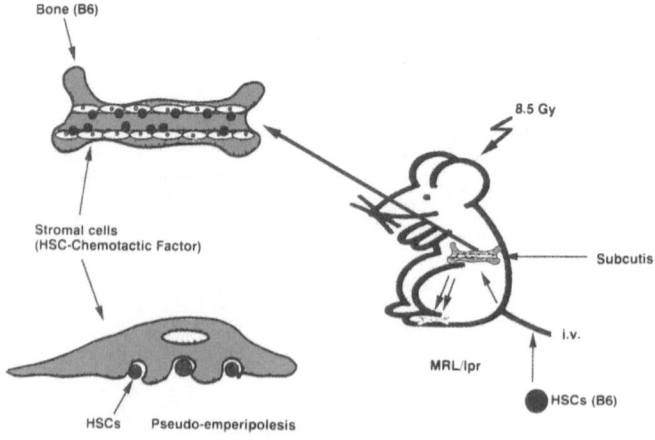

Fig. 14 BMT plus bone grafts in [B6 → MRL/lpr] mouse. The MRL/lpr mouse is lethally (8.5Gy) irradiated and then reconstituted with T cell-depleted B6 bone marrow cells. The mouse is subcutaneousy engrafted with B6 bone fragments. Stromal cells present in the B6 bones produce a HSC-chemotactic factor, which results in the migration of B6 HSCs into the engrafted bones. MHC-matched donor-derived stromal cells and HSCs stimulate each other and proliferate, and both migrate into the MRL/lpr bone marrow. The bone marrow in the MRL/lpr mouse is thus replaced by both B6-derived stromal cells and hemopoietic cells.

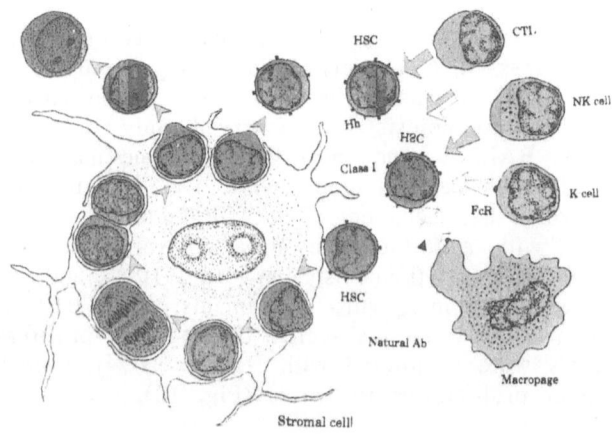

Fig. 15 Protection of P-HSCs by stromal cells from attack by host cells. Stromal cells embrace the P-HSCs (pseudo-emperipolesis) and protect them from the host cells such as CTLs, NK cells, K cells and macrophages.

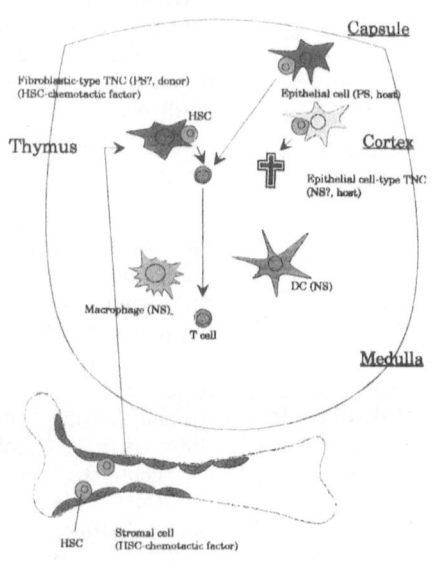

Fig. 16 Hypothesis for negative selection (NS) and positive selection (PS) after BMT plus bone grafts. Bone marrow stromal cells migrate into the thymus, where they engage in positive selection as thymic nurse cells (TNCs).

MHC restriction between P-HSCs and stromal cells

We have thus found that donor-derived stromal cells play a crucial role in successful BMT across MHC barriers. This finding prompted us to examine whether there is MHC restriction between P-HSCs and stromal cells. As shown in Fig. 17, hemopoiesis was observed only in the bone marrow engrafted with the BALB/c bone when BALB/c bone marrow cells (T cell-depleted and adherent cell-depleted) were i.v. injected into irradiated C3H/HeN mice which had been engrafted with bones of C3H/HeN, B6, and BALB/c mice or with a teflon tube as a control. This finding strongly suggests that an MHC restriction exists between P-HSCs and stromal cells in vivo. This was confirmed in in vitro experiments; when B10 (H-2^b) P-HSCs were cocultured with B10 stromal cells, the P-HSCs proliferated, whereas when B10 P-HSCs were cocultured with B10D2 (H-2^d) stromal cells, the P-HSCs showed poor proliferative responses (Fig. 18).

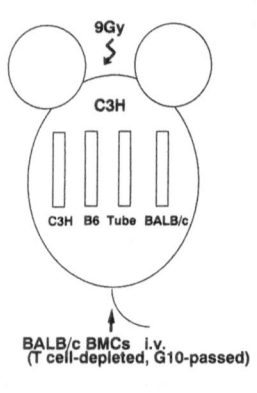

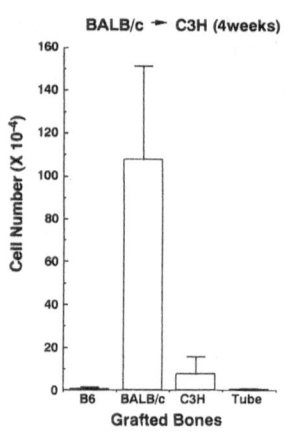

Fig. 17 In vivo MHC restriction between P-HSCs and stromal cells. Hemopoiesis is observed only in the bone marrow of the BALB/c bone which has been engrafted subcutaneously, when BALB/c BMCs (T cell-deplered and adherent cell-depleted) are i.v. injected into the irradiated (9Gy) C3H/HeN mouse.

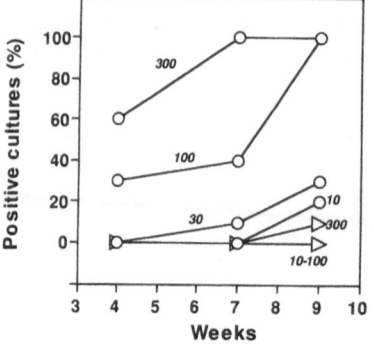

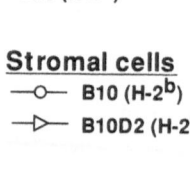

Stem cells
B10 (H-2^b)

Stromal cells
—○— B10 (H-2^b)
—▷— B10D2 (H-2^d)

Fig. 18 In vitro MHC restriction between P-HSCs and stromal cells. When B10 (H-2^b) P-HSCs (300 or 100 cells) are cocultured with B10 stromal cells, the P-HSCs proliferate. In contrast, When B10 P-HSCs are cocultured with B10D2 (H-2^d) stromal cells, the P-HSCs (10 to 300 cells) show poor proliferative responses.

New concept of "stem cell disorders"

We have shown that both systemic and organ-specific autoimmune diseases are "stem cell disorders". It is now accepted that leukemia and preleukemia are "stem cell disorders" [41]; in 1987, we presented a case report (T-cell acute lymphoblastic leukemia relapsing as acute myelocytic leukemia and terminating possibly as chronic myelocytic leukemia), and proposed that leukemia originates in a P-HSC [42]. Here we would like to propose a new concept of "stem cell disorders" including autoimmune diseases: i) stem cell aplasia (aplastic anemia), ii) monoclonal abnormal stem cell proliferative syndrome (leukemia and preleukemia), and iii) polyclonal abnormal stem cell proliferative syndrome (autoimmune diseases).

Qualitative differences between normal and abnormal P-HSCs

The next question was whether there are any qualitative differences between normal and abnormal P-HSCs. To answer this question, we first carried out BMT between normal and autoimmune-prone mice using partially purified P-HSCs. Transplantation of bones plus abnormal P-HSCs obtained from autoimmune-prone mice induced autoimmune diseases in normal mice, as did transplantation of T cell-depleted bone marrow cells. However, transplantation of bones plus normal P-HSCs could not reconstruct hemopoiesis in autoimmune-prone mice due to graft rejection (manuscript in preparation), although transplantation of T cell-depleted bone marrow cells from normal mice can be used to prevent and treat autoimmune diseases in autoimmune-prone mice [5-7], as described above. This finding suggests that abnormal P-HSCs are more resilient than normal P-HSCs; the former can proliferate in MHC-mismatched microenvironments, while the latter cannot. This was also confirmed in in vitro experiments. As shown in Fig. 19, abnormal P-HSCs can proliferate in collaboration with MHC-incompatible stromal cells, although normal P-HSCs can do so only in collaboration with MHC-compatible stromal cells, not MHC-incompatible stromal cells (manuscript in preparation).

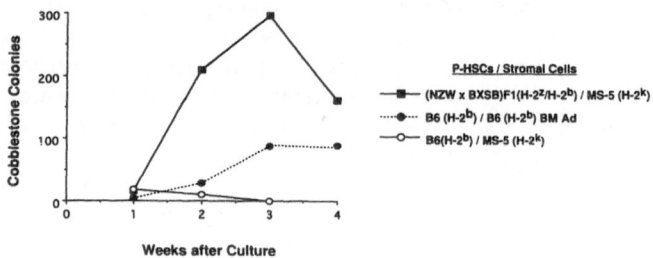

Fig. 19 No MHC restriction between abnormal P-HSCs and stromal cells. Abnormal P-HSCs obtained from W/BF1 mice show a significantly highter responsiveness in coculture with MHC-incompatible stromal cells than do normal B6 P-HSCs cocultured with B6 stromal cells.

Immunological aging

Two factors are involved in immunological aging: the thymus and P-HSCs. It is conceivable that the thymus determines immunological aging, since P-HSCs have the capacity to self-renew eternally. We have very recently confirmed this using two kinds of animal models.

The first is the MRL/+ mouse, a late-onset autoimmune animal model, which shows SLE, chronic pancreatitis and sialoadenitis more than 10 months after birth [43]. Using this mouse, we have found that BMT plus embryonal thymus grafts can be used to treat autoimmune diseases in old recipients, although BMT alone cannot rescue the recipients even if fetal liver cells are used as a source of active P-HSCs [44].

The other is the SAMP1 mouse, a substrain of an animal model for the senescence-accelerated mouse (SAM), which shows premature thymic involution and the symptoms of aging such as allopecia at the age of 5 months [45,46]. The mice also show immunological dysfunctions (T cells, B cells and APCs) [47], which result in the development of amyloidosis probably due to bacterial infection. Using this mouse strain, we have found that BMT plus thymus grafts can be used to prevent not only the aging but also the development of amyloidosis (manuscript in preparation).

In humans, it is well known that the success rate of BMT in patients more than 45 years old is low. We believe that this is due to the atrophy of the thymus, and that transplantation of the embryonal thymus in conjunction with BMT should become a valuable strategy for older patients with various diseases.

Tolerance induction in triple chimeras

For human application of thymus grafts, we examined the induction of tolerance using triple chimeric mice. BALB/c nu/nu (H-2^d) mice were lethally (7Gy) irradiated and then reconstituted with T cell-depleted bone marrow cells of C3H/HeN (H-2^k) mice. The mice were engrafted with B6 (H-2^b) embryonal thymuses (Fig. 20). As shown in Fig. 21, the triple chimeric mice accepted the skins of BALB/c, B6, and C3H/HeN mice, but rejected the third party skin of DBA/1(H-2^q) mice (manuscript in preparation). This finding suggests that newly-developed T cells are tolerant of not only MHC determinants of P-HSCs and the thymus but also MHC determinants of the microenvironment (stromal cells). These findings suggest that MHC-mismached embryonal thymus graft in conjunction with BMT can be used to treat older patients.

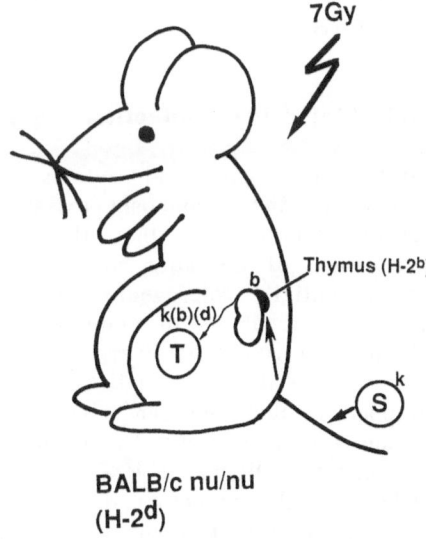

Fig. 20 Experimental design in triple chimeric mice. The BALB/c nu/nu (H-2d) mouse is lethally (7Gy) irradiated and then reconstituted with T cell-depleted C3H/HeN (H-2^k) BMCs. The mouse is engrafted with the B6 (H-2^b) embryonal thymus.

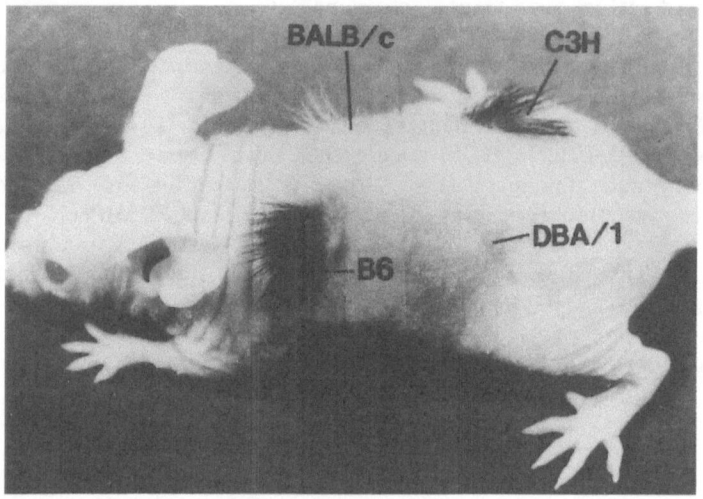

Fig. 21 Skin grafts in triple chimeric mice.   The BALB/c nu/nu triple chimeric mouse accepts the skins of BALB/c, C3H/HeN and B6 mice, but rejects the third party skin of the DBA/1 (H-2q).

Mechanism underlying portal vein tolerance induction

It is well known that liver allografts in humans and rodents are not susceptible to rejection even without using any immunosuppressants [48]. It has been postulated and recently demonstrated that this inherent tolerogenicity of the liver is a consequence of migration and perpetuation within the host lymphoid tissues of potentially tolerogenic donor-derived ("chimeric") leukocytes, in particular, the precursors of chimeric dendritic cells (DC) [49].   We have recently found that HSCs are likely to be trapped in the liver after injection from either the portal vein or tail vein, and that allogeneic HSCs which have been trapped in the liver can induce tolerance [50].   As shown in Fig. 22, persistant tolerance could be maintained by portal venous plus intra-venous injections of allogeneic HSCs.   We have recently clarified the mechanism underlying the induction of tolerance by portal vein injection of allogeneic HSCs (manuscript in preparation); as shown in Fig. 23, allogeneic HSCs which have been trapped in the liver differentiate into natural suppressor cells (NSCs), resulting in suppression of immunological functions non-specifically.   Allogeneic HSCs induce not only suppressor T cells in the recipients but also clonal anergy in the recipient CTLs (CD8+ T cells).   These findings suggest that HSCs can induce tolerance, and that the injection of allogeneic HSCs via the portal vein may prevent the rejection of organ allografts.

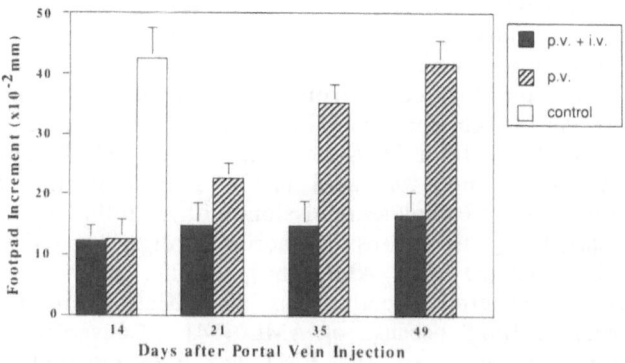

Fig. 22 Induction of persistent tolerance by portal venous (p.v.) plus intra-venous (i.v.) injections. Tolerance is gradually attenuated by one shot from the portal vein of allogeneic HSCs. However, persistent tolerance can be maintained by p.v. plus i.v. injections; i.v. injections were carried out every other week to recruit allogeneic HSCs.

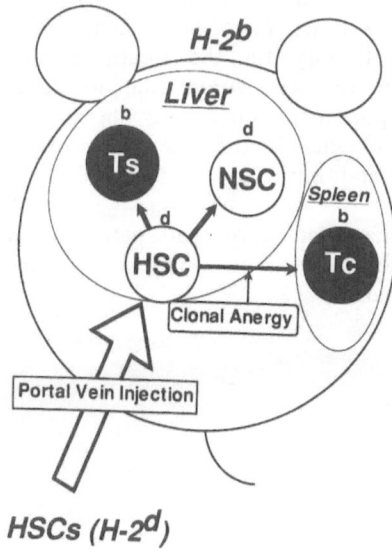

HSCs (H-2^d)

Fig. 23 Mechanisms underlying portal vein tolerance induction. When BALB/c (H-2^d) HSCs are injected into B6 (H-2^b) mice from the portal vein, the HSCs are trapped in the B6 liver, where they differentiate into natural suppressor cells (NSCs). The NSCs non-specifically suppress immunological functions. The allogeneic HSCs induce not only suppressor T cells (Ts) in the recipients but also clonal anergy in the cytotoxic T-lymphocytes (Tc) of the recipients.

Prospective BMT and organ transplantation

Using various animal models, we have demonstrated that BMT can be used to treat not only systemic but also organ-specific autoimmune diseases, and that autoimmune diseases can be induced in normal mice by transplanting bone marrow cells from autoimmune-prone mice. These findings have recently been confirmed in humans. Seven cases of RA have received allogeneic BMT from HLA-identical siblings, all because of severe aplastic anemia supervening after gold and/or D-penicillamine therapy [51-53]. Two patients are in complete remission with a follow-up of six years. It was also reported that two cases of psoriasis vulgaris were resolved after BMT: one was associated with AML [54], and the other with CML [55]. Stable remission of ulcerative colitis has also been reported in a young woman who received BMT because of AML [54]. Conversely, the adoptive transfer of autoimmune diseases after BMT has been reported. Grau et al. and others reported six cases of myasthenia gravis (MG) occurring after allogeneic BMT [56,57]. Other adoptive, post-transplant autoimmune diseases include autoimmune thyroiditis [58,59], IDDM [60-63], and Graves' disease [64]. Recently, Marmont has reviewed these data in humans [65].

In humans, BMT across MHC-barriers has had a low success rate as a consequence of i) GVHR due to contamination with T cells from the peripheral blood and ii) graft rejection. We have provided evidence that, in mice, no such problems are associated with BMT. GVHR can be prevented if T cell-depleted bone marrow cells are used. Graft rejection can be prevented by bone grafts and transplantation of NSCs. It is certain that similar conditions to permit successful BMT in humans will be realized in the near future. When such conditions have been achieved, we can expect BMT to become a valuable strategy for the treatment of patients with autoimmune diseases. Furthermore, we would like to suggest that organ allografts of heart, kidney, pancreas, etc., may be accomplished without using long-term immunosuppressants if the organ is obtained from the same donor as the bone marrow and both are transplanted at the same time.

Finally, we would like to emphasize that more than half the intractable diseases recognized by the Health and Welfare of Japan will be treated by BMT or BMT plus organ grafts (see Table).

Intractable Diseases

(according to the Ministry of Health and Welfare of Japan)

  1) Behçet Syndrome
○ 2) Multiple sclerosis
○ 3) Myasthenia gravis
○ 4) Systemic lupus erythematosus
  5) SMON
◎ 6) Aplastic anemia
  7) Sarcoidosis
  8) Amyotrophic lateral sclerosis
○ 9) PSS, DM and PM
◎ 10) Idiopathic thrombocytopenic purpura (ITP)
○ 11) Polyarteritis nodosa
◎ 12) Ulcerative colitis
  13) Aortitis syndrome
  14) Buerger's disease
◎ 15) Pemphigus
  16) Spinocerebellar degeneration
◎ 17) Crohn's disease
  18) Fulminant hepatitis
◎ 19) Malignant rheumatoid arthritis
  20) Parkinson's disease
  21) Amyloidosis
  22) Ossification of the posterior longitudinal ligament
  23) Huntington's chorea
  24) Occlusive diseases in Willis' circle
○ 25) Wegener's granulomatosis
○ 26) Idiopathic cardiomyopathy (diastolic)
  27) Shy-Drager syndrome
◎ 28) Bullous diseases
◎ 29) Psoriasis vulgaris
  30) Diffuse spinal canal stenosis
○ 31) Primary biliary cirrhosis
○ 32) Severe Acute Pancreatitis
  33) Idiopathic necrosis of the femoral head
○ 34) Mixed connective tissue diseases
◎ 35) Primary immunodeficiency
  36) Idiopathic interstitial pneumonia

○ possibly curable, ◎ definitely curable

ACKNOWLEDGEMENTS

These experiments were carried out in collaboration with researchers who appear in the references of this paper. I would like to express my deep appreciation to them.

I would also like to thank Ms. Yoshiko Shinno and Ms. Yuki Matsui for their skillful technical assistance, and Mr. Hilary Eastwick-Field and Ms. Keiko Ando for preparing this manuscript.

This work was supported by a grant from the Japanese Ministry of Health and Welfare; the Ministry of Education, Science, and Culture, Japan; the "Traditional Oriental Medical Science Program" of the Public Health Bureau of the Tokyo Metropolitan Government; the Mochida Memorial Foundation for Medical and Pharmaceutical Research (1986); the Naito Foundation (1986); the Mitsubishi Foundation (1986); the Suzuken Memorial Foundation (1987); the Takeda Science Foundation (1989); Yasuda Igaku Kinen Zaidan (1990); the Foundation for Rheumatic Diseases (1990), and the Science Research Promotion Fund of the Japan Private School Promotion Foundation, Japan.

REFERENCES

1. Theofilopoulos AR, Dixon FJ (1985) Murine models of systemic lupus erythematosus. Adv Immunol 37: 269-358
2. Morton JI, Siegel BV (1974) Transplantation of autoimmune potential. I. Development of antinuclear antibodies in H-2 histocompatible recipients of bone marrow from New Zealand Black mice. Proc Natl Acad Sci USA 71: 2162-2165
3. Akizuki M, Reeves JP, Steinberg AD (1978) Expression of autoimmunity by NZB/NZW marrow. Clin Immunol Immunopathol 10: 247-250
4. Jyonouchi H, Kincade PW, Good RA, Fernandes GJ (1981) Reciprocal transfer of abnormalities in clonable B lymphocytes and myeloid

progenitors between NZB and DBA/2 mice. J Immunol 127:1232-1238

5. Ikehara S, Good RA, Nakamura T, Sekita K, Inoue S, Maung Maung Oo, Muso E, Ogawa K, Hamashima Y (1985) Rationale for bone marrow transplantation in the treatment of autoimmune diseases. Proc Natl Acad Sci USA 82:2483-2487

6. Ikehara S, Ohtsuki H, Good RA, Asamoto H, Nakamura T, Sekita K, Muso E, Tochino Y, Ida T, Kuzuya H, Imura H, Hamashima Y (1985) Prevention of type I diabetes in nonobese diabetic mice by allogeneic bone marrow transplantation. Proc Natl Acad Sci USA 82: 7743-7747

7. Ikehara S, Yasumizu R, Inaba M, Izui S, Hayakawa K, Sekita K, Toki J, Sugiura K, Iwai H, Nakamura T, Muso E, Hamashima Y, Good RA (1989) Long-term observations of autoimmune-prone mice treated for autoimmune disease by allogeneic bone marrow transplantation. Proc Natl Acad Sci USA 86:3306-3310

8. Ikehara S, Kawamura M, Takao F, Inaba M, Yasumizu R, Soe Than, Hisha H, Sugiura K, Koide Y, Yoshida TO, Ida T, Imura H, Good RA (1990) Organ-specific and systemic autoimmune diseases originate from defects in hematopoietic stem cells. Proc Natl Acad Sci USA 87: 8341-8344

9. Yasumizu R, Sugiura K, Iwai H, Inaba M, Makino S, Ida T, Imura H, Hamashima Y, Good RA, Ikehara S (1987) Treatment of type 1 diabetes mellitus in non-obese diabetic mice by transplantation of allogeneic bone marrow and pancreatic tissue. Proc Natl Acad Sci USA 84: 6555-6557

10. Oyaizu N, Yasumizu R, Inaba-Miyama M, Nomura S, Yoshida H, Miyawaki S, Shibata Y, Mitsuoka S, Yasunaga K, Morii S, Good RA, Ikehara S (1988) (NZW × BXSB)F1 mouse, a new model of idiopathic thrombocytopenic purpura. J Exp Med 167: 2071-2022

11. Miyama-Inaba M, Kuma S, Inaba K, Ogata H, Iwai H, Yasumizu R, Muramatsu S, Steinman RM, Ikehara S (1988) Unusual phenotype of B cells in the thymus of normal mice. J Exp Med 168: 811-816

12. Good RA, Martinez C, Gabrielsen AE Clinical considerations of the thymus in immunobiology. In: The Thymus in Immunobiolog. Good RA, Gabrielsen AE (eds). Hoeber-Harper, New York, 1964; pp 3-48

13. Mackay IR, Gail P (1963) Thymic germinal centres and plasma cells in systemic lupus erythematosus. Lancet 2: 667

14. Ikehara S, Tanaka H, Nakamura T, Furukawa F, Inoue S, Sekita K, Shimizu J, Hamashima Y, Good RA. (1985) The influence of thymic abnormalities on the development of autoimmune diseases. Thymus 7: 25-36

15. Nakamura T, Ikehara S, Good RA, Inoue S, Sekita K, Furukawa F, Tanaka H, Maung Maung Oo, Hamashima Y (1985) Abnormal

stem cells in autoimmune-prone mice are responsible for premature thymic involution.   Thymus   7: 151-160

16. Adachi Y, Inaba M, Inaba K, Soe Than, Kobayashi Y, Ikehara S   (1993) Analyses of thymic abnormalities in autoimmune-prone (NZW × BXSB)F1 mice.   Immunobiol 188: 340-354

17. Nakamura T, Good RA, Inoue S, Maung Maung Oo, Hamashima Y, Ikehara S (1986)   Successful liver allografts in mice by combination with allogeneic bone marrow transplantation.   Proc Natl Acad Sci USA   83: 4529-4532

18. Hang LM, Izui S, Dixo FJ (1981)   (NZW x BXSB F1) hybrid. A model of acute lupus and coronary vascular disease with myocardial infarction.   J Exp Med   154: 216-221

19. Adachi Y, Inaba M, Amoh Y, Yoshifusa H, Nakamura Y, Suzuki H, Akamatu S, Nakai S, Haruna H, Adachi M, Ikehara S   (1995) Effect of bone marrow transplantation on anti-phospholipid antibody syndrome in murine lupus mice. Immunobiol 192: 218-230

20. Estess P, Begovich AB, Koo M, Jones PP, McDevitt HO (1986) Sequence analysis and structure function of murine q, k, u, s, and f haplotype I-Aβ cDNA clones. Proc Natl Acad Sci USA 83: 3594-3598

21. Koide Y, Yoshida TO (1989) The unique nucleotide sequence of the Aβ gene in the NOD mouse is shared with its nondiabetic sister strains, the ILI and the CTS mouse.   Int Immunol 2: 189-192

22. Nishimoto H, Kikutani H, Yamamura K, Kishimoto T (1989) Prevention of autoimmune insulitis by expression of I-E molecules in NOD mice.   Nature 328: 432-434

23. Reich EP, Sherwin RS, Kanagawa O, Janeway CA., Jr (1989)   An explanation for the protective effect of the MHC class II I-E molecule in murine diabetes.   Nature 341: 326-328

24. Acha-Orbea H, McDevitt HO (1987)   The first external domain of the nonobese diabetic mouse class II I-Aβ chain is unique.   Proc Natl Acad Sci USA   84: 2435-2439

25. Todd JA, Bell JI, McDevill HO (1987) HLA-DQβ gene contributes to susceptibility and resistance to insulin-dependent diabetes mellitus. Nature 329: 599-604

26. Visser JWM, Bauman JGJ, Mulder AH, Eliason JF, de Leeuw AM (1984) Isolation of murine pluripotent hemopoietic stem cells. J Exp Med 159: 1576-1590

27. Miyama-Inaba M, Ogata H, Toki J, Kuma S, Sugiura K, Yasumizu R, Ikehara S (1987)   Isolation of murine pluripotent hemopoietic stem cells in the Go phase. Biochem Biophys Res Commu 75: 1809-1812

28. Ishida T, Inaba, Hisha H, Sugiura K, Adachi Y, Nagata N, Ogawa R, Good RA, Ikehara S (1994)   Requirement of donor-derived stromal cells in the bone marrow for successful allogeneic bone marrow transplantation: complete prevention of recurrence of autoimmune diseases in MRL/MP-lpr/lpr mice by transplantation of bone marrow plus bone (stromal cells) from the same donor. J Immunol 152: 3119-3127

29. Hisha H, Nishino T, Kawamura M, Adachi S, Ikehara S (1995) Successful bone marrow transplantation by bone grafts in chimeric-resistant combination. Exp Hematol 23: 347-352

30. Soe Than, Ishida H, Inaba M, Fukuba Y, Seino Y, Adachi M, Imura H, Ikehara S (1992) Bone marrow transplantation as a strategy for treatment of non-insulin-dependent diabetes mellitus in KK-Ay mice. J Exp Med 176: 1233-1238

31. Nishimura M, Toki J, Sugiura K, Hashimoto F, Tomita T, Fujishima H, Hiramatsu Y, Nishioka N, Nagata N, Takahashi Y, Ikehara S (1994) Focal segmental glomerular sclerosis, a type of intractable chronic glomerulonephritis, is a stem cell disorder. J Exp Med 179: 1053-1058

32. Yasumizu R, Miyawaki S, Sugiura K, Nakamura T, Ohnishi Y, Good RA, Hamashima Y, Ikehara S (1990) Allogeneic bone marrow plus liver transplantation in C57BL/KsJ spm/spm mouse, an animal model of Niemann-pick disease. Transplantation 49: 759-764

33. Vellodi A, Hobbs JR, Hugh-Jones K (1987) Bone marrow transplantation for Niemann-Pick disease, type B. Bone Marrow Transplantation 2 (suppl 1): 128

34. Ogata H, Bradley WG, Inaba M, Ogata N, Ikehara S, Good RA (1995) Long-term repopulation of hematolymphoid cells with only a few hemopoietic stem cells in mice. Proc Natl Acad Sci USA 92: 945-5949

35. Okada S, Nakauchi H, Nagayoshi K, Nishikawa S, Nishikawa S-I, Miura Y, Suda T (1991) Enrichment and characterization of murine hematopoietic stem cells that express c-kit molecule. Blood 78: 1706-1712

36. Katayama N, Shih JP, Nishikawa S, Kinaa T, Clark SC, Ogawa M (1993) Stage-specific expression of c-kit protein by murine hematopoietic progenitors. Blood 82: 2353-2360

37. Sugiura K, Inaba M, Ogata H, Yasumizu R, Inaba K, Good RA, Ikehara S (1988) Wheat germ agglutinin-positive cells in a stem cell-enriched fraction of mouse bone marrow have potent natural suppressor activity. Proc Natl Acad Sci USA 85: 4824-4826

38. Sugiura K, Ikehara S, Inaba M, Haraguchi S, Ogata H, Sardiña EE, Sugawara M, Ohta Y, Good RA (1992) Enrichment of murine bone marrow natural suppressor activity in the fraction of hematopoietic progenitors with interleukin 3 receptor-associated antigen. Exp Hematol 20: 256-263

39. Izumi-Hisha H, Soe Than, Ogata H, Inaba M, Ikehara S, Kawai M (1991) Monoclonal antibodies against a preadipose cell line (MC3T3-G2/PA6) which can support hemopoiesis. Hybridoma 10: 103-112

40. Cherry, Yasumizu R, Toki J, Asou H, Nishino T, Komatsu Y, Ikehara S (1994) Production of hemopoietic stem cell-chemotactic factor by bone marrow stromal cells. Blood 83: 964-971

41. Lichtman MA Classification and clinical manifestations of the hemopoietic stem cell disorders. In: Hematology: Hemopoietic stem cell disorders: Classification and manifestations. Williams WJ,

Beutler E, Erslev AJ. Lichtman MA (eds). New York-Toronto: McGraw-Hill Publishing Company, 1990; pp 148-157

42. Shimizu J, Hamashima Y, Tsuda H, Akiyama Y, Mikawa H, Ikehara S (1987) A case report: T-cell acute lymphoblastic leukemia relapsing as acute myelomonocytic leukemia and terminating possibly as chronic myelocytic leukemia. Am J Hematol 24: 199-205

43. Kanno H, Nose M, Itoh J, Taniguchi Y, Kyogoku M (1992) Sponaneous development of pancreatitis in the MRL/Mp strain of mice in autoimmune mechanism. Clin Exp Immunol 89: 68-73

44. Hosaka N, Nose M, Kyogoku M, Nagata N, Miyahsima S, Good RA, Ikehara S Aging of the thymus is a critical factor in successful bone marrow transplantation: bone marrow transplantation plus fetal thymus grafts as a strategy for treatment of autoimmune diseases in old MRL/+ mice. Proc Natl Acad Sci USA in press

45. Takeda T, Hosokawa M, Takeshita S, Irino M, Higuchi K, Matsushita T (1981) A new murine model of accelerated senescence. Mech Ageing Dev 17: 183-194

46. Higuchi K, Matsubara A, Hashimoto K, Honnma A, Takeshita S, Hosokawa M, Yasuhira K, Takeda T (1983) Isolation and characterization of senile amyloid-related antigenic substance (SAS_{SAM}) from mouse serum: Apo SAS_{SAM} is a low molecular weight apoprotein of high density lipoprotein. J Exp Med 158: 1600-1614

47. Haruna H, Inaba M, Inaba K, Taketani S, Sugiura K, Fukuba Y, Doi H, Toki J, Tokunaga R, Ikehara S (1995) Abnormalities of B cells and dendritic cells in SAMP1 mice. Eur J Immunol 25: 1319-1325

48. Starzl TE, Demetris AJ, Murase N, Ildstad S, Ricordi C, Trucco M (1992) Cell migration, chimerism, and graft acceptance. Lancet 339: 1579-1582

49. Lu L, Rudert WA, Qian S, McCaslin D, Fu Fumin, Rao AS, Trucco M, Fung JJ, Starz TE, Thomson AW (1995) Growth of donor-derived dendritic cells from the bone marrow of murine liver allograft recipients in response to granulocyte/macrophage colony-stimulating factor. J Exp Med 182: 379-387

50. Zhang Y, Yasumizu R, Sugiura K, Hashimoto F, Amoh Y, Lian Z, Cherry, Nishio N, Ikehara S (1994) Fate of allogeneic or syngeneic cells in intravenous or portal vein injection: possible explanation for the mechanism of tolerance induction by portal vein injection. Eur J Immunol 24: 1558-1565

51. Baldwin JL, Storb R, Thomas ED, Mannik M (1977) Bone marrow transplantation in patients with gold-induced marrow aplasia. Arthr Rheum 20: 1043-1048

52. Jacobs P, Vincent MD, Martell RW (1986) Prolonged remission of severe refractory rheumatoid arthritis following allogeneic bone marrow transplantation for drug-induced aplastic anaemia. Bone Marrow Transpl 1: 237-239

53. Lowenthal RM, Cohen ML, Atkinson K, Biggs JC (1993) Apparent cure of rheumatoid arthritis by bone marrow transplantation. J Rheumatol 20: 137-140

54. Eedy DJ, Burrows D, Bridges JM, Jones FG (1990) Clearance of severe psoriasis after allogeneic bone marrow transplantation. Br Med J   300: 908-909

55. Liu Yin JA, Jowitt SN (1992)   Resolution of immune-mediated diseases following allogeneic bone marrow transplantation for   leukaemia. Bone Marrow Transpl   9: 31-33

56. Grau JM, Casademont J, Monforte R, Marin P, Granena A, Rozman C, Urbano-Marquez A (1990)   Myasthenia gravis after allogeneic bone marrow transplantation: report of a new case and pathogenetic considerations.   Bone Marrow Transpl 5: 435-437

57. Melms A, Faul C, Sommer N, Wietholter H, Muller CA, Ehninger G (1992) Myasthenia gravis after BMT: identification of patients at risk?   Bone Marrow Transpl 9: 78-79

58. Wyatt DT, Lum L, Casper J, Hunter J, Camitta B (1990)   Autoimmune thyroiditis after bone marrow transplantation.   Bone Marrow Transpl 5: 357-361

59. Aldouri MA, Ruggier R, Epstein O, Prentice HG (1990)   Adoptive transfer of hyperthyroidism and autoimmune thyroiditis following allogeneic bone marrow transplantation for chronic myeloid leukaemia.   Br J Haematol   74: 118-119

60. Hagopian W, Lernmark A   Autoimmune diabetes mellitus.   In: The Autoimmune Diseases II. Rose NR, Mackay IR (eds). San Diego-Toronto: Academic Press, 1992; pp 235-278

61. Lampeter EF, Homberg M, Quabeck K, Schaffer UW, Wernet P, Bertrams J, Grosse-Wilde H, Gries FA, Kolb H (1993)   Transfer of insulin-dependent diabetes between HLA-identical siblings by bone marrow transplantation.   Lancet 341:   1243-1244

62. Vialettes B, Maraninchi D, San Marco MP, Birg F, Stoppa AM, Mattei-Zevaco C, Thivolet C, Hermitte L, Vague P, Mercier P (1993) Autoimmune polyendocrine failure ---- Type I (insulin-dependent) diabetes mellitus and hypothyroidism ---- after allogeneic bone marrow transplantation in a patient with lymphoblastic leukaemia. Diabetologia 36: 541-546

63. Lampeter EB (1993)   Discussion remark to Session 24: BMT in autoimmune diseases.   Exp Hematol   21: 1153-1156

64. Holland FJ, McConnon JK, Volpé R, Saunders EF (1991)   Concordant Graves' disease after bone marrow transplantation: implication for pathogenesis.   J Clin Endocrinol Metab 72: 837-840.

65. Marmont AM (1994)   Immune ablation followed by allogeneic or autologous bone marrow transplantation: a new treatment for severe autoimmune diseases?   Stem Cells   12: 125-135